RURAL WOMEN'S HEALTH

Edited by Beverly D. Leipert, Belinda Leach,
and Wilfreda E. Thurston

A woman in a remote northern Aboriginal community is tormented over the suicide of her neighbour, in the wake of other suicides and violence in her community. Mennonite women in an Ontario farming community insist that their environment is safe, even as serious contaminants are measured in their water supply. In a northern British Columbia community, women who volunteer as home care providers worry about reduction of government funding and access to health care, and about the shortage of new volunteers to replace them when they burn out. These are a few of the stories told in the chapters of this book.

This ground-breaking collection of essays identifies priority issues that must be addressed to ensure rural women's well-being, and offers innovative ideas for improvement and further research. Rural women play a critical role within their families and communities, and the health of these women has been a marginalized area of study. Rural Canada itself is often taken for granted or trivialized as an 'escape' or as a problem, a setting fraught with natural disasters and loss of infrastructure, rather than as an important source of food, drinking water, and other natural resources that city-dwellers rely on. This volume, by focusing on the Canadian context, will provide direction for discussion of practices, policies, and scholarship that promote rural women's well-being. It integrates perspectives from health practitioners, rural residents, and scholars in a variety of fields, including nursing, sociology, anthropology, and geography. *Rural Women's Health* fills an important gap in the literature, and complements existing projects in other countries, including the United States, Australia, and England, thus also providing an opportunity for comparative study.

BEVERLY D. LEIPERT is an associate professor in the Arthur Labatt Family School of Nursing at the University of Western Ontario.

BELINDA LEACH is a professor and associate dean (research) in the College of Social and Applied Human Sciences at the University of Guelph.

WILFREDA E. THURSTON is a professor in the Faculty of Medicine and the Faculty of Veterinary Medicine at the University of Calgary.

RURAL WOMEN'S HEALTH

Edited by Beverly D. Leipert, Belinda Leach, and Wilfreda E. Thurston

UNIVERSITY OF TORONTO PRESS
Toronto Buffalo London

RA 771.7 .C3 R88 2012 (handwritten)

ISBN 978-1-4426-4539-4 (cloth)
ISBN 978-1-4426-1348-5 (paper)

Printed on acid-free, 100% post-consumer recycled paper with vegetable-based inks.

Library and Archives Canada Cataloguing in Publication

Rural women's health / edited by Beverly D. Leipert, Belinda Leach, and Wilfreda E. Thurston.

Includes bibliographical references.
ISBN 978-1-4426-4539-4 (bound).   ISBN 978-1-4426-1348-5 (pbk.)

1. Rural women – Health and hygiene – Canada.   2. Rural women – Medical care – Canada.   3. Rural health – Canada.   4. Women's health services – Canada.   I. Leipert, Beverly   II. Leach, Belinda, 1954–   III. Thurston, Wilfreda Enid, 1953–

RA771.7.C3R88 2012   362.1'042570820971   C2012-903358-8

University of Toronto Press acknowledges the financial assistance to the publication of this book by the Social Sciences and Humanities Research Council–funded research programs of Dr Beverly Leipert and Dr Belinda Leach and the College of Social and Applied Sciences, University of Guelph.

University of Toronto Press acknowledges the financial assistance to the publication of this book by the Institute for Public Health and the Faculty of Medicine of the University of Calgary.

University of Toronto Press acknowledges the financial assistance to its publishing program of the Canada Council for the Arts and the Ontario Arts Council.

 Canada Council   Conseil des Arts
for the Arts   du Canada

 ONTARIO ARTS COUNCIL
CONSEIL DES ARTS DE L'ONTARIO

University of Toronto Press acknowledges the financial support of the Government of Canada through the Canada Book Fund for its publishing activities.

We dedicate this book to the rural women and rural health care providers who so creatively and courageously attend to the health of rural families, communities, and themselves.

Contents

Acknowledgments

Thank you to Kathy Dirk, Calgary, Clare Morgan, Guelph, and Tamara Landry and Robyn Plunkett, London, for their coordination of chapters and communication among authors and for their editorial assistance with the preparation of the manuscript at different stages in the process. Thanks to Robyn also for her very helpful organizational and editorial assistance in the final stages of manuscript preparation. We also acknowledge and thank the Rural Women Making Change Research Alliance, the Department of Community Health Sciences at the University of Calgary, the College of Social and Applied Human Sciences at the University of Guelph, the Faculty of Health Sciences at the University of Western Ontario, and the Social Sciences and Humanities Research Council for funding various aspects of the research, preparation, and publication of this project. Thank you also to the Institute for Public Health, University of Calgary, for financial support.

RURAL WOMEN'S HEALTH

Introduction:
Connecting Rural Women's Health across Time, Locales, and Disciplines

Beverly D. Leipert, Belinda Leach,
and Wilfreda E. Thurston

This is the first Canadian book to focus on rural women's health, an emerging field of scholarship within the last two decades. This book represents the diversity of interest and expertise in the topic by its inclusion of scholars, students, practitioners, and rural women from a wide variety of disciplines and locations across the country. It also includes chapters from Australia and the United States that illustrate great overlap in rural women's experiences in countries historically relevant to Canadian policy development, and one from England that raises new questions about the urbanization of rural spaces.

The purpose of the book is to present a Canadian perspective on the nature of rural women's health, while respecting and considering internal and regional diversity; to demonstrate an interdisciplinary and determinants-of-health focus on rural women's health; to formulate a basis from which to approach future policy analysis and research; and to provide a resource for senior undergraduate and graduate students, researchers, health care practitioners, and policymakers.

The book documents how rural women play a critical role in rural family and community health, while their own health needs are often marginalized. Because of its diversity and depth, the book will be of relevance to an international audience interested in rural, gender, and health studies, to name a few. As a resource for training and research, this book will encourage additional exploration of policy-relevant topics. As an overview of important issues facing rural populations, it will provide current practitioners and policymakers with a gendered analysis of information that can be used in shaping how they address the well-being of rural populations.

This ground-breaking collection identifies priority issues that must be addressed to ensure rural women's well-being and offers innovative theoretical and methodological ideas for improvement and further research. Readers will learn of true and often troubling stories of Canadian rural women. A woman in a remote northern Aboriginal community anguishes over the suicide of her neighbour, compounded by other suicides and violence, and is eventually able to label her suffering as post-traumatic stress disorder. Mennonite women in an Ontario farming community insist that their environment is safe, even as serious contaminants are measured in their water supply. In a northern British Columbia community, women who volunteer as home care providers worry that reduced government funding limits access to hospital and other care, and that there is a shortage of new volunteers to replace them when they burn out. And in Australia, a woman fights for official recognition of her 'invisible' health condition that will bring her social supports, even as her rural location makes that support difficult to access. These are some of the stories told in the chapters of this book. They are stories of rural women's health and of women's efforts to protect the health of their families and communities. They are stories of the resilience, insight, and action that we, the editors, consider profoundly important to understanding rural women's health. These stories are influenced by different disciplines of research and practice, often several at a one time, illustrating how central interdisciplinary scholarship is to this field.

It is fashionable these days to either dismiss rural Canada as nothing more than a playground, a place for urban dwellers to visit to escape the stressors of urban life, or as a problem, a setting fraught with natural disasters and loss of infrastructure, such as schools and hospitals. Yet many Canadians obtain their drinking water from rural areas, large amounts of the food we eat are produced there, and some of the country's most valuable resources are located in rural areas.

In using a determinants-of-health framework to understand health, we included chapters that address the social, psychological, environmental, and political factors that contribute to a person's or community's capacity to pursue a full life. In taking a population health perspective, we recognized that the well-being of rural communities also affects the well-being of the far larger percentage of the population who reside in towns and cities. Any assessment of the overall health of Canadians and Canadian society must carefully and systematically include an evaluation of the health of those who live and work in rural and remote areas, including rural women. This requires addressing the gap in a gendered analysis of rural life and of the policies that affect it.

The following sections discuss the theoretical frameworks that informed development of this book: gender, determinants of health, and primary health care. We then provide some background information on rural women's health that is needed to place the various chapters in context, and specifically consider the histories of Aboriginal peoples, rural work, the environment, and marital relations, as well as looking at the issues that dominate rural policy in this decade, globalization and the changing nature of the rural economies and environments.

Gender as a Theoretical Lens

Health researchers and practitioners continue to show a great deal of confusion mixed with apathy about the meaning of 'gender' and its role in ending health inequities. The Institute of Gender and Health of the Canadian Institutes of Health Research has done much in Canada to increase consistency in the use of the term and continues to promote health research that explicates the role of gender (see http://www.cihr-irsc.gc.ca/e/32019.html). Gender is one of the twelve determinants of health according to the policy of Health Canada (Public Health Agency of Canada, 2010). Those who were involved in the women's health movements of the 1980s and 1990s, however, know that the inclusion of gender in the Canadian official list of determinants and the establishment of an institute that might draw attention to women's health needs were outcomes of hard-fought political battles. While gender research does not apply solely to women, women's health research springs from a gender research agenda because women's health is disproportionately harmed by gendered policies (Phillips, 2005). It was not a foregone conclusion that women's particular needs would receive attention, even after the successes of the earlier women's movement (Hankivsky & Canadian Women's Health Network, 2005; Working Group on the CIHR, 2000), and as this book reveals, it is not a foregone conclusion today.

We view gender as a social institution, that is, as a set of processes that are coordinated and take place in many sites of society with clusters of rules and mechanisms for maintaining the institution that are sustained over time (DeVault & McCoy, 2001; Giddens, 1984). Sex, a biological characteristic, is a key aspect of the gendering of society, but is insufficient as a variable for indicating gender in health research. Thurston and Vissandjee (2005) demonstrate how gender, culture, and migratory experience interact to affect the health of immigrant women, but their ecological model can be applied to understanding the role of gender in every woman's health. As Hankivsky, Cormier, and deMerisch (2009) demonstrate, gender intersects with all of the other determinants of a population's health, as well as having analytic value as a variable in itself. Lorber (1994, 1997) has demonstrated this analytic value in relation to health, and the chapters in this book also highlight these intersections.

The impacts of gender differ over the life course; therefore gender analysis needs to take life course into account (Vespa, 2009). Porter and Beausoleil (chapter 9) discuss how three generations of Newfoundland and Labrador women deal with hegemonic gendered messages that are sexist, ageist, and ableist. Etowa and colleagues (chapter 15) consider how both life course and place intersect for African Nova Scotia women. Novik (chapter 16) reveals the importance of relationships in the lives of older Ukrainian women. These chapters show that gender and rurality interact to create a sense of place that incorporates social relationships and social processes over the life course (Thurston & Meadows, 2003).

Thurston and Meadows (2003) found that there was great diversity in what rurality meant to women and to their lives. With chapters from many parts of Canada and internationally, this book demonstrates how geography and gender intersect and interact. The experiences of farm women (see McIntyre and Rondeau, chapter 6, and Heather and colleagues, chapter 13), for instance, may be quite different from those of their non-agricultural rural neighbours. Gerrard and Woodland (chapter 14) reveal that intergenerational farming is one source of stress for some farm women; nevertheless, farm and non-farm women will experience many of the opportunities and constraints of gender as a social institution in the same way (Gerrard, Thurston, Scott, & Meadows, 2005; Thurston & Meadows, 2004). Little (chapter 19) and Pini and Soldatic (chapter 20) reveal that in other countries rurality and gender interact to affect women in both health and illness situations.

Frameworks for Health and Health Care

Health is recognized globally as more than the absence of illness and injury, rather, it is seen to be a resource for everyday living (World Health Organization [WHO], 1986). This perspective on health is consistent with two key health philosophies and approaches: the determinants of health (Raphael, 2004) and primary health care (WHO, 1978, 1986).

The determinants of health, acknowledged as critical to the advancement of health (Commission on the Social Determinants of Health, 2008), are the conditions in which people are born, grow, live, work, and age. Determinants include factors such as income and economics, education, social exclusion, food security, and health care services (Raphael, 2004). These determinants are shaped by the distribution of money, power, and resources at global, national, and local levels, which are themselves influenced by policy choices. As we and others (e.g., Leipert & George, 2008; Pederson & Raphael, 2006) have argued, women's health needs to be a focused area of analysis. Wanless, Mitchell, and Wister (2010) recommend that, due to its complexity, rural residence needs to be integrated as a unique dimension within the determinants-of-health framework. This is consistent with a growing body of research showing that place has a strong influence on a population's health.

The determinants of health that are social in nature explain most health inequities – the unfair and avoidable differences in health status seen within and between people, communities, and countries. Responding to increasing concern about these persisting and widening inequities, WHO (Commission on the Social Determinants of Health, 2008) has provided important recommendations on how to reduce them:

- improve daily living conditions,
- tackle the inequitable distribution of power, money, and resources, and
- measure and understand the problem and assess the impact of action.

The chapters in this book attest to the importance of the WHO recommendations for obtaining equity in rural women's health, addressing such issues as social exclusion, gender equity, and empowerment (Haworth-Brockman et al., chapter 2; Leipert, Landry, and Leach, chapter 3; Sutherns and Haworth-Brockman, chapter 1); food security (McIntyre and Rondeau, chapter 6; Kubik and Fletcher, chapter 7); housing (Montgomery et al., chapter 12); daily living conditions (Dyck, Stickle, and Hardy, chapter 10; Illauq, chapter 11; Porter and Beausoleil, chapter 9); and understanding the problems and assessing the impact of action (Haworth-Brockman et al., chapter 2; Sutherns and Haworth-Brockman, chapter 1). In addition, many of the chapters suggest ways that policies and programs could reduce inequities. This important information can assist governments, policymakers, and practitioners to move beyond the present persistent fixation on the provision of illness and treatment services as the way to improve rural women's health to a more effective multidimensional interdisciplinary position that addresses the determinants of rural women's health.

Primary health care, a philosophy and framework that is well accepted in Canada and elsewhere (Smith, Jacobson, & Yiu, 2008), acknowledges the role of health care providers from diverse disciplines and is guided by the principles of universal accessibility to appropriate health care, public participation in health-related decision making, health promotion, appropriate technology, and intersectoral cooperation (WHO, 1978, 1986). The ultimate goal of primary health care is better health for all. WHO (1978) has identified five key means to achieving that goal:

- reducing exclusion and social disparities in health (universal coverage reforms),
- organizing health services around people's needs and expectations (service delivery reforms),
- integrating health into all sectors (public policy reforms),
- pursuing collaborative models of policy dialogue (leadership reforms), and
- increasing stakeholder participation.

Recent commissions (e.g., the Mental Health Commission [Romanow, 2002]) and political discussions, if they address rural health care at all, have taken a limited view of rural health care. Rural people are rarely consulted or included in health care decisions that affect them directly, which often results in rural communities receiving inadequate and inappropriate health care. There are critical and growing shortages of physicians and nurses in rural areas; nurse practitioners and midwives are for the most part not present or not adequately supported in most rural communities; and alternative care providers, such as naturopathic practitioners and nutritionists, are difficult to find in rural settings. Health system development in rural Canada is still focused almost exclusively on providing treatment for acute and chronic conditions and addressing physician shortages, as if this were the gold standard for health care.

Care providers such as midwives, nurse practitioners, public health nurses, social workers, massage therapists, naturopathic physicians, and nutritionists, who have a focus on and expertise in illness prevention and health promotion as well as treatment over the life course, are often better suited to address the multifaceted nature of rural women's health and provide the appropriate primary health care (Health Canada, 2005; Leipert, 1999). The chapters in this book clearly reveal that a more inclusive and broader multidisciplinary approach to primary health care is needed to effectively address rural women's health and to reduce inequities.

Several chapters, such as those of Sutherns and Haworth-Brockman (chapter 1) and Haworth-Brockman and colleagues (chapter 2) highlight that health promotion and illness and injury prevention programs, social inclusion, and empowerment through meaningful representation, are key to the advancement of rural women's health in Canada. Leipert, Landry, and Leach (chapter 3) note that enhancing government support for rural women's organizations would facilitate the inclusion of the perspectives of rural women, thereby increasing the effective development of rural health care policies and practices and providing opportunities and empowerment.

The chapters in this book present a rich mosaic of rural women's experiences as they relate to health. In the following section we provide background to this mosaic with historical, socio-cultural, economic, and other information that may help the reader to draw the pieces of the mosaic together and more clearly understand the complexities of rural women's health. Background information will address the colonization of Aboriginal peoples, illustrating how this is gendered, and how immigration policies have shaped rural populations over time, along with factors in the physical and social environments. More recent history, captured by the term 'globalization,' is discussed in terms of changing economics, employment opportunities, and geographies.

The History of Colonization of Aboriginal People and Women's Health

Aboriginal scholars in particular have shown that rural Canada cannot be understood until the history and lives of Aboriginal peoples are understood. It is important to note that the very terms used to refer to the indigenous peoples of Canada, that is, those who were here before colonization, perpetuate misunderstanding. As Monture and McGuire (2009, p. 2) explain:

> It is always important to understand that the words Aboriginal, Native, Indigenous, or Indian are colonial words imposed upon many diverse nations ... Generally, Aboriginal draws its meaning from Canada's constitution where we are defined as the 'Indian, Inuit, and Métis.' Indians are called 'status' Indians. So those who are not registered under the Act do not have status, and frankly we find that reference to others disturbing.

Thus, even the descriptive term used for populations has political implications for rights and responsibilities. For the purposes of this chapter we will refer mainly to Aboriginal peoples, recognizing there is great diversity across the country.

At least four generations of Canadians have grown up in and been schooled in an environment that largely ignored the history and role of Aboriginal peoples of Canada (Newhouse, Voyageur, & Beavon, 2005). Kirmayer, Tait, and Simpson (2009) report that there were an estimated seven million indigenous people in Canada before Europeans made contact; in the 2006 census, there were 1.2 million. From the time of contact, violence and disease and policies of assimilation, relocation, and removal began to destroy the indigenous population. As Moffit (chapter 17) notes, memories of the loss of whole communities still resonate with Aboriginal people and contribute to their present-day health. Aboriginal people were relegated to rural lands and largely excluded from the rest of Canadian society. While residential schools often attempted to change Aboriginal men into agricultural workers, there is little to date in the published literature about Aboriginal farmers and ranchers.

Prior to World War II the Canadian government, through successive Indian Acts, attempted to control every aspect of Aboriginal peoples' lives through oppressive laws and institutions:

> From 1927 until 1951, Indians were prevented from accessing legal counsel to undertake action in defence of their treaty and other rights. They were also hampered in efforts to form organizations that could advance their rights. Band council funds were subject to government control ... development of Indian leadership was held back by the control Indian

agents exercised over reserves and by abysmal levels of Indian education. (Cassidy, 2005, p. 39)

The goals of the Indian Act were assimilation of the Aboriginal peoples into Eurocentric values, and the processes employed were seldom questioned. This included enforcing gender inequality; for instance, a non-Aboriginal woman could gain Aboriginal status by marrying an Aboriginal man, but an Aboriginal woman lost her status if she married a non-Aboriginal man. Aboriginal women still have no matrimonial property rights under the Indian Act (Native Women's Association of Canada, 2007). Thus, the experiences of rural Aboriginal women differ significantly from those of their non-Aboriginal neighbours.

Feminist historians have identified that the process of colonization imposed other gendered rules upon Aboriginal peoples. Carter (1996) reveals, for instance, that the mobility of Aboriginal women was more severely restricted than that of Aboriginal men and that rules concerning food distribution took away women's previous roles in managing communal food supplies. Interestingly, Carter's work also reveals that Aboriginal women resisted and managed the rules that oppressed them and their communities, albeit with varying success. The roles and images for Aboriginal women portrayed by the dominant cultures were predominately those of 'beasts of burden or fetching maidens' (Guthrie Valaskakis, 2005, p. 130). As Dyck, Stickle, and Hardy (chapter 10) show, the outcomes of these colonization practices are still being felt today in the interpersonal violence that Aboriginal women experience.

Researchers have consistently concluded that Aboriginal women are at greater risk of spousal violence (including stalking) than non-Aboriginal women (Statistics Canada, 1993, 2005). In fact, a general social survey found that Aboriginal women were three times more likely to be victims of spousal violence than non-Aboriginal women (21% vs. 7%) and more than twice as likely to experience emotional abuse (36% vs. 17%) (Statistics Canada, 2005). Aboriginal women report sustaining more frequent and more severe injuries than non-Aboriginal victims (43% vs. 31%) and also report higher rates of fear for their life as a result of the violence (33% vs. 22%) (Statistics Canada, 2005). Furthermore, Aboriginal children are at greater risk of witnessing violence and experiencing physical and sexual abuse than non-Aboriginal children (LaRocque, 1994; Ristock, 2002). Several reports have noted that the alarming rate of interpersonal violence in Aboriginal communities demands urgent study and action (e.g., Stout, Kipling, & Stout, 2002).

Aboriginal women experience barriers to personal empowerment and to services, including the impacts of colonization and racism that are linked to higher rates of alcohol and substance abuse, and disruption of family systems due to residential school abuse (Brownridge, 2003; Perrault & Proulx, 2000). The complicated dynamics of racism and discrimination as well as cultural values and beliefs frequently make it difficult for Aboriginal women to disclose abuse to both formal services (police, shelters, and health care professionals) and informal supports (family and relatives). Further, many Aboriginal women living in northern and remote communities are faced with the additional challenge of finding services specific to Aboriginal cultures (McGillivray & Comaskey, 2000; Thomlinson, Erickson, & Cook, 2000). As Illauq (chapter 11) reveals, the consequences for many northern communities have been high rates of trauma and what she refers to as 'community-level post-traumatic stress disorder.' Tanner (2009, p. 249) links the 'social suffering' experienced by northern communities to the sedentarization that was imposed by the Canadian government and the impact of replacing existing social structures with external controls. He discusses a healing movement that places the needs of wounded individuals within the context of community or collective healing and care, arguing that although psychology and psychiatry may be of help to many, placing them within Aboriginal world views may be necessary for healing and prevention. This is in keeping with the recent demand for cultural competence of all health workers and cultural safety in all settings (Nursing Council of New Zealand, 2005; Smylie, 2001). Anderson and colleagues (2003) note that full adoption of cultural safety will lead to better care for everyone.

Histories of Rural Work, the Environment, and Marital Relations

The contemporary position of rural women derives from the historical processes of Canada's settlement by immigrants that accompanied the history of colonization discussed above. In rural areas the change settlement brought took place relatively slowly, as new settlers moved gradually westward deeper into the country. Patterns of settlement were shaped by multiple factors: the opportunities and constraints presented by particular environments; pull factors such as government policies of support for homesteaders; push factors (poverty, economic and religious persecution) that propelled people to leave their original country; and the inevitable chain migration, as new immigrants followed family members and relied on their support when they arrived. The result of push and pull factors of immigration for rural areas has been tremendous diversity in regional economies and population characteristics.

While southern Ontario, the Prairies, and the interior of British Columbia were primarily settled for agricultural development, other areas, such as Newfoundland and Nova Scotia, were established for the extraction of lumber, fish, and minerals. British and Irish immigrants settled in Upper Canada early and through the nineteenth century. Later in the nineteenth century, waves of Ukrainians, Germans, Mennonites, and Poles, among others, settled in rural areas across Canada, particularly in the Prairies, shaping the cultural landscape with the industries, agricultural practices, social and labour relations, and cultural activities they brought with them. As Stiles and colleagues show (chapter 18) in their study of leisure activities, the variation in community identity that arises from historical and geographical factors has real effects on present-day health promotion. Little (chapter 19) further explores this with the notion of therapeutic landscapes, and Thien (chapter 22) examines the intersections of emotion and place.

The diversity of regional economies has contributed to diversity in gendered divisions of labour. Extraction industries, especially in single-industry communities, exhibited some of the greatest job segregation (Lucas, 1971); men engaged in the heavy manual labour while women were permitted only to take the limited support jobs (such as cooking for work crews and, in the twentieth century, office jobs). However, women were more likely to be unable to find paid work (Luxton, 1980). Industries like fishing accommodated more flexibility in gendered expectations. Although most commonly men worked the boats while women worked on shore in fish plants cleaning and canning, men often also worked in the fish plants and both engaged in informal income generation to supplement erratic fishery incomes (MacDonald & Connelly, 1990). Agriculture, as a household-based enterprise, demanded intra-familial cooperation as well as everyone's labour at particular times, but still constructed distinct gendered work spheres, often spatially divided between field and household (Cebotarev, Blacklock, & McIsaac, 1986; Ghorayshi, 1989).

However, gendered divisions of labour in agriculture often varied according to the commodity being produced (Machum, 2006), the ways that technological innovations were adopted (Cohen, 1988), and the background and circumstances of the population. Silverman (1985) has argued, for instance, that women who originally farmed in the western regions of the country were largely working class, immigrant, poor, and not well educated. Enduring gender identities generally emerged and were associated with gendered divisions of labour, as men took on the heavy labour of clearing the bush and building dwellings and barns, while women were expected to garden, care for animals and people, and cook and clean.

All of this had consequences both for the health of women and their families and for how health issues were addressed. Men and women alike worked with limited resources and in a frequently hostile natural environment. Segregated work, however, exposed men and women to different health hazards; for men, accidents, and for women, isolation and the complications of childbirth in locales far from medical assistance, were some of the most serious health challenges that confronted rural residents. Alongside these issues, in the late nineteenth and early twentieth centuries, urban concerns about rural public health led to educational outreach programs that targeted farm women, implemented most famously through the Women's Institutes and in some provinces by rural public health nurses (Mill, Leipert, & Duncan, 2002). The objectives were to improve family health through education about such topics as the safe handling of food and care of ill family members, but the approaches used reinforced gendered divisions and traditional understandings of gender roles (Kechnie, 2004; Mill, Leipert, & Duncan, 2002).

As Moffit (chapter 17) and several other authors in this text attest, for many women in rural areas the gendered division of roles has not changed very much. As Porter and Beausoleil (chapter 9) argue, reproductive issues also continue to be significantly under-resourced. Settlement patterns have not been matched with accompanying adequate and accessible population health care systems with adequate resources recognizing the diverse needs of rural populations (see, for example, Dabrowska and Wismer, chapter 8; Etowa et al., chapter 15).

Deep-rooted gender identities have also entrenched differential and unequal social and economic resources between rural men and women. Ideologies of self-reliance that developed out of these experiences still resonate in rural peoples' reluctance to seek support from outsiders (Leipert & George, 2008), including governments, a situation that often disadvantages women without family networks or economic resources. For women who married into farming before the 1970s, the marriage contract constituted an employment contract, regulating 'farm assets

and debt through divorce, credit and bankruptcy, and inheritance legislation' (Carbert, 1995, p. xii; see also Clapton, 2008) that benefitted men.
These inequitable laws were partly remediated by changes in the divorce laws in the 1970s, but inequities still abound, often fuelled by
cultural and historical practices and values in rural areas that favour
male farmers and the maintenance and inheritance of the family farm
by male siblings (Forbes-Chilibeck, 2005).

Globalization and the Changing Nature of Rural Economies and Environments

Despite popular notions that rural communities have remained un-
changed since the early days of settlement, in reality they constantly
confront and initiate change. In recent decades that change has been
largely driven by the global economy. In the context of global markets
for agricultural commodities, large-scale farming is increasing and
family farms are experiencing serious debt crisis. The consequences
reach far beyond the farm gate (see McIntyre and Rondeau, chapter 6;
Heather et al., chapter 13). Food security has become a global concern,
with local and national implications, as the agribusiness community
attempts to contend with the food requirements of growing urban
populations while addressing short- and long-term environmental and
health effects of intensive farming (see Kubik and Fletcher, chapter 7).
Food and agriculture are intimately connected to the health of urban
and rural populations and to men and women (Winson, 1993), but in
different ways, as the chapters in this book elaborate.

Despite the longstanding economic significance of Canada's natural
resources (Innis, 1930), some of those resources have declined in competitiveness because other world regions can produce them more
cheaply, for example, nickel and wood. Meanwhile others, like water,
oil, and diamonds, have taken on renewed value. Established rural
manufacturing regions, such as in southern Ontario and Quebec, have
been largely eclipsed by lower-wage parts of the world (Winson &
Leach, 2002), but regions closer to transportation routes, such as
Saskatchewan, have been revitalized by new industrial investment
(Yates & Leach, 2007). Some regions that have lost economic opportunities in the global economy have turned to marketing tourism and leisure pursuits to maintain a local economy. In western and northern
Canada the well-being of Aboriginal communities is often threatened
by resource and industrial development.

Such economic changes have altered the occupational structure in many rural areas by creating new opportunities while closing off old ones. Women and men have benefitted differentially from the changes in available work. Evidence from the early stages of globalization showed that despite increasing participation rates for women in the paid workforce in rural regions, the pay structure changed very little, with women still holding the lower levels of pay (Phillips, 1977). Broadly, with the exception of skilled technical positions in resource development regions, job creation in most rural areas has been in the low-paid segments of the service sector (Winson & Leach, 2002). As a result of government cutbacks and restructuring (including the closure of rural hospitals and clinics), rural areas have in fact lost some of the better-paying and stable jobs, especially for women, that were previously available in health care, education, and government services (Leach, 1999).

All of these changes reshape rural social relations. Migrants from outside of Canada are bringing their labour to rural communities, while resident rural young people find expanded opportunities elsewhere and leave. Simultaneously urbanites and younger retirees seek out new and at times cheaper places to raise families and experience a different lifestyle (Barrett, 1994), while resident rural elderly and infirm may decide to move to cities for easier access to care (see Pini & Soldatic, chapter 20, for example). These and many other transformations have shifted local demographics in terms of class, age, ethnicity, religion, education, and race, and all with gendered implications.

The shifting demographics and economic opportunities resulting from these broadly adopted structural adjustments often lead to rural depopulation and closure of businesses in rural areas, and have been accompanied by government decisions to curtail or cancel rural services, especially in the realm of regulation. Some of the consequences for rural (and urban) health, which are discussed by Fiske and colleagues (chapter 2) and Dyck and colleagues (chapter 10), may be seen in health crises such as BSE (bovine spongiform encephalitis), the H1N1 virus ('swine flu'), and the Walkerton water contamination incident. Other consequences may only just be beginning to emerge, such as increased cancer rates associated with the use of chemicals in farming (see Brophy et al., chapter 5).

Global concerns about the degradation of the environment take on particular urgency in rural areas. For one thing, climate change, which can lead to reduced average rainfall and catastrophic climate events such as windstorms and tornados, affect local ecosystems, changing the kinds of flora and fauna that are found and affecting the land's capacity for particular forms of agriculture. Furthermore, the push to find new and to intensify old sources of energy has both acute and chronic environmental effects, as tar sands leave dangerous residue ponds and wind farms shift wind patterns and misdirect birds and bats in their ambit. Thus, globalization and the changing nature of rural environments have significant impacts upon the health of rural women in Canada. This book also reveals that these experiences of rural Canadian women are similar in many ways to those of women in the United States and Australia (see Bushy, chapter 4, and Pini & Soldatic, chapter 20).

Rural Women's Health Research Methodologies, Methods, and Future

As this is the first book to address Canadian rural women's health, it is important to note that various methodologies and approaches to research are needed to understand the population health needs of rural peoples. Together, the chapters point to ways forward for the development of future research.

The chapters in this book highlight the utility and importance of using a diverse array of research methods when exploring rural women's health. Authors in this book have used a variety of quantitative and qualitative methods, from surveys to ethnographic interviews, to address an array of rural women's health topics. In addition, several authors note that significant knowledge may be discovered vicariously and that researchers of rural women's health topics need to be conscious of research assumptions and responsive to unexpected findings. For example, Brophy and colleagues (chapter 5) highlight how unanticipated, yet vital, information about breast cancer was revealed in a study exploring rural occupations, and how researchers' assumptions about the age at which occupations begin needed to be transcended in order to detect important rural women's health information.

Both large- and small-scale quantitative studies remain important to understanding women's health. Demographics, for instance, help in understanding the social context, and epidemiological studies can identify health concerns as well as individual and community strengths. Brophy and colleagues (chapter 5), for example, highlight the importance of being sensitive to data relevant to rural women's health within large quantitative research data sets in order to reveal important, and sometimes embedded and obscure, information regarding rural women's health.

As authors in this book reveal, qualitative research methods reveal important experiential, contextual, personal, and socio-cultural information that has significant implications for understanding the past, present, and future of rural women's health in Canada. Illauq (chapter 11), for example, reveals personal and community experiences within a remote Aboriginal community and how these experiences can serve to both perpetuate and address health issues for rural and remote women. On a national level, Leipert, Landry, and Leach (chapter 3) used telephone interviews and face-to-face focus groups to explore the state of rural women's organizations across the country, as a means to identifying socio-political influences upon these organizations and the consequences of these influences. The qualitative methodologies of these and other authors in this book importantly reveal rural women's health needs, resources, and agency within their contexts, whether they be homes, communities, or national or international arenas.

The importance of gender analysis in both qualitative and quantitative research is highlighted by all of the chapters in this text. At the very least, sex-disaggregated data should be examined to determine experiences and issues that are gender specific (for example, see Thurston, Blundell-Gosselin, & Rose, 2003). However, as authors in this text reveal, research must move beyond this essential investigation in order to comprehensively and accurately understand the complex contexts, experiences, and health needs and resources of rural women. Effective health promotion planning depends on such rich research that specifically adopts a gender analysis lens (Leipert, 1999, 2010; Thurston, Blundell-Gosselin, & Vollman, 2003).

Research about rural women's health is in its infancy in Canada, as well as in other comparatively high-income countries (see Bushy, chapter 4). Although the amount of rural research in Canada is growing (Kulig, 2010), a concentrated and cohesive focus on rural women's health is lacking. Several factors are responsible for this limited focus. Funding for rural research is very limited, with no dedicated funds at the national level for rural research or for rural women's health research. As a result, rural women's health researchers must compete for funding with other researchers whose topics and methodologies are frequently more familiar, valued, and supported. Nonetheless, the chapters in this book reveal that significant rural women's health research is being conducted by researchers with diverse backgrounds on an array of topics, using various approaches and methods. Such research and researchers provide a rich basis for rural women's health research in Canada and bode well for the future development of research methods, programs, and advocacy that advance rural women's health and scholarship.

Conclusion

The book is organized in five sections bringing together chapters with overlapping themes, such as community action, the environment, approaches to population health, and theorizing rurality and gender together. This enables readers to identify chapters that may be of special interest; however, there is a great deal to be learned from each chapter, and readers are encouraged to explore what each has to offer to a full and interdisciplinary understanding of rural women's health. As we have said, however, not everything can be covered in one text, and there is much that remains to be studied in rural health, particularly for women.

Based on the contributions to this book we propose a research agenda for the future:

- *Geographical and socio-cultural needs and resources, inequities, and strengths:* Research is needed to identify and describe health-related differences in rural settings across Canada ('from sea to sea to sea') and in diverse cultures including Aboriginal, African Canadian, Mennonite, Ukrainian, and other groups and understanding how social class affects rural populations.
- *Diversity issues in rural women's health:* More information is required about the needs and strengths of rural women with disabilities, mental health issues, and ageing experiences, and of the health issues of rural girls and youth.
- *Knowledge translation and political advocacy*: Research is needed regarding health literacy, the benefits and challenges of technology for rural women, and accessible and acceptable methods for research and health information dissemination. Knowledge that can help to empower rural women, policy makers, and others to advance rural women's health agendas is also vital.
- *Rural health care:* Appropriate, acceptable, and accessible health care is often not available to rural women. More research, from the

perspectives of rural women and rural health care providers, would facilitate the enactment of such care.

- *Research development:* More rural women's health research needs to be developed and funded. This research should promote and support interdisciplinary collaborations, meaningful inclusion of rural women, the development of rural women's health research methodologies and methods (for example, photovoice [Leipert, 2010]), and the development of theories relevant to rural women's health. In addition, enhanced and focused advocacy is needed for increased and dedicated rural women's health research funding. A rural women's health champion, or champions, in universities, government, and local communities could help to identify key rural women's health issues, lead and engage in research that addresses rural women's health issues, and advocate for increased and sustained funding for rural women's health research.

References

Anderson, J., Perry, J., Blue, C., Browne, A., Henderson, A., Khan, K.B., Kirkman, S.R., Lyman, J., Semeniuk, P., & Smye, V. (2003). 'Rewriting' cultural safety within the postcolonial and postnational feminist project: Toward new epistemologies of healing. *Advances in Nursing Science, 26*(3), 196–214.

Barrett, S. (1994). *Paradise.* Toronto: University of Toronto Press.

Brownridge, D.A. (2003). Male partner violence against Aboriginal women in Canada. *Journal of Interpersonal Violence, 18*(1), 65–84.

Carbert, L. (1995). *Agrarian feminism.* Toronto: University of Toronto Press.

Carter, S. (1996). First Nations women of prairie Canada in the early reserve years, the 1870s to the 1920s: A preliminary inquiry. In C. Miller & P. Chuchryk (Eds.), *Women of the First Nations: Power, wisdom, and strength* (pp. 51–75). Winnipeg: University of Manitoba Press.

Cassidy, M. (2005). Treaties and Aboriginal-government relations, 1945–2000. In D.R. Newhouse, C.J. Voyageur, & D. Beavon (Eds.), *Hidden in plain sight: Contributions of Aboriginal peoples to Canadian identity and culture* (pp. 38–60). Toronto: University of Toronto Press.

Cebotarev, N., Blacklock, W.M., & McIsaac, L. (1986). Farm women's work patterns. *Atlantis, 11*(2), 1–22.

Clapton, M.S. (2008). Murdoch v. Murdoch: The organizing narrative of matrimonial property law reform. *Canadian Journal of Women and the Law, 20*(2), 197–230.

Cohen, M. (1988). The decline of women in Canadian dairying. In A. Prentice & S. Mann Trofimenkoff (Eds.), *The neglected majority* (pp. 61–83). Toronto: McClelland and Stewart.

Commission on the Social Determinants of Health (2008). *Closing the gap in a generation: Health equity through action on the social determinants of health.* Geneva: World Health Organization.

DeVault, M.L., & McCoy, L. (2001). *Institutional ethnography: Using interviews to investigate ruling relations.* Thousand Oaks, CA: Sage.

Forbes-Chilibeck, E. (2005). Have you heard the one about the farmer's daughter? Gender bias in the intergenerational transfer of farm land on the Canadian prairies. *Canadian Woman Studies, 24*(4), 26–35.

Gerrard, N., Thurston, W.E., Scott, C.M., & Meadows, L.M. (2005). Silencing of women in Canada: The effects of the erosion of support programs for farm women. *Canadian Woman Studies, 24*(4), 59–66.

Ghorayshi, P. (1989). The indispensable nature of wives' work for the farm family enterprise. *Canadian Review of Sociology and Anthropology, 26*, 571–95.

Giddens, A. (1984). *The constitution of society: Outline of the theory of structuration.* Berkeley: University of California Press.

Guthrie Valaskakis, G. (2005). *Indian country: Essays on contemporary Native culture.* Waterloo, ON: Wilfrid Laurier University Press.

Hankivsky, O., Cormier, R., deMerich, D., and Chou, J. (2009). *Intersectionality: Moving women's health research and policy forward.* Vancouver: Women's Health Research Network.

Hankivsky, O., & Canadian Women's Health Network. (2005). Women's health in Canada: Bejing and beyond. Winnipeg: Canadian Women's Health Network. Retrieved from www.cwhn.ca/resources/pub/beijingBeyond.pdf.

Health Canada. (2005). *Baseline natural health products survey among consumers.* Retrieved from www.hc-sc.gc.ca/dhp-mps.alt_formats/hpfb-dgpsa/pdf/pubs/eng_cons_survey_e.pdf.

Innis, H. (1930). *The fur trade in Canada.* New Haven: Yale University Press.

Kechnie, M. (2004). *Organizing rural women: The Federated Women's Institutes of Ontario, 1897–1919.* Montreal: McGill-Queen's University Press.

Kirmayer, L.J., Tait, C.L., & Simpson, C. (2009). The mental health of Aboriginal peoples in Canada: Transformations of identity and community. In L.J. Kirmayer & G.G. Valaskakis (Eds.), *Healing traditions: The mental health of Aboriginal peoples in Canada* (pp. 3–35). Vancouver: UBC Press.

Kulig, J. (2010). Rural health research in Canada: Assessing our progress. *Canadian Journal of Nursing Research, 42*(1), 7–11.

LaRocque, E.M. (1994). *Violence in Aboriginal communities.* Ottawa: Royal Commissions on Aboriginal Peoples.

Leach, B. (1999). Transforming rural livelihoods: Gender, work and restructuring in three Ontario communities. In S. Neysmith (Ed.), *Restructuring caring labour: Discourse, state practice and everyday life* (pp. 209–25). Toronto: Oxford University Press.

Leipert, B. (2010). Rural and remote women and resilience: Grounded theory and photovoice variations on a theme. In C. Winters and H. Lee (Eds.), *Rural nursing: Concepts, theory, and practice* (3rd ed., pp. 105–29). New York: Springer.

Leipert, B. (1999). Women's health and the practice of public health nurses in northern British Columbia. *Public Health Nursing, 16*(4), 280–9.

Leipert, B., & George, J. (2008). Determinants of rural women's health: A qualitative study in southwest Ontario. *Journal of Rural Health, 24*(2), 210–18.

Lorber, J. (1994). *Paradoxes of gender.* New Haven: Yale University Press.

Lorber, J. (1997). *Gender and the social construction of illness.* Thousand Oaks, CA: Sage.

Lucas, R. (1971). *Minetown, milltown, railtown: Life in Canadian communities of single industry.* Toronto: University of Toronto Press.

Luxton, M. (1980). *More than a labour of love: Three generations of women's work in the home.* Toronto: Women's Press.

MacDonald, M., & Connelly, P. (1990). Class and gender in Nova Scotia fishing communities. In B. Fairley, C. Leys, & J. Sacouman (Eds.), *Restructuring and resistance: Perspectives from Atlantic Canada* (pp. 131–49). Toronto: Garamond.

Machum, S. (2006). Commodity production and farm women's work. In B.B. Bock & S. Shortall (Eds.), *Rural gender relations: Issues and case studies* (pp. 47–62). Wallingford: CABI Publishing.

McGillivray, A., & Comaskey, B. (2000). 'Everybody had black eyes': Intimate violence, Aboriginal women and the justice system. In J. Proulx & S. Perrault (Eds.), *No place for violence: Canadian Aboriginal alternatives* (pp. 39–57). Halifax: Fernwood Publishing and RESOLVE.

Mill, J., Leipert, B., & Duncan, S. (2002). A history of public health nursing in Alberta and British Columbia, 1918–1939. *The Canadian Nurse, 98*(1), 18–23.

Monture, P.A., & McGuire, P.D. (2009). Introduction. In P.A. Monture & P.D. McGuire (Eds.). *First Voices: An Aboriginal women's reader* (p. 2). Toronto: INANNA Publications and Education.

Native Women's Association of Canada. (2007). *Violence against Aboriginal women and girls.* Retrieved from www.nwac-hq.org/en/documents/nwac-vaaw.pdf.

Newhouse, D.R., Voyageur, C.J., & Beavon, D. (2005). Introduction. In D.R. Newhouse, C.J. Voyageur, & D. Beavon (Eds.), *Hidden in plain sight: Contributions of Aboriginal peoples to Canadian identity and culture* (pp. 3–13). Toronto: University of Toronto Press.

Nursing Council of New Zealand. (2005). *Guidelines for cultural safety, the Treaty of Waitangi and Maori health in nursing education and practice.* New Zealand: Nursing Council of New Zealand.

Pederson, A., & Raphael, D. (2006). Gender, race, and health inequalities. In D. Raphael & M. Rioux (Eds.), *Staying alive: Critical perspectives on health, illness, and health care* (pp. 159–91). Toronto: Canadian Scholars Press.

Perrault, S., & Proulx, J. (2000). Introduction. In J. Proulx & S.Perrault, (Eds.), *No place for violence: Canadian Aboriginal alternatives* (pp. 13–21). Halifax: Fernwood Publishing and RESOLVE.

Phillips, P. (1977). Women in the Manitoba labour market: A study of their changing economic role. In H.C. Klassen (Ed.), *The Canadian West: Social change and economic development* (pp. 79–93). Calgary: University of Calgary/Comprint.

Phillips, S.P. (2005). Defining and measuring gender: A social determinant of health whose time has come. *International Journal of Equity in Health, 4*(11), doi: 10.1186/1475-9276-4-11.

Public Health Agency of Canada. (2010). *What determines health?* Retrieved from http://www.phac-aspc.gc.ca/ph-sp/determinants/index-eng. php#determinants.

Raphael, D. (Ed.). (2004). *Social determinants of health: Canadian perspectives.* Toronto: Canadian Scholars Press.

Ristock, J. (2002). Responding to lesbian relationship violence: An ethical challenge. In L.M. Tutty & C. Goard (Eds.), *Reclaiming self: Issues and resources for women abused by intimate partners* (p. 98–116). Halifax: Fernwood Publishing.

Romanow, R. (2002). *Building on values: The future of health care in Canada.* Saskatoon: Commission on the Future of Health Care in Canada. Retrieved from http://www.cbc.ca/healthcare/final_report.pdf.

Silverman, E.L. (1985). Women's perceptions of marriage on the Alberta frontier. In D.C. Jones & I. MacPherson (Eds.), *Building beyond the homestead: Rural history on the Prairies* (pp. 49–64). Calgary: University of Calgary Press.

Smith, D., Jacobson, L., & Yiu, L. (2008). Primary health care. In L. Stamler & L. Yiu (Eds.), *Community health nursing: A Canadian perspective* (2nd ed., pp. 111–24). Toronto: Pearson Prentice Hall.

Smylie, J. (2001). A guide for health professionals working with Aboriginal peoples: Health issues affecting Aboriginal peoples. *Journal of the Society of Obstetricians and Gynecologists, 1*, 1–15.

Statistics Canada. (1993). *Violence against women survey.* Ottawa : Statistics Canada.

Statistics Canada. (2005). *Family violence in Canada: A statistical profile.* Ottawa: Canadian Centre for Justice Statistics, Statistics Canada.

Stout, M.D., Kipling, G.D., & Stout, R. (2002). Aboriginal women's health research. *Canadian Women's Health Network, 4/5*(4/1), 11–12.

Tanner, A. (2009). The origins of Northern Aboriginal social pathologies and the Quebec Cree Healing Movement. In L.J. Kirmayer & G.G. Valaskakis (Eds.), *Healing traditions: The mental health of Aboriginal peoples in Canada* (pp. 249–71). Vancouver: UBC Press.

Thomlinson, E., Erickson, N., & Cook, M. (2000). Could this be your community? In J. Proulx & S. Perrault (Eds.), *No place for violence: Canadian Aboriginal alternatives* (pp. 22–38). Halifax: Fernwood Publishing and RESOLVE.

Thurston, W.E., Blundell-Gosselin, H.J., & Rose, S. (2003). Stress in male and female farmers: An ecological rather than an individual problem. *Canadian Journal of Rural Medicine, 8*(4), 247–54.

Thurston, W.E., Blundell-Gosselin, H.J., & Vollman, A.R. (2003). Health concerns of male and female farmers: Implications for health promotion planning. *Canadian Journal of Rural Medicine, 8*(4), 239–46.

Thurston, W.E., & Meadows, L.M. (2003). Rurality and health: Perspectives of mid-life women. *Rural and Remote Health, 3.* Retrieved from http://www.rrh.org.au/publishedarticles/article_print_219.pdf.

Thurston, W.E., & Meadows, L.M. (2004). Embodied minds, restless spirits: Mid-life rural women speak of their health. *Women & Health, 39*(3), 97–112.

Thurston, W.E., & Vissandjee, B. (2005). An ecological model for understanding culture as a determinant of women's health. *Critical Public Health, 15*(3), 229–42.

Vespa, J. (2009). Gender ideology construction: A life course and intersectional approach. *Gender & Society, 23*(3), 363–87.

Wanless, D., Mitchell, B., & Wister, A. (2010). Social determinants of health for older women in Canada: Does rural-urban residency matter? *Canadian Journal on Aging, 29*(2), 233–47.

Winson, A. (1993). *The intimate commodity: Food and the development of the agro-industrial complex in Canada.* Toronto: Garamond.

Winson, A., & Leach, B. (2002). *Contingent work, disrupted lives: Labour and community in the new rural economy.* Toronto: University of Toronto Press.

Working Group on the CIHR, Gender and Women's Health Research. (2000). *A women's health research institute in the Canadian Institutes of Health Research.* Available from British Columbia Centre of Excellence on Women's Health.

World Health Organization. (1978). *The declaration of Alma Ata.* Geneva: WHO.

World Health Organization. (1986). *Ottawa charter for health promotion.* Geneva: WHO.

Yates, C., & Leach, B. (2007). Industrial work in a post-industrial age. In V. Shalla & W. Clement (Eds.), *Work in tumultuous times: Critical perspectives* (pp. 163–91). Montreal: McGill-Queen's University Press.

PART ONE

Research, Policy, and Action

Beverly D. Leipert

Chapters that focus on research, policy, and action begin this text as essential bases for the consideration of policy, practice, and research issues and topics addressed throughout its pages. This section reveals from an interdisciplinary perspective important determinants of health issues and accomplishments of rural women. Margaret Haworth-Brockman and colleagues note the many research, policy, and action achievements of the Prairie Women's Health Center of Excellence over the past years, and further reveal the need to build on and continue this important work into the future. Rebecca Sutherns and Margaret Haworth-Brockman take a more national view of achievements related to rural women's health research and policy. Although much has been accomplished, these authors reveal that attention by governments, research funders, and policy makers to rural health and women's health remains fixated at the margins. This circumstance seems to have become entrenched across Canada recently, as Leipert, Landry, and Leach note in their research about rural women's organizations throughout the country. Participants in their study stated that fewer funds and less interest in rural and women's issues and organizations have become the norm in most provinces. Bushy, too, in her description of health issues of rural women in the United States, notes that economic, social, geographic, environmental, and cultural factors create some unusual barriers to health for rural women. Clearly the voices and perspectives of rural women have been vital to their health and the health of their communities, and must be included and promoted in future health, research, government, and policy endeavours.

1 Looking Back and Forging Ahead: Rural Women's Health Research and Policy in Canada

Rebecca Sutherns and Margaret Haworth-Brockman

'I need to know the lay of the land' – a profoundly rural expression and a highly appropriate one to describe this chapter, as it explores the research and policy landscape for rural women's health in Canada since the mid-1990s.

Why begin with research and policy? It has been said that research defines a discipline, not only by generating new knowledge but also by framing the very ways in which questions are asked and by delineating what is not known. The quantity, breadth, and depth of scholarship also point to the level of enthusiasm and investment in a particular field of inquiry. Policy too acts as an indicator of the salience and energy behind a topic, gauging the extent to which research findings have percolated into real-life decisions that guide behaviour. Many of the contributions in this book demonstrate the critical significance of scholarship about rurality, gender, and health to national health policy. By examining both research and policy related to rural women's health in Canada in this chapter, we provide a preliminary 'lay of the land' – an assessment of the contours, vitality, and relevance of the field itself.

Background

The description of a landscape is never neutral; it is always infused with the perspectives and preferences of one's guides. We bring particular lenses to this overview, including a commitment to gender-based analysis, an understanding that health is about far more than physicians and medical services, and an acknowledgement that 'rural' is part of a dynamic, contextually specific continuum with both spatial and social dimensions (See Bushy, chapter 5 in this volume). We also bring a solid belief that the health of rural women in Canada is worthy of renewed attention.

We begin our tour by examining trends in scholarship – Canadian research funded and/or published over the past decade addressing rural women's health. We then assess three broad examples of policy responses to the needs of rural women in Canada at federal, provincial, and local levels. We conclude by making a case both for and against the mainstreaming of rural women's health, asserting that specialists and generalists are both needed to ensure that rural women's health is better protected and promoted.

Scholarship

This section explores the support for and trends within recent Canadian research related to rural women's health. This literature review relies heavily on three published annotated bibliographies on rural, remote, and Aboriginal women's health in Canada (Bennett, 2005; Sutherns, McCallum, & Haworth-Brockman, 2007; Sutherns, Wakewich, Parker, & Dallaire, 2003) as well as an overview by Leipert (2005), which were supplemented by more recent topic-specific individual sources.

The process of searching for relevant scholarship itself yielded important insights about the contours of this field. The three main search terms, 'rural', 'women,' and 'health,' are each vast, individually generating an unmanageable number of documents, even when limited by the additional term 'Canada.' Yet using all three terms together proved inadequate, in part because it excludes other relevant terms, such as 'farm' or 'gender,' or the plethora of health-related words. Moreover, any or all of those terms may be used purely as descriptive demographic categories (e.g., 'The sample included men and women, urban and rural residents') rather than as the subject of the analysis itself. When only two of the three terms were central to an article, its relevance to rural women's health was variable. For instance, 'women's health' work may have no focus on rurality at all. 'Rural health' papers may be very relevant to women, yet when women's concerns are not made explicit, they are often not implicit in the research either. 'Rural women' tended to be a more useful category. So as in real life, rural women's health proved elusive to uncover in scholarship.

In terms of supporting scholarship by and about rural women, the Centres of Excellence for Women's Health (CEWH) and the Canadian Institutes for Health Research (CIHR) figure prominently. From 2001 to

2003, the CEWH thoroughly examined the influences of gender and rurality on women's health across Canada to generate an agenda for policy making and further research. That national study (Sutherns, McPhedran, & Haworth-Brockman, 2004) and its follow-up by the Prairie Women's Health Centre of Excellence (PWHCE) are discussed in chapter 3 of this volume. The Atlantic Centre's 'On the Margins' program among rural black women in Nova Scotia also emerged from the national study, and the CEWH have continued to support rural women's health research in innovative ways.

When CIHR was established in 2000, rural and northern health was not selected as a separate institute but was identified as an important cross-cutting theme requiring its own strategic research initiative. A National Steering Committee was struck, national consultations were held, a five-year strategic framework (2002–2007) was outlined, and rural health networking funds were released. Multi-year funding for rural health was made available in 2004, with grants awarded in the areas of rural maternity care, young women's health, social dimensions of rural health, and the role of pharmacists in improving rural health care, as well as two initiatives focused on public health nurses and improving northern accessibility to care. Yet since then, rural issues have not garnered significant attention within CIHR; online CIHR articles on rural health have not been updated since 2006 and directed funding has all but disappeared. The Institute of Gender and Health, for example, has had no explicit focus on rural women's issues, and the word 'rural' is not used even once in its strategic directions document through to 2012, although its 2008 'pillars' do include northern health and anti-violence work, which should have direct rural relevance.

As for other funding sources, in June 2009 the Social Sciences and Humanities Research Council reported that their Committee for Health Studies had been abolished and all health-related research proposals should be directed to CIHR. In Ontario, there has been a groundbreaking endowed chair position in rural women's health research at the University of Western Ontario since 2003, but the position was vacated in 2009 and had not yet been filled as of mid-2010. Limited funding for Aboriginal women's research is available through Pauktuutit (a longstanding Inuit women's advocacy group), the Native Women's Association of Canada, and the National Aboriginal Health Organization.

As for research quantity and thematic content, the body of research on rural women's health is very limited. Social-scientific approaches continue to dominate, especially small-scale, single-issue studies, with few studies exploring rural health status or disease prevalence rates. Longitudinal or statistical data related to rural women remain rare. One major exception is the DesMeules and Pong (2006) study entitled *How Healthy Are Rural Canadians? An Assessment of Their Health Status and Health Determinants.*

Access to appropriate rural maternity care remains the most thoroughly researched theme (see, for example, Couchie & Sanderson, 2007; Kornelsen & Grzybowski, 2006; Kornelsen, Moola, & Grzybowski, 2009; Van Wagner et al., 2007). Scarcity of rural physicians has also dominated the literature over the past ten years, including discussions of supply and demand projections and barriers to rural practice (Reid, Grava-Gubins, & Carroll, 2000). More recently, the focus of rural access has broadened to include the importance of local and culturally sensitive care. Other frequently published topics have included rural access to health care services, some aspects of Aboriginal women's health, the impacts of health reform, and rural nursing (Bennett, 2005; Sutherns et al., 2007; Sutherns et al., 2003). Work since 2006 has shown some concentration in the area of rural seniors, including chronic illness, home care, and long-term care (Allan & Cloutier-Fisher, 2006; Clark & Leipert, 2007; Skinner et al., 2008; see also Bushy, chapter 5 of this volume, for comparable US data) as well as the importance of gender and place (Melville Whyte & Havelock, 2007). Harris and Wathen have focused on rural women's health-information-seeking behaviours (Harris & Wathen, 2007; Harris, Wathen, & Fear, 2006; Wathen & Harris, 2007). Rural experiences of breast cancer (most notably a literature review by Bettencourt, Schlegel, Talley, & Molix, 2007) and intimate partner violence (Riddell, Ford-Gilboe, & Leipert, 2009; Thurston, Patten, & Lagendyk, 2006) are also becoming better documented. *Canadian Woman Studies* devoted an entire issue to rural women in Canada in 2005. Despite containing numerous excellent articles, the journal is currently difficult to access electronically, limiting its lasting impact.

Gaps identified in previous literature reviews that have begun to be addressed include the interplay between various social determinants of rural women's health (Caldwell & Arthur, 2009; Frankish et al., 2007; Hankivsky & Christoffersen, 2008; Leipert & George, 2008) and the experience of immigrant and/or minority subpopulations of rural women (Etowa, Wiens, Bernard, & Clow, 2007; Kulig, Wall, Hill, & Babcock, 2008). Some work on rural children and youth is emerging, particularly in the areas of obesity, nutrition, fitness (Bruner, Lawson,

Pickett, Boyce, & Janssen, 2008; Galloway, 2006, 2007; Martz, 2008; Salvadori et al., 2008), and sexual health (Langille et al., 2009; Poon & Saewyc, 2009). Further research is needed to explore why certain topics have received more research attention than others, but this is usually the result of the complex interplay between priorities reflected in research funding, research training, government policy, local needs, professional agendas, and media attention.

Even the organizations that gather and galvanize researchers appear to be waning. The most prominent and promising groupings are the Canadian Rural Health Research Society (CRHRS) and the Society of Rural Physicians of Canada (SRPC). The trajectory of the CRHRS is well documented in MacLeod, Dosman, Kulig, and Medves (2007), which underscores the ongoing challenges of effective collaboration in a competitive research environment. They confirm that 'the rural health research community in Canada remains small and widely dispersed, with few senior researchers'; when gender is added, that pool is even smaller. While some Canadian researchers (such as Denise Cloutier-Fisher, Stefan Grzybowski, Jude Kornelsen, Judith Kulig, Belinda Leach, Beverly Leipert, Martha MacLeod, Nadine Wathen, and Wilfreda Thurston) continue to focus on rural women's health, many have seen their funding cut and their priorities shift accordingly. The SRPC has contributed significantly to the field of rural health research through its online library and its publication of the *Canadian Journal of Rural Medicine* (CJRM). Although obstetrics have been thoroughly covered, gender analysis within the CJRM is rare, and the vast majority of the articles in its library were written in the late 1990s. As a voluntary organization comprising already over-stretched rural doctors, the SRPC has struggled to maintain the momentum that propelled its efforts a decade ago.

There appears to have been considerably more energy behind rural women's health issues in the late 1990s and early 2000s than we see today. The declining trend noted in the 2003–2006 literature review (Sutherns et al., 2007) has continued. We have noted an overall deterioriation in terms of leadership, dedicated expertise, research productivity, funding sources and opportunities, and organizations that could be supportive of rural women's health research.

While this trend is worrisome, there is still reason for some optimism. Even though rural women's health is not currently the subject of much direct attention, those concerns can be repackaged to adapt to new realities and attract renewed investment in inventive ways. For instance, ageing, mental health, the environment, anti-violence education, diabetes, or health record management are timely health issues that are well supported and directly relevant to the well-being of rural women. Creativity is required to make those connections clear.

Another opportunity exists in the fact that the findings from well-funded research supported over the last ten years should now be in the public domain. It is time to put into action the learning from those studies. Whether it be through using national research to inform local workshops and capacity-building tools as PWHCE has done (see Haworth-Brockman et al., chapter 3 of this volume), remote provision of mental health services to mothers in Nova Scotia by Patrick McGrath and his team,[1] or the Rural Women Making Change program energized by Belinda Leach and others,[2] a lack of published research activity may not necessarily indicate a lack of progress or action.

A final reason for optimism resides in the resilience of rural residents themselves. In Seaforth, Ontario, Canada's first community-driven, privately funded rural health research centre was established in 2008. It is already pioneering research projects, attracting the attention of skilled researchers and practitioners, and winning national awards. In the Arctic, innovative models of northern maternity care are being piloted and replicated with great success (Van Wagner et al., 2007). Throughout northern Ontario, research interns are being placed in rural communities in a program developed through a federal, provincial, and educational partnership. So there are clearly innovative models of research that hold promise for rural women.

Policy

Assessing trends in policy changes is a broader exercise. We will make it more manageable by highlighting examples of rural women's health policy decisions at three levels of health authority: federal bureaucratic infrastructure, gender in rural health planning in the Province of Manitoba, and the impact of health reforms on rural women's local access to health care, looking particularly at hospital closures and the centralization of maternity care.

Rural Women's Health in the Federal Government[3]

Generally speaking, conservative governments are not known for their investment in social services to benefit marginalized populations. This pattern has held true under the current leadership, which has been characterized by an ideological project-based approach rather than commitment to longer-term strategies and programs, with little attention to gender equity or a strong social safety net. This tendency is exacerbated in Canada by historical tensions around federal/provincial responsibility for health and social services funding, particularly complex in the case of First Nations women (Bent, Havelock, & Haworth-Brockman, 2007), along with high turnover within federal bureaucracies, which has limited institutional memory and continuity of expertise.

As for federal investment in women's issues, one clear example of weakened capacity is the cutting of administrative, research, and advocacy funding to Status of Women Canada (SWC) in 2006 and the ensuing demise of women's groups across the country (see Leipert et al., chapter 4 in this volume). More recently, the federal government has shown some renewed leadership in the area of gender-based analysis (GBA). Having committed to implementing GBA throughout its departments and agencies in 1995, its adherence to that standard was limited and patchy, as evidenced by a scathing 2009 Auditor General's report in which only four of sixty-eight federal initiatives were found to have integrated GBA effectively in policy development. As a result, the Privy Council Office and the Treasury Board of Canada Secretariat have committed to work closely with SWC to perform their GBA 'challenge function' more effectively, and government-wide GBA performance will now be evaluated annually (Office of the Auditor General of Canada, 2009).

More specifically regarding women's health, some federal bureaucrats have asserted that although women's health is less politically visible than it used to be, solid gender-based work is continuing nonetheless, having been mainstreamed into the fabric of federal political life. Others affirm that the prominence of women's health in the 1980s and 1990s has dropped off considerably over the past decade – a casualty of substitution as other marginalized groups have successfully competed for scarce federal funding. Some might argue that women's health is a victim of its own success, as substantial gains in gender equity through the women's movements of the 1960s to 1990s have led to a drop in the sense of urgency that could justify a dedicated investment in women's health, resulting in resources being diverted elsewhere.

As for the priority given to rural issues federally, the establishment of the Rural Secretariat has promoted engagement with rural issues within the federal bureaucracy, and its funding has recently been extended to

2013. Unfortunately the Secretariat focuses almost exclusively on economic issues, with virtually no attention paid to gender and/or health. While pressure from elected officials on behalf of their rural constituents can at times push rural issues higher on the agenda, urban concerns still have far greater political traction. Even accessing federal information on rural issues electronically is problematic, with sites billed as information portals for rural Canadians offering limited lists of outdated resources, incomplete timelines, and broken links.[4]

In the years 1997–2002, roughly corresponding to the period of increased attention to rural health in research circles as well, a federal Office of Rural Health was established, along with a Ministerial Advisory Council on Rural Health. Both of these bodies proved to be short-lived, closing shop with very little public attention not long afterwards. It is telling that the two federal documents identified at the top of the list from a mid-2009 Internet search of 'federal rural health in Canada' are dated 2002 and 2000. The downward trend in rural health scholarship has therefore been paralleled by a lack of federal policy leadership.

Not surprisingly then, rural women's health has garnered very little direct federal attention in recent years. Health Canada's support of the CEWH, and in turn the decisions of those centres to support rural women, has represented perhaps its most important investment. Yet there remains no clear lead organization to champion rural women's health issues in Canada.

Gender in Rural Health Planning in Manitoba

A second example of rural women's health policy, this time at a provincial level, is the Manitoba Department of Health, which has supported GBA and a focus on women's health for many years.

With the release of the Women's Health Strategy in conjunction with the provincial Status of Women office in 2001, Manitoba Health supported a number of developments, including formal policy recognition of gender as a determinant of health, a commitment to health services accessibility regardless of place of residence, and the development of a guide, in partnership with PWHCE, showing how GBA can be used to interpret health surveillance data. Following the release of the GBA guide (Donner, 2003), Manitoba Health funded training workshops in those regional health authorities (RHAs) that requested them.

At the same time, University of Manitoba's Manitoba Centre for Health Policy, which produces annual deliverables for Manitoba Health, was more routinely developing reports with sex-disaggregated data. For instance, it published a significant report in 2005 entitled *Sex Differences in Health Status, Health Care Use and Quality of Care: A Population-Based Analysis for Manitoba's Regional Health Authorities* (Fransoo et al., 2005).

To maintain the momentum, Manitoba Health then agreed to support the development of a Profile of Women's Health, which paid attention to comparisons and descriptions of women's health in rural parts of the province wherever possible. Further analyses compared women's health across and between regions, by districts within regions, by age, and by First Nations or Aboriginal identity (Donner, Isfeld, Haworth-Brockman, & Forsey, 2008). This project brought health researchers into frequent contact with health planners and policy makers at regional and provincial levels to share what was being learned. In advance of the profile's release, Manitoba Health contracted for new, targeted workshops in RHAs. These workshops served a dual purpose of drawing attention to both women's health and the importance of GBA.

Benefiting from good working relationships with health care providers (RHAs) and health researchers (PWHCE), Manitoba Health has followed through on its commitment to propel new knowledge and application of GBA with the intent of improving the health of rural women in the province. A revised Women's Health Strategy is slated to be released in 2011.

Local Health Reforms

A third lens through which to view rural women's health policy is a trend that is at once local, national, and even international in scope: the effects of recent health reforms on rural women's local access to care. Broadly speaking, these reforms have included movements away from institutionally based care and towards privatization, centralization, and cost cutting. (Ironically, these reforms have come about as part of *de*centralization of administration in some parts of Canada.) We illustrate with two examples: rural hospital closures and the centralization of rural maternity care.

The best-documented example of shutting down rural hospitals in Canada is the 1993 closures of 52 of Saskatchewan's 112 small hospitals.

While some have argued that this decision has proven to make good financial, medical, and political sense, as evidenced in part by the re-election of that provincial government (Lepnurm & Lepnurm, 2001; Liu, Hader, Brossart, White, & Lewis, 2001), others have asserted that the relative safety and efficiency of rural hospitals has been lost (Hutten-Czapski, 2009) and have enumerated the additional psychological, economic, and community costs of closures that are rarely factored into decision making. These include higher unemployment and lower per capita income, higher costs to access care, higher stress on providers and patients, less patient education, and a fundamental shift in the way communities are perceived (James, 1999). Similar costs have been documented throughout the industrialized world (e.g., Holmes, Slifkin, Randolph, & Poley, 2006; Petrucka & Wagner, 2003).

With women as the primary navigators, users, and providers of health care, men and women are clearly affected differently by rural hospital closures. Hospitals are often the major employers in small communities, employing predominantly women. Women generally have less access to financial resources to pay for the increased costs of care that is either privatized or available at a distance, including lost wages, transportation, meals, parking, childcare, and home medical supplies. Fewer hospital beds have meant more community-based and home care – responsibilities which usually fall to women. When such services are underfunded, resulting in poorer care, overcrowding, and delays, women's stress levels are especially high (National Coordinating Group on Health Care Reform and Women, 2002). The experiences of rural women therefore clearly need to be considered when evaluating the outcomes of policy decisions related to small hospitals.

As small hospitals close or offer fewer services, rural women become less able to give birth in their home communities. This trend has been well documented in the Canadian literature from a variety of angles, including the safety of birth in small hospitals (Iglesias, Grzybowski, Klein, Gagné, & Lalonde, 1998; Kornelsen & Grzybowski, 2008), the challenges of recruiting and retaining obstetric professionals in small communities (Reid et al., 2000), the need for collaborative models of maternity care (Peterson, Medves, Davies, & Graham, 2007; Sutherns, 2004), the desirability of being able to give birth close to home (Kornelsen et al., 2009; Lynch, Thommasen, Anderson, & Grzybowski, 2005; Zelek, Orrantia, Poole, & Strike, 2007), and women's resistance to being forced to travel to larger centres to have their babies (Kornelsen & Grzybowski, 2006). Although a thorough treatment of this field is clearly beyond the scope of this chapter, we raise it here to draw attention to the fact that many other formal and informal policy decisions that affect the sustainability of rural maternity care, such as health professional education, recruitment incentives, transportation infrastructure, childcare, obstetric care protocols, and on-call schedules, have far-reaching and profound effects on the lives of rural women. Gender-based analysis with a rural lens is therefore critical in effective policy development and analysis.

Implications

The trends within research and scholarship and policy at various levels are variable but overall are not moving in encouraging directions for rural women's health in Canada. What can be done to solidify a more positive direction for this important field of inquiry and practice?

Debate and policy attention continue to vacillate between specialized focus and mainstreaming to advance the causes of marginalized populations. Should there be a gender specialist on staff or should everyone become gender specialists? We find ourselves back in that same conversation here, but armed with the knowledge that effective research, policy, and action always require both.

Because 'rural women's health' does not presently benefit from a high degree of currency in research and policy circles, promoting it requires adapting the rural women's health agenda to new opportunities in areas such as disease-specific or place-based research. Although much more fragmented, this approach provides opportunities to think creatively about how to keep rural women's health issues on the radar of those in power, even if that requires calling those issues by new names. Doing so situates rural women's health within the mainstream even if it is not known as such.

But responding to opportunities to repackage rural women's health does not take us far enough. A failure to focus explicitly and directly on rural women's health means we lose things of critical importance. For example, rurality and gender remain important determinants of health, not just tick boxes on demographic surveys. We need to understand them, separately and together. New research affirms that various social determinants of health interact differently depending on the health outcome in question (Wilson, Eyles, Elliott, & Keller-Olaman, 2009), so targeted research is required. Second, although the attention paid to rural women may be in decline, their needs have not lessened over that time.

Being female and living rurally means combatting a double layer of disadvantage. Without explicit attention being paid to rural women, there will be a tendency, borne out by decades of experience, for their concerns to be forgotten. Third, lessons learned through the women's movement and anti-racism efforts, among others, indicate that marginalized populations require structural support – government funding and attention – to overcome barriers that might otherwise be seen as individual-level choices or deficiencies. Finally, Canada has a role to play in this field. Its significant rural population and history, relative wealth, and reputation for promoting justice and human rights mean that Canada is a country strongly placed to take leadership in ensuring equitable access to health for men and women, regardless of where they live.

Conclusion

So the lay of the land is highly variable. On the whole, the trends are not moving in encouraging directions for rural women's health. With many other competing interests vying for attention and investment, the downsizing of support for rural and gender-focused issues, and the lack of rural women's health champions, it is perhaps not surprising that rural women's health has struggled to build and maintain momentum in scholarship and policy. Integrating rural women's health concerns into other current issues, as well as raising their profile directly in other ways, are both required. Opportunities for creativity and examples of innovation do exist, and they inspire us to move forward. As one federal employee and long-time gender advocate wisely reminded us, 'It is a battle. It always has been. Gains that should take five years seem to take fifteen when it comes to women's health. But stick with it. It's worth it in the end.'

Notes

1 http://www.bringinghealthhome.com.
2 http://www.rwmc.uoguelph.ca.
3 We are grateful to Christine Burton, Monique Charron, Gail Erickson, Beverly Leipert, and Wilfreda Thurston, whose expertise informed this section.
4 http://www.hc-sc.gc.ca/hl-vs/jfy-spv/rural-rurale-eng.php and http://www.rural.gc.ca.

References

Allan, D., & Cloutier-Fisher, D. (2006). Health service utilization among older adults in British Columbia: Making sense of geography. *Canadian Journal on Aging, 25*(2), 219–32.

Bennett, M. (2005, December). *Annotated bibliography of Aboriginal women's health and healing research*. Commissioned by the Aboriginal Women's Health and Healing Research Group, Vancouver.

Bent, K., Havelock, J., & Haworth-Brockman, M. (2007). *Entitlements and health services for Métis and First Nations women in Manitoba and Saskatchewan*. Winnipeg: Prairie Women's Health Centre of Excellence.

Bettencourt, B.A., Schlegel, R.J., Talley, A.E., & Molix, L.A. (2007). The breast cancer experience of rural women: A literature review. *Psycho-Oncology, 16*(10), 875–87.

Bruner, M.W., Lawson, J., Pickett, W., Boyce, W., & Janssen, I. (2008). Rural Canadian adolescents are more likely to be obese compared with urban adolescents. *International Journal of Pediatric Obesity, 3*(4), 205–11.

Caldwell, P., & Arthur, H. (2009). The influence of a 'culture of referral' on access to care in rural settings after myocardial infarction. *Health and Place, 15*(1), 180–5.

Clark, K., & Leipert, B. (2007). Strengthening and sustaining social supports for rural elders. *Online Journal of Rural Nursing and Health Care, 7*(1), 13–26.

Couchie, C., & Sanderson, S. (2007). A report on best practices for returning birth to rural and remote Aboriginal communities. *Journal of Obstetrics and Gynaecology Canada, 29*(3), 250–60.

DesMeules, M., & Pong, R. (2006). *How healthy are rural Canadians? An assessment of their health status and health determinants*. Ottawa: Canadian Institute of Health Information. Retrieved from http://secure.cihi.ca/cihiweb/displayPage.jsp?cw_page=GR_1529_E.

Donner, L. (2003). *Including gender in health planning: A guide for regional health authorities*. Winnipeg: Prairie Women's Health Centre of Excellence. Retrieved from http://www.pwhce.ca/gba.htm.

Donner, L., Isfeld, H., Haworth-Brockman, M., & C. Forsey. (2008). *A profile of women's health in Manitoba*. Winnipeg: Prairie Women's Health Centre of Excellence. Retrieved from http://www.pwhce.ca/profile/mbWomensHealthProfile.htm.

Etowa, J., Wiens, J., Bernard, W., & Clow, B. (2007). Determinants of Black women's health in rural and remote communities. *Canadian Journal of Nursing Research, 39*(3), 56–76.

Frankish, C.J., Moulton, G.E., Quantz, D., Carson, A.J., Casebeer, A.L., Eyles, J.D., Labonte, R., & Evoy, B.E. (2007). Addressing the non-medical determinants of health: A survey of Canada's health regions. *Canadian Journal of Public Health, 98*(1), 41–7.

Fransoo, R., Martens, P., Burland, E., Prior, H., Burchill, C., Chateau, D., & Walld, R. (2005). *Sex differences in health status, health care use and quality of care: A population-based analysis for Manitoba's Regional Health Authorities.* Winnipeg: Manitoba Centre for Health Policy.

Galloway, T. (2006). Obesity rates among rural Ontario schoolchildren. *Canadian Journal of Public Health, 97*(5), 353–6.

Galloway, T. (2007). Gender differences in growth and nutrition in a sample of rural Ontario schoolchildren. *American Journal of Human Biology, 19*(6), 774–88.

Grzybowski, S., Kornelsen, J., & Schuurman, N. (2009). Planning the optimal level of local maternity service for small rural communities: A systems study in British Columbia. *Health Policy, 92*(2), 149–57.

Hankivsky, O., & Christoffersen, A. (2008). Intersectionality and the determinants of health: A Canadian perspective. *Critical Public Health, 18*(3), 271–83.

Harris, R., & Wathen, N. (2007). 'If my mother was alive I'd probably have called her.' Women's search for health information in rural Canada. *Reference and User Services Quarterly, 47*(1), 67–79.

Harris, R.M., Wathen, C.N., & Fear, J.M. (2006). Searching for health information in rural Canada. Where do residents look for health information and what do they do when they find it? *Information Research, 12*(1). Retrieved from http://informationr.net/ir/12-1/paper274.html.

Holmes, G.M., Slifkin, R.T., Randolph, R.K., & Poley, S. (2006) The effect of rural hospital closures on community economic health. *Health Services Research, 41*(2), 467–85.

Hutten-Czapski, P. (2009). Rural health under attack (editorial). *Canadian Journal of Rural Medicine. 14*(2), 41.

Iglesias, S., Grzybowski, S., Klein, M.C., Gagné, G.P., & Lalonde, A. (1998). Rural obstetrics. Joint position paper on rural maternity care. Joint Working Group of the Society of Rural Physicians of Canada (SRPC), The Maternity Care Committee of the College of Family Physicians of Canada (CFPC), and the Society of Obstetricians and Gynaecologists of Canada (SOGC). *Canadian Family Physician, 44*, 831–43.

James, A.M. (1999). Closing rural hospitals in Saskatchewan: On the road to wellness? *Social Science and Medicine, 49*(8), 1021–34.

Kornelsen, J., & Grzybowski, S. (2006). The reality of resistance: The experiences of rural parturient women. *Journal of Midwifery and Women's Health, 51*(4), 260–5.

Kornelsen, J.A., & Grzybowski, S.W. (2008). Obstetric services in small rural communities: What are the risks to care providers? *Rural and Remote Health, 8*, 943. Retrieved from http://www.rrh.org.au/publishedarticles/article_print_943.pdf.

Kornelsen, J., Moola, S., & Grzybowski, S. (2009). Does distance matter? Increased induction rates for rural women who have to travel for intrapartum care. *Journal of Obstetrics and Gynaecology Canada, 31*(1), 21–7.

Kulig, J.C., Wall, M., Hill, S., & Babcock, R. (2008). Childbearing beliefs among low-German-speaking Mennonite women. *International Nursing Review, 55*(4), 420–6.

Langille, D.B., Flowerdew, G., Aquino-Russell, C., Strang, R., Proudfoot, K., & Forward, K. (2009). Gender differences in knowledge about chlamydia among rural high school students in Nova Scotia, Canada. *Sexual Health, 6*(1), 11–14.

Leipert, B. (2005). Rural women's health in Canada: An overview and implications for policy and research. *Canadian Woman Studies, 24*(4), 109–16.

Leipert, B.D., & George, J.A. (2008). Determinants of rural women's health: A qualitative study in southwest Ontario. *Journal of Rural Health, 24*(2), 210–18.

Lepnurm, R., & Lepnurm, M.K. (2001). The closure of rural hospitals in Saskatchewan: Method or madness? *Social Science and Medicine, 52*(11), 1689–1707.

Liu, L., Hader, J., Brossart, B., White, R., & Lewis, S. (2001). Impact of rural hospital closures in Saskatchewan, Canada. *Social Science and Medicine, 52*(12), 1793–1804.

Lynch, N., Thommasen, H., Anderson, N., & Grzybowski, S. (2005). Does having cesarean section capability make a difference to a small rural maternity service? *Canadian Family Physician, 51*, 1238–9.

MacLeod, M.L.P., Dosman, J.A., Kulig, J.C., & Medves, J.M. (2007). The development of the Canadian Rural Health Research Society: Creating capacity through connection. *Rural and Remote Health, 7*, 622. Retrieved from http://www.rrh.org.au/publishedarticles/article_print_622.pdf.

Martz, D. (2008). *Saskatchewan rural youth healthy lifestyles and risk behaviour.* Winnipeg: Prairie Women's Health Centre of Excellence. Retrieved from http://www.pwhce.ca/program_rural_youth.htm.

Melville Whyte, J., & Havelock, J. (2007). *Rural and remote women and the Kirby-Keon report on mental health: A preliminary gender-place analysis.* Winnipeg: Prairie Women's Health Centre of Excellence.

National Coordinating Group on Health Care Reform and Women. (2002). *Women and health care reform.* Toronto: Author. Retrieved from http://www.womenandhealthcarereform.ca/publications/women-hcren.pdf.

Office of the Auditor General of Canada. (2009, Spring). Gender-based analysis. In *Report of the Auditor General of Canada to the House of Commons* (pp. 1–40). Ottawa: Minister of Public Works and Government Services CanadaPeterson, W.E., Medves, J.M., Davies, B.L., & Graham, I.D. (2007). Multidisciplinary collaborative maternity care in Canada: Easier said than done. *Journal of Obstetrics and Gynaecology Canada, 29*(11), 880–6.

Petrucka, P.M., & Wagner, P.S. (2003). Community perception of rural hospital conversion/closure: Re-conceptualising as a critical incident. *Australian Journal of Rural Health, 11*(5), 249–53.

Poon, C.S., & Saewyc, E.M. (2009). Out yonder: Sexual-minority adolescents in rural communities in British Columbia. *American Journal of Public Health, 99*(1), 118–24.

Reid, A.J., Grava-Gubins, I., & Carroll, J.C. (2000). Family physicians in maternity care. Still in the game? Report from the CFPC's Janus Project. *Canadian Family Physician, 46,* 601–11.

Riddell, T., Ford-Gilboe, M., & Leipert, B. (2009). Strategies used by rural women to stop, avoid, or escape from intimate partner violence. *Health Care for Women International, 30*(1–2), 134–59.

Salvadori, M., Sontrop, J.M., Garg, A.X., Truong, J., Suri, R.S., Mahmud, F.H., Macnab, J.J., & Clark, W.F. (2008). Elevated blood pressure in relation to overweight and obesity among children in a rural Canadian community. *Pediatrics, 122*(4), e821–e827.

Skinner, M.W., Rosenberg, M.W., Lovell, S.A., Dunn, J.R., Everitt, J.C., Hanlon, N., & Rathwell, T.A. (2008). Services for seniors in small-town Canada: The paradox of community. *Canadian Journal of Nursing Research, 40*(1), 80–101.

Sutherns, R. (2004). Adding women's voices to the call for sustainable rural maternity care. *Canadian Journal of Rural Medicine, 9*(4), 239–44.

Sutherns, R., McCallum, M., & Haworth-Brockman, M. (2007). A thematic bibliography and literature review of rural, remote and northern women's health in Canada 2003–2006. *Resources for Feminist Research, 32*(3/4), 142–78.

Sutherns, R., McPhedran, M., & Haworth-Brockman, M. (2004). *Rural, remote and northern women's health: Policy and research directions – Summary report.* Winnipeg: Prairie Women's Health Centre of Excellence. Retrieved from http://www.pwhce.ca/ruralAndRemote.htm.

Sutherns, R., Wakewich, P., Parker, B., & Dallaire, C. (2003). *Rural, remote and northern women's health in Canada: Policy and research directions – A literature review and thematic bibliography.* Retrieved from http://www.pwhce.ca/pdf/rr/RRN_SecE_E.pdf.

Thurston, W.E., Patten, S., & Lagendyk, L.E. (2006). Prevalence of violence against women reported in a rural health region. *Canadian Journal of Rural Medicine, 11*(4), 259–67.

Van Wagner, V., Epoo, B., Nastapoka, J., & Harney, E. (2007). Reclaiming birth, health, and community: Midwifery in the Inuit villages of Nunavik, Canada. *Journal of Midwifery and Women's Health, 52*(4), 384–91.

Wathen, C.N., & Harris, R.M. (2007). 'I try to take care of it myself.' How rural women search for health information. *Qualitative Health Research, 17*(5), 639–51.

Wilson, K., Eyles, J., Elliott, S., & Keller-Olaman, S. (2009). Health in Hamilton neighbourhoods: Exploring the determinants of health at the local level. *Health and Place, 15*(1), 374–82.

Zelek, B., Orrantia, E., Poole, H., & Strike, J. (2007). Home or away? Factors affecting where women choose to give birth. *Canadian Family Physician, 53*(1), 78–83.

2 Rural Women's Research and Action on the Prairies

Margaret Haworth-Brockman, Rachel Rapaport Beck, Joanne Havelock, Harpa Isfeld, Noreen Johns, Diane Martz, Lynn Scruby, and Jayne Whyte

> PWHCE has made a significant difference in the lives of rural women. Often rural women feel left out in any discussion of policies affecting their health, but it is clear that PWHCE wants their voices to be heard. (Merrill, 2007, p. 15)

Prairie Women's Health Centre of Excellence (PWHCE) is a policy-oriented research centre with fifteen years' experience fostering, developing, and creating new research with community and academic partners. It has a mandate for the provinces of Saskatchewan and Manitoba, but PWHCE's work is often national or international in scope. There is some overlap among the organization's four primary areas of focus – women in poverty; Aboriginal women; women who live in rural, remote, and northern communities; and gender in health planning – but there has been a considerable number of new projects in each of these areas. It is through research at PWHCE that new information and resulting action in communities and policy directions emerge.

The health influences of living in a rural, remote, or northern location are multiple. Unfortunately, little research has been conducted on this important social determinant of health, particularly for women (see Sutherns & Haworth-Brockman, chapter 1). PWHCE and the other Centres of Excellence for Women's Health recognized this gap in knowledge more than a decade ago and undertook to conduct a national, comprehensive study to explore what rural and remote-dwelling women had to say about the health issues that concerned them. The final report, *Rural, Remote and Northern Women's Health: Policy and Research Directions* (Sutherns, McPhedran, & Haworth-Brockman,

2004), was released in June 2004. That groundbreaking work helped turn the tide of attention more to rural and remote women's health, at least for a time.

This chapter will focus on work with rural women supported and conducted by PWHCE,[1] beginning with the 2004 pan-Canadian project, and how this work led to changes in policy and community action. Some of PWHCE's work arose directly from the results and recommendations of the national study, ultimately benefitting from the new knowledge generated and the greater understanding of the issues relating to women who live rurally, remotely, and in the north in Manitoba and Saskatchewan. Other projects were enriched by PWHCE's commitment to including aspects of rural women's health, particularly related to the health and health issues of Aboriginal women. Indeed, rural women's perspectives have become one of the 'lenses' in PWHCE's ongoing program of research and policy.

Learning from Rural, Remote, and Northern Women

> It was energizing to have such a variety of women come together to share their insights, and for many of the women [it was] a first opportunity to discuss their concerns in a national forum. (participant, quoted in Sutherns et al., 2004, p. C8)

The national project *Rural, Remote and Northern Women's Health: Policy and Research Directions* (Sutherns et al., 2004) was intended to address two key areas where research was needed: an understanding of the health needs of women living in rural, remote, and northern parts of Canada; and a gender analysis of rural health policy and research. Women across the country, from the high Arctic to the prairies, to the coasts of Canada and points between, participated throughout the project to inform the development of future research and to make policy recommendations to improve their health and health services.

Qualitative methods were used to honour the expertise of the women, their daily lives providing context and meaning to the research. In addition, the multiple voices and perspectives of community, academe, and government gave a breadth of knowledge and expertise to the report. A number of women commented that they had never before been asked to contribute to research or been asked their opinions about health policy.

Eight key interrelated findings emerged from the comprehensive. literature review, pan-Canadian focus groups, policy forums, and the final national consultation:

1. Rurality is a powerful determinant of women's health, as both a geographical and a sociocultural influence.
2. Rural Canada is not homogeneous.
3. Consistent rural health priorities are discernable in the face of diversity.
4. Rural women are largely invisible to policy makers.
5. The health care system is perceived as underfunded and deteriorating.
6. Efforts to restructure that system have exacerbated rather than improved an already vulnerable system.
7. Poverty and financial insecurity, primarily resulting from unemployment, job insecurity, low wages, or seasonal work, are key determinants of health for rural women and their families.
8. Health is perceived as being synonymous with, and distinct from, health care.

Three key policy recommendations for new directions were provided by the women who participated in the project:

1. Factor gender, place, and culture into all health policy,
2. Define health policy as more than health care services, and
3. Improve health by improving access.

These findings and recommendations remain relevant. In the years that followed, PWHCE was able to lead and support numerous community and academic projects, building on the national agenda from the report findings, and working with women to make the recommendations meaningful to them.

A Community Kit to Bring Research Back to Women

No one is more important in this process than you. No one will have more passion about improving rural women's health than rural women. No one has more insight into the challenges or the solutions. (Sutherns & Fish, 2004, p. 1)

At the request of participants and in follow-up to one of the recommendations made in the national project, PWHCE's first step was to commission a Community Kit. The kit was intended to assist women to make changes in their home communities. Recognizing that 'one size does not fit all,' as the national project illuminated, the kit encourages women living in rural, remote, or northern regions of Canada to identify issues that are important to them and to help strategize about the best course of action to take in terms of influencing policy.

The plain-language Community Kit has several components that guide both formal and ad hoc community groups through the process of 'helping to make change happen.' The Community Kit was distributed widely in Canada and received accolades from Literacy Partners in Canada. It became the starting place for PWHCE's ensuing work with women in Saskatchewan.

The Rural Women's Issues Committee of Saskatchewan

Is it possible to reinforce to young women the positive things that living rurally can give to themselves and their families? Let them have a positive choice in 'Why I live where I do!' (Johns & Havelock, 2006, p. 16)

Building on the intent and content of the kit, PWHCE sought to develop greater investment in rural women's health, using women's own leadership and local knowledge to set the directions and actions needed. In the autumn of 2004, PWHCE's Regina office began working directly with rural women in Saskatchewan to see how the national report's recommendations could be of use to them. A Rural Women's Health workshop held in Young, Saskatchewan, in November 2004 was a place for women to discuss follow-up action for the group. As a result of that first meeting, the Rural Women's Issues Committee of Saskatchewan (RWICS) was born, with the intent of becoming a stand-alone women's organization. The group was successful in securing grants from the Women's Program of Status of Women Canada in 2005 and 2006 from the Empowering Rural Women's Voices project, and, combined with continued infrastructure from PWHCE, the Centre for Rural Studies and Enrichment in Muenster, Saskatchewan, and the support of passionate volunteer committee members, RWICS was able to bring many women together over four years.

Working with RWICS, PWHCE ran six similar workshops in a number of communities in the southern half of Saskatchewan (funds and opportunity restricted the RWICS to southern Saskatchewan). A provincial policy forum was held in Muenster in 2006, and a final workshop on rural women and leadership was held in Davidson in 2009. Over the course of the meetings women made more than 370 suggestions for personal, local, provincial, national, or international actions that could improve the well-being of rural women and their communities. Where possible, local women's groups determined and acted upon the recommendations from the original national project that had been clarified and refined in the RWICS workshops.

The need for leadership training and support for strong women's organizations whose perspectives would be heard on issues affecting rural Canada was raised at the workshops time and again. The final RWICS gathering in Davidson was a place to continue to encourage reclaiming rural women's leadership. Participants also agreed that it was time for Saskatchewan rural women to work with women in the cities, to create better understanding of rural women's situations and to achieve common goals.

Along with hosting the workshops, RWICS established and maintained a website[2] and produced and distributed reports about each workshop to participants and policy makers. Through good working relationships with reporters, RWICS received local and provincial media coverage in agriculture and women's health publications. RWICS members were invited to participate in research and policy forums related to health, agriculture, and the status of women, and there was ongoing interest in the work of RWICS from policy makers.

The mandate of RWICS was to bring rural women together to discuss issues relevant to rural women and to envision the future. Too often rural women are excluded from discussions and feel geographically and socially isolated. While Saskatchewan has a long history of women organizing to effect change, this tradition has been more difficult to uphold in recent years, particularly for rural and farm women. In part this is the result of increasing demands on farm women, the 'triple workload,' including on-farm and off-farm work in addition to running households, child rearing, and community responsibilities. A further barrier has been the systematic reduction and removal of funding for women's groups and gatherings. Not surprisingly, women's groups have not flourished. Unfortunately, after four years of working together, federal changes to PWHCE funding and cuts to Status of Women

Canada left RWICS without financial and staff support. Without a mandate to provide ongoing support to community groups PWHCE had to reduce its own involvement and could not step in to help. Given the constraints of organizing women across a wide geographical area without a major funder, RWICS had to cease its activities. This is truly unfortunate for rural women, who for a time were collectively heard by community groups, media, and policy makers.[3]

Gender and Place in Women's Mental Health

> Isolation can be geographic (distance from neighbours and services) but also social (alone because of the symptoms and stigma of mental illness). (Whyte & Havelock, 2007, p. 6)

Building on the growing body of evidence and support from rural women, PWHCE commissioned a gender and place analysis of a ground-breaking federal report on mental health. The Senate Standing Committee on Social Affairs, Science and Technology report on mental health, mental illness, and addictions, *Out of the Shadows at Last*, was released by senators Kirby and Keon in 2006. The report documents the needs of those affected by mental illness and suggests changes required to bring meaningful improvements to the lives of people requiring mental health services in Canada. In response, PWHCE published *Rural and Remote Women and the Kirby-Keon Report on Mental Health: A Preliminary Gender-Place Analysis*, developed by Jayne Whyte with Joanne Havelock (2007), who reviewed the Senate report 'Highlights and Recommendations' with a gender-place lens focused on women in rural and remote areas of Saskatchewan.

Mental health issues have been long neglected, and the attention generated by the Kirby-Keon report and its suggestions for change were welcomed. Despite federal commitments to gender-based analysis (GBA), the Senate report makes no mention of gender. Three pillars – choice, community, and integration – were identified in the Kirby report as key to strengthening care and services for individuals with mental illness. Whyte and Havelock illustrated how these pillars could be strengthened by a gender-place analysis. In smaller or farming communities there may be access to only one care giver, and having a 'choice' requires travelling to a larger centre. Choice of a care giver who is experienced and sensitive to the unique needs of lesbian, Aboriginal, immigrant, or disabled women can be impossible to obtain. 'Community' may be experienced as both a strength and a burden to a woman seeking care in a rural area where anonymity is a challenge, if not impossible. The culture of farm communities can be very supportive and cooperative, but there can also be significant stigma felt by those who 'do not pull their own weight.' Finally, 'integration' can happen more quickly in smaller communities; however, the constant change in personnel, who often work in a rural area for a short time or only occasionally, disrupts continuity of care and the development of trust between clients and health care workers.

Women in all environments play a fundamental role in caring for others, and in doing so face a number of gender-specific stresses and challenges as they take on multiple roles in their families and communities. The care that women provide for friends and family must be recognized and integrated into workforce planning and in meeting the needs of rural and remote women through providing respite care to prevent further stress and related mental and physical illness.

Whyte and Havelock's analysis helped to reiterate the importance of gender and place to local health planning and policy. Their document is an example of how attention to women and to GBA can be applied in health policy at any level.

Including Low-Income Women with Children

> It's really just the sense of community that you find here [at the Family Resources Center]; the moms really become their own supports. (Scruby & Rapaport Beck, 2007, p. 21)

Women who participated in the national project consistently reported that precarious and inadequate income was among the most important influences on their physical and mental health (Sutherns et al., 2004). As women living in poverty have been a focus for research and policy analysis at PWHCE, it was natural that new work considered the interactions of gender, poverty, and rural living. In an exploration of the role of Family Resource Centres (FRCs) as supports for low-income women, PWHCE collaborated with Dr Lynn Scruby of the University of Manitoba in a community-based research project (Scruby & Rapaport Beck, 2007).

FRCs provide support, programming, and a shared setting for families across Canada, yet are often overlooked by researchers. Scruby and Rapaport Beck conducted several focus groups at four FRCs in

Manitoba, two in the city of Winnipeg and two in rural Manitoba, to investigate how best to contribute to participant-led program changes at FRCs and to provide policy advice for provincial and local governments. In an unanticipated development as the project progressed, the staff at the FRC in one of the rural Manitoba sites found that they were facing a demographic shift in their participant base: a significant number of German Mennonite farmers had recently moved to the area and were increasingly finding themselves facing poverty in their new country. To assist the FRC and to create more responsive research, the researchers included this group and conducted a focus group in German with on-site English translation for the researchers and note taker. All stakeholders in the project were able to benefit from the knowledge gained from this situation and the addition of this subpopulation to the focus groups.

The 'big picture' emerged from the focus groups, and interestingly, the issues were common in both urban and rural settings. Six key policy areas and twenty-one recommendations emerged from discussions with women, including access to programs and services, housing, childcare, food security, education, FRCs as safe and nurturing environments, and the need to foster partnerships.

Rural women in the study spoke specifically about their isolation and lack of access to programs and services, including food banks, transportation, and legal aid. Reaching these and other services often requires travel from a home community, which can be both time consuming and expensive, particularly when children must come along or if they require care while they remain at home. The greater costs of services, particularly telephone and transportation, in rural areas add to women's isolation and become barriers to services. However, the rural women did have some advantages over low-income women in the city. The women at the rural FRCs typically had a higher level of education and income than their urban counterparts, as well as lower housing costs. Socially, the benefits of being in a small town or rural environment allow for an informal referral process in that each person in a community is known to one another, and information about services is shared through word of mouth.

The researchers reaffirmed that rurality is a powerful social determinant of health for women and, likewise, geography is an important contributor to women's experiences. That is, rural women felt invisible to policy makers, living at such great distances from where decisions are made. The women in this study felt their low incomes hindered their involvement in advocating for change that could improve their circumstances; living away from large towns and the capital increased their feelings of powerlessness.

The Bovine Spongiform Encephalitis (BSE) Crisis on the Prairies

> She's the one that gets the phone calls from the bank...from the fertilizer place. She's the one that gets the mail ... The wives probably are the ones that do the books ... So the stress is on her. Then she has to go and try buy groceries, and she has no money to buy groceries and how are you going to feed your children, especially if you're a young family? (Enarson, Martz, Haworth-Brockman, McLachlan, Amaratunga, & Thurston, 2007, n.p.)

In 2006, PWHCE was invited to participate in new research about the effects of BSE on farm families, based out of the universities of Calgary and Ottawa. PWHCE's first contribution was a review of the international literature (McCallum, Sutherns, & Haworth-Brockman, 2006). Only a handful of articles were discovered that related to the interactions of coping with BSE and personal or community health. As suspected, most of the research on BSE has been quantitative and there was almost no gender analysis.

Subsequently, project researchers recruited and surveyed farm families in several provinces, including Saskatchewan and Manitoba. The goal of the research was to examine the health of farm families and determine how the discovery of BSE in Canadian cattle had affected these families and their communities. PWHCE conducted interviews in Saskatchewan and looked at the human toll of the BSE crisis on farmers, ranchers, and communities, employing a gender-based analysis.

Declining rural populations, depressed agricultural economies, and the shifting and eliminating of access to markets in other countries are all part of the complex history of and context for the BSE crisis in Canada. A distinct cultural climate of self-sufficiency and resilience in farming families and communities was threatened and strained with the coming of BSE. The multigenerational aspect of farming in Canada creates a great deal of pressure on farm families; they do not want to give up farming after decades of shared sacrifice and work within the family.

BSE created stressors that specifically affected the health of girls and women, including overwork (on- and off-farm); substance abuse; increased 'emotion work' with partners, children, and parents; and increased potential for interpersonal violence. As well, social pressures to be 'the good wife and mother' with a 'successful marriage' under such stressful conditions took their toll. BSE often contributed to increased labour (for the family, on- and off-farm, and in the community), increased numbers of single-headed households (young, old, divorced), increased outmigration (in to town and out of province), and stretched kin networks (grandparenting) and smaller farm households. The intent of the researchers was to return to the participants with their findings, but to date the project has not had the funds to do so. Without an organization like RWICS, there are few opportunities to meet with rural women collectively.

Risky Behaviours and Lifestyles among Saskatchewan Rural Youth

> Drinking and partying become the social activities of the whole community. What alternative do we provide for youth? (key informant, Youth at Risk, quoted in Martz & Wagner, 2008)

In an effort to encourage healthy lifestyles and curb risky behaviour in rural youth in Saskatchewan, an investigation was undertaken to identify behaviour in this under-researched population. *Saskatchewan Rural Youth Healthy Lifestyles and Risk Behaviour Project* (Martz & Wagner, 2008) had a number of partners, including PWHCE. Issues facing rural female and male youth in western Canada have been a neglected area of research and must be better studied in order to effectively serve the young women and men in rural areas.

A series of key informant interviews were held with rural youth service providers working in health, education, and justice sectors. Additionally, university students were trained to administer a questionnaire survey of young people in grades seven to twelve (ages twelve to eighteen years). In all, thirty-four schools participated with a range of 7–71% student participation. Over 950 surveys were included for analysis, involving 31% of students in the target age group in one rural school division in Saskatchewan. Through these surveys, as well as the key informant interviews, a wide range of issues were raised, including sexuality, tobacco and alcohol use, drug use (illegal, prescription, and non-prescription), healthy eating and weight, physical activity, gambling, personal safety, and depression. The results were presented to youth focus groups to check for accuracy. A gender-based analysis was a critical part of the research, and the results were presented to the focus groups to gain understanding as to why the differences between results for female and male youth persisted in many areas.

Alcohol use and associated drinking and driving emerged as a major issue in this study of rural youth. Although young females were as likely as young males to binge drink, females start drinking later, drink less often, and are less likely to drink and drive than males. Female youth reported starting smoking at a younger age than male youth but were much less likely to use other tobacco products. Female and male youth were not significantly different in their age of initiation and frequency of use of marijuana or in their use of other illegal drugs; however, female youth were more likely to see drug and alcohol use as a problem. This Saskatchewan study showed that female youth were more likely to report sad feelings and thoughts of suicide, although between 2000 and 2005 suicide accounted for an average of 23% of deaths for male youths in Canada and 18% of deaths for female youths (Statistics Canada, 2007). Females were more likely to use seat belts and less likely to be threatened, injured, or involved in a physical fight. Over half of the youth had engaged in sexual intercourse by age seventeen; there were no significant differences in the proportions of female and male youth who reported having had sex, the age they first had sex, or the likelihood that they used alcohol or drugs before sex. With rates of sexually transmitted infections rapidly increasing among youth, a significant health issue arises in the finding that only 71% of sexually active youth used a condom the last time they had sex. Female youth were more likely to report they had been forced to have sex. They were also found to be much more likely to describe themselves as overweight, to want to lose weight, and to fast, vomit, or take laxatives to lose or keep from gaining weight. At the same time, they were less physically active than their male counterparts.

The key informants and participants raised a number of critical health issues specific to rural living: there is little support and few resources for dealing with youth substance abuse in rural settings; attitudes prevalent in rural communities, such as denial, fear of isolation, and stigmatization, often hinder health service access; lack of transportation makes access to health services difficult; and limited opportunities for and choices of activities for young people create a situation for youth to make poor choices.

As the study demonstrated, not only does gender interact with rural living, but age is a critical health determinant as well.

Gender in Health Planning

Gender-based analysis (GBA) is a method of analysis which assesses the differences and similarities between and among men and women. It is used to demonstrate the differences and similarities in health status, health care utilization, and health needs of men and women. (Donner, Isfeld, Haworth-Brockman, & Forsey, 2008, p. 6)

Over time, PWHCE's work has involved rural women and incorporated their needs wherever possible. This has been the case in the areas of gender-based analysis (GBA) in health planning and related work in women's health indicators. The application of GBA makes for more effective and responsive health policy for both women and men.

As part of its ongoing collaboration with the Manitoba department of health, PWHCE developed a plain-language guide to GBA for regional health planners (Donner, 2003). The guide was distributed to all eleven regional health authorities (RHAs) in Manitoba, and Manitoba Health sponsored local workshops to work on topics of priority to the individual regions. Based on the success of the guide and workshops, Manitoba Health commissioned PWHCE to develop a full profile of women's health in Manitoba.

A Profile of Women's Health in Manitoba (Donner et al., 2008) is a GBA of health administration and surveillance data, drawing upon other existing research and knowledge relating to the influences and intersections of age, geographical location (RHA), income, and Aboriginal identity. Urban-to-rural comparisons are made wherever possible. The report is comprehensive in its scope, examining over 150 health indicators relating to health status, health services use, socio-economic influences, health system preferences, and lifestyle choices, for a more complete picture of women's health throughout the province.

The profile has generated a number of related projects, including further GBA training throughout Manitoba. Training in RHAs was critical to making the information in the profile accessible to the key target audience – health care planners throughout the province. Across Manitoba, 110 planners and programmers took part in workshops that were developed to share the results of the profile pertaining to the RHAs and to build upon and reinforce existing skills in GBA that would ultimately support its use in regional community health assessments. Given all that PWHCE has learned in our work with rural women, we tailored each RHA workshop to their local concerns and priorities. Workshop participants came away from the experience feeling re-energized and committed to GBA as an organizing principle in their work and its role in health planning.

Because of the attention paid to rural women's health, and how this does or does not differ from the health of women who live in urban areas, the profile and attendant workshops have been significant assets to Manitoba Health in drawing continued attention to rural and remote women's health, including how RHAs conduct and use their community assessments.

Aboriginal Women's Health Research at PWHCE

The Aboriginal population of Manitoba and Saskatchewan makes up a significant proportion of the total population of the two provinces. It is essential to understand the complex health needs of First Nations and Métis women who reside throughout the Prairie provinces (a small population of Inuit women also live in the prairies) as part of rural women's health. As noted at the beginning of this chapter, Aboriginal women's health has been a fundamental focus for PWHCE. Naturally, it is entwined with the work concerning rural, remote, and northern women's health – one very often includes the other. PWHCE has endeavoured to work with Aboriginal women, communities, and governing bodies to develop that information.[4] Each of these projects was undertaken with the blessing of local community leaders with the aim to bring forward the ideas, visions, and voices of the women they represented.

There are a number of complicating factors related to any discussion of Aboriginal women's health in Canada. The first relates to language. Often the term 'Aboriginal' is used as an umbrella without differentiation between the groups – First Nations with and without Indian Status, Métis, and Inuit peoples. These differences are important in health research because of their varied entitlements and access to health services. The PWHCE paper *Entitlements and Health Services for First Nations and Métis Women in Manitoba and Saskatchewan* provides a history and legal description of these differences and addresses implications in the realm of health care, 'because terminology, identity and legal status have direct bearing on who receives what health benefits' (Bent, Havelock, & Haworth-Brockman, 2007, p. 1).

Discussion

In the last decade, research on women's experience of rurality as a social determinant of health has grown. New work that includes gender considerations has important social policy implications.

The projects reviewed in this chapter each highlighted the influence of rural living in women's lives, and women often reported feeling ignored by policy makers. Through research and the development and maintenance of community groups, the voices of marginalized groups and individuals can be heard. Community groups that operate across large geographic areas face multiple and expensive barriers; without financial support they cannot survive, as Leipert et al. have described in chapter 3 of this book. Rural women involved in these projects placed a high value on the opportunities they had to hold meetings in person, but the costs and time needed for travel were difficult to sustain. Consistent and sufficient core funding for agencies and community groups will best serve the needs of those who are geographically distant from policy discussions and decisions.

PWHCE has been in a privileged position to undertake the many research projects described in this chapter. Moving those research projects into policy advice and community action is a responsibility that will continue for the organization. Exploring and understanding issues and concerns specific to rural women is a valuable undertaking and is critical to the advancement of their health, and the health of rural families and communities. Policy makers must be reminded that women and men experience health and health policy differently and that an effective gender-based analysis necessarily includes a place analysis, particularly in a country as diverse (geographically and otherwise) as Canada.

Conclusion

Since 2002, PWHCE has significantly added to the breadth of knowledge on Aboriginal and rural, remote, and northern women's health through new research with community and academic partners. Recognition of the importance of applying gender-based analysis in health planning has been a major step forward for provincial governments and women in Manitoba and Saskatchewan. With GBA, the importance to women and their health of place and culture, as well as the impacts of living rurally, can become better understood in all their complexities and contexts.

Women find themselves in multiple roles on any given day – farming, raising children, working outside the farm, caring for parents or others, and volunteering in their communities. These not only take time, they take energy, leaving women with not enough hours in the day. The fostering of relationships and partnerships built on women's shared experiences becomes less possible. In addition, women living in rural Manitoba and Saskatchewan report feeling invisible to policy makers, whose decisions have so much effect on their lives. The need to recapture this important aspect of women's lives helped to foster the Rural Women's Issues Committee of Saskatchewan. Born from the efforts of the national project, *Rural, Remote and Northern Women's Health*, RWICS brought women together to work for change in the prairies.

Research that encourages change and action is most relevant to rural women (Sutherns et al., 2004). And policy built from research that successfully brings forward voices that were previously unheard can be most effective. PWHCE has been providing this forum for researchers, policy makers and, most importantly, women in these two provinces to create positive change. With sufficient, consistent, and sustained federal and other funding, PWHCE looks forward to continuing this important work.

Notes

1 All reports referred to in this chapter can be accessed at www.pwhce.ca.
2 See the RWICS website: http://www.ruralwomensask.ca.
3 Since this chapter was first written, the Women's Information Network of Saskatchewan (WIN-S; www.winsask.net3) was incorporated as a not-for-profit, involving many of the same women who had participated in RWICS. The group aims to enhance communication between rural and urban women across the province.
4 www.pwhce.ca/program_aboriginal.htm.

References

Bent, K., Havelock, J., & Haworth-Brockman, M. (2007). *Entitlements and health services for First Nations and Métis women in Manitoba and Saskatchewan*. Winnipeg: Prairie Women's Health Centre of Excellence.

Donner, L. (2003, rev. 2005). *Including gender in health planning: A guide for Regional Health Authorities*. Winnipeg: Prairie Women's Health Centre of Excellence.

Donner, L., Isfeld, H., Haworth-Brockman, M., & Forsey, C. (2008). *A profile of women's health in Manitoba*. Winnipeg: Prairie Women's Health Centre of Excellence.

Enarson, E., Martz, D., Haworth-Brockman, M., McLachlan, S., Amaratunga, C., & Thurston, W. E. (2007). *'Just another nail on the coffin': Living with BSE on the Canadian Prairie*. Presented at the Canadian Risks and Hazards Network, Vancouver, November 2007.

Johns, N., & Havelock. J. (2006). *Rural women's health workshop: Christopher Lake, Saskatchewan October 27-28, 2006*. Winnipeg: Prairie Women's Health Centre of Excellence.

Kirby, M.J.L., & Keon, W.J. (2006). *Out of the shadows at last: Transforming mental health, mental illness and addiction services in Canada*. Ottawa: Standing Senate Committee on Social Affairs, Science and Technology.

Martz, D., & Wagner, A. (2008). *Saskatchewan rural youth healthy lifestyles and risk behaviour project*. Fact Sheet (Health Canada DSCIF Study #6558-08-2005/3480566). Saskatoon: University of Saskatchewan.

McCallum, M., Sutherns, S., & Haworth-Brockman, M. (2006). *Bovine Spongiform Encephalitis (BSE): An annotated review of the international literature*. Winnipeg: Prairie Women's Health Centre of Excellence.

Merrill, A. (2007). *Fertile ground, healthy harvest: A decade of Prairie Women's Health Centre of Excellence*. Winnipeg: Prairie Women's Health Centre of Excellence.

Scruby, L., & Rapaport Beck, R. (2007). *Including low-income women with children: Program and policy directions*. Winnipeg: Prairie Women's Health Centre of Excellence.

Statistics Canada. (2007). *Deaths, by selected grouped causes, age group and sex, Canada, provinces and territories, annual* (Table 102-0551; 269280 Series). Retrieved from http://cansim2.statcan.ca/cgi-win/cnsmcgi.exe?Lang=E&RootDir=CII/&ResultTemplate=CII/CII_pick&Array_Pick=1&ArrayId= 102-0551.

Sutherns, R., & Fish, S. (2004). *Rural, remote and northern women's health: Policy and research directions: Community kit*. Winnipeg: Prairie Women's Health Centre of Excellence.

Sutherns, R., McPhedran, M., & Haworth-Brockman, M. (2004). *Rural, remote and northern women's health: Policy and research directions*. Winnipeg: Prairie Women's Health Centre of Excellence.

Whyte, J., & Havelock, J. (2007). *Rural and remote women and the Kirby-Keon report on mental health: A preliminary gender-place analysis*. Winnipeg: Prairie Women's Health Centre of Excellence.

3 Closing the Gap:
Rural Women's Organizations
and Rural Women's Health in Canada

*Beverly D. Leipert, Tamara Landry,
and Belinda Leach*

Rural women experience unique and significant physical, mental, and social health challenges. Physical health issues include increased incidence of cancer (Brophy et al., 2006), shorter life expectancies (Canadian Institute for Health Information [CIHI], 2006), increased risk of violence and abuse (Hornosty & Doherty, 2003), and physical health issues related to lack of health resources, low income, rural stress, hunger, and homelessness (Kubik & Moore, 2003). Mental health issues of rural women include depression, despair, and psychological distress related to rural socio-economic circumstances and isolation, and limited availability and lack of anonymous mental health resources (Leipert, 2006; Sutherns, McPhedran, & Haworth-Brockman, 2004). Social health issues are related to limited social support, and lack of understanding of rural women's social support needs, including support that is tailored to the diverse needs of women in rural locations, for example women who are elderly, disabled, single mothers, lesbian, and of various cultural backgrounds (Clark & Leipert, 2007; Leipert, 2010). This holistic approach to women's health issues, that recognizes the contribution of social and economic factors to health outcomes, is captured in the social determinants of health framework (Raphael, 2008).

Rural areas are significantly under-resourced with regard to health information and services as well as a plethora of other assets and services that urban Canadians take for granted (CIHI, 2006). It is in this context that rural women seek services and resources to close the gap between what is available to them as rural residents and what they need as full Canadian citizens. Our research suggests that over the past thirty years rural women's organizations (RWOs) have been one of the few resources providing women in rural communities with support around a range of issues, including their own and their family's health and well-being. RWOs encompass a diverse set of mandates and missions among which health information and health services, conventionally defined, occupy only a relatively small number. While some RWOs are privately funded, many are heavily dependent on provincial and federal funding.

In this chapter we present findings from our national study conducted in 2008 that explored the effects of financial cutbacks on rural women's health and well-being and on RWOs themselves. Our research findings indicate that women have frequently used an available RWO as an entry point for assistance on issues that go far beyond the mandates of the organizations they are consulting. We argue that RWOs have provided an essential resource for rural women that implicitly and appropriately adopts a social determinants of health approach to women's needs. We argue further that cuts to funding for RWOs in recent years, which in some cases have led to the demise of entire organizations, have grave implications for the health and well-being of rural women.

Purpose and Objectives of the Study

The purpose of this research was to determine the utility and accessibility to rural women of RWOs that strive for women's equality and the advancement of their health, and how funding cutbacks to RWOs affect rural women's access to RWOs and thus affect their health and well-being.[1] Study objectives were to (1) determine ways that rural women access RWOs, (2) identify the nature and reasons for rural women's access to RWOs, and (3) explore effects of recent financial cutbacks to RWOs on those organizations and on the health and well-being of rural women.

Review of the Literature

A social determinants of health approach has come to characterize the contemporary moment for health research and health delivery in Canada (Health Canada, 1996) and in other parts of the world (World Health Organization, 2008). The social determinants approach is significant in that it shifts attention away from individual behaviours and lifestyle choices, such as smoking, diet, and exercise, towards socio-economic factors that can be addressed through public policy. However, as Leipert and George (2008) note, much of the concern regarding social determinants, both as a research tool and as a framework for service delivery, is that they are viewed through an urban lens and largely fail to consider how the determinants might be nuanced to apply to rural people and rural environments.

A growing body of literature considers rural women's lives in order to highlight the ways in which women experience the rural environment differently from men and to draw attention to the importance of gender itself as a key determinant of health (for example, see Sutherns and Haworth-Brockman, chapter 1, and Haworth-Brockman et al., chapter 2 in this text). Traditional rural pursuits (farming, hunting, logging for men; horticulture, preserving food, and practising skilled handicrafts for women) that are quite fiercely defended even in the face of rapid change in urban settings lead to strong and enduring rural gender identities (Leach, 2011). Young rural girls often grow up with greater limits on their freedom than boys, with the effect of closing down social opportunities for girls (Dunkerley, 2004). As they get older some young women will leave to pursue educational opportunities, but many will stay behind and not gain the qualifications associated with better-paid jobs (Corbett, 2007), with life-long negative consequences for their income and social and employment security. Economic restructuring in the past twenty-five years in Canada has reduced well-paid rural employment opportunities for women (e.g., in the public sector, teaching, and nursing) and increased those in the lower-paid jobs of the service sector (Leach, 1999). Women living on farms may be especially vulnerable economically as family farming becomes an increasingly precarious endeavour (Heather, Skillen, Young, & Vladicka, 2005). Women may be perceived to have a weaker financial claim on family farms that they marry into, their economic fate linked to intergenerational family relations that are not easily disentangled (Machum, 2006). As women lose male partners due to death or for other reasons, they are often unable to move from a deteriorating rural home – both because rural rental accommodation is scarce and because supply in rural housing markets is highly constrained (Bruce, 2003). Rural women's access to a range of economic resources and an acceptable quality of life is further complicated by very limited public transportation (Fuller & O'Leary, 2008) and limited or no childcare (Gott, 1997), the latter of which is still predominantly considered the domain of women.

Thus, women in rural areas contend with a particular set of socio-economic circumstances, but services that would help them negotiate these have always been far more limited than for urban residents. This situation has worsened in the last two decades, as urban-based efficiency models have led to the closure of many rural services (Halseth & Ryser, 2006).

It is in this context that RWOs became a valuable resource for women. In the early twentieth century, the Women's Institutes (WI) set up by the Ontario Department of Agriculture targeted women for education in the public health aspects of farming. WIs then followed in the other Canadian provinces and internationally. By the 1920s grassroots rural women had taken hold of the organization and began to shape it according to their own agendas (Kechnie, 2003). In the early 1970s farm women organized into autonomous groups separate from mainstream farmer's organizations, spurred by incidents such as the notorious Murdoch divorce case,[2] the developing women's movement, and the deepening farm crisis (Shortall, 1994). Furthermore, 'equality seeking' women's organizations were eligible to pursue government funding through the Secretary of State's Women's Program established in 1973 and since 1995 housed in Status of Women Canada. This program encouraged farm women's organizations to broaden their mandates and provided the means to establish a range of organizations, including women's health centres, anti-violence shelters and rape crisis centres, and women's employment resource centres.

It is important to note that the *Report of the Royal Commission on the Status of Women*, published in 1970, had recognized the crucial role that women's organizations were playing in fighting discrimination, providing appropriate services, and seeking alternatives to existing policies and programs (Riddell-Dixon, 2001). In the 1980s the government's funding strategy for women's organizations and for women's programs came under attack. Federal and provincial support programs for farm women have been decimated under successive governments (Gerrard, Thurston, Scott, & Meadows, 2005). Under pressure from non-feminist women's organizations and conservatives more generally, there has been a sustained diversion of funds from the Women's Program, along with its reorganization around project rather than program funding (Canadian FAFIA, 2008).

For women's organizations in rural communities these cuts have been devastating. The shift to project funding has undermined the organizations' ability to maintain staff and infrastructure. Stretched to provide services with diminishing resources and ever-increasing accountability measures, as well as increasing reliance on private fundraising in competition with other similarly cash-strapped organizations, many women's organizations have reluctantly ceased operations or curtailed their services. Leach, Hawkins, and Pletsch (2009) argue that the elimination of many organizations and the reduction in others' capacity constitute a triple blow to women in rural communities: they diminish the visibility of women's issues and the possibility of making change, as well as leaving women without the assistance they desperately need. It is in the context of these shifts in government funding to women's organizations that our study of RWOs' support for rural women's health and well-being took place.

Methodology

RWOs were recruited by word of mouth, by contacting RWOs known to the authors, and by sending an email message about the research to women's groups, women's health researchers, and rural women across the country who the authors believed would be interested in this research. Inclusion criteria for the RWOs were that they (1) had as their mandate the striving for women's equality, (2) supported rural women's health in some capacity, and (3) had been in existence for a minimum of five years. Examples of RWOs that participated in this research included rural women's resource centers, rural shelters, and rural women's farm groups and employment and training centres. Individual interviews were conducted with directors and other former and present personnel of RWOs in nine provinces; in one province a focus group was conducted with personnel of one RWO. Interested respondents were invited to contact the first author collect by phone or by email. There is representation in the study from all of the provinces in Canada except Quebec, where the authors had limited contacts and where contacts did not respond to recruitment efforts.

Data Collection

Sixteen women were interviewed by telephone and an additional five women participated in a focus group setting. The one-to-one interviews were thirty to sixty minutes in length and were audio-recorded. An open-ended interview guide was used to elucidate reasons for accessing RWOs, including health reasons, and effects of cutbacks on RWOs and on the health and well-being of rural women. Participants were also encouraged to provide any additional information that they felt was important. After completing the interview, each participant received an honorarium to express appreciation for her time and expertise.

To analyse the data, each of the seventeen audio-recordings was transcribed verbatim, and content analysis (Reinharz & Kulick, 2007) of the transcribed interview data was conducted by a minimum of two researchers to determine themes that addressed the purpose and objectives of the study. During analysis, attention was paid to identifying both expressed and hidden meanings in participants' comments and to locating relevant socio-political contextual information (Reinharz & Kulick, 2007). Analysis was enriched by regular meetings of the research team to discuss analysis process and findings. NVIVO™ (1999), a computer qualitative data management program, assisted in the data retrieval and analysis process.

The twenty-one women who participated in this study represented nineteen RWOs[3] and had rich experience with RWOs, both past and present. This experience included serving as board members, directors, volunteers, and other personnel of RWOs. Participants were farm women, counsellors, outreach workers, social workers, a public health nurse, a former teacher, a policy analyst, women with degrees in agriculture, horticulture, and sociology, and women with limited or no post-secondary education. As a result of interviews with these participants, several themes emerged.

Missions of Rural Women's Organizations and Services They Provide

The missions or mandates of the RWOs varied and included advocacy and consulting, counselling, education and training, outreach, providing housing and shelter, promoting farming and agriculture, and improving the overall status of women. RWOs whose mission was advocacy and consulting provided services to women such as counselling for women (and sometimes to men when there were no services available for males), lobbying efforts for equality issues, and policy development. Counselling services provided by RWOs focused on financial advice, social support, violence and abuse, and addiction disorders. RWOs also provided education and training that helped women to gain knowledge and skills in accounting, homemaking, assertiveness/leadership, volunteering, and agriculture and farming. Outreach services provided to women by RWOs focused on various topics such as sexual health and coping skills, adult literacy, rural health and safety, and health-related topics. Housing and shelter services provided by RWOs offered emergency shelter for women and children leaving violent or abusive relationships and temporary housing for women transitioning from an emergency shelter to a new residence. RWOs supported farming through the farm stress telephone support line and offered rural-related courses for women on topics such as cattle management and farm bookkeeping. RWOs also lobbied on behalf of rural women to bring their concerns to politicians, met with provincial premiers and government departments, and either arranged visits themselves or were invited by organizations to represent women's perspectives on agricultural and farm issues. In addition, RWOs provided women with opportunities to participate in research projects that addressed the social determinants of women's health, gender analysis and health planning, and policy issues. Participation in these research projects allowed RWOs to accurately represent women on equality issues, in public policy, and regarding needs in their communities.

RWOs also provided community-based services and support to women through transportation services and transportation and childcare subsidies, victim assistance and witness abuse programs, abuse/ assault hotlines, lending libraries, drop-in clinics/centres, childcare resources and referrals, and the hosting of community events.

A significant aspect of the services RWOs provided to women is that for most rural communities, the RWO was the only resource available to provide these services. Housing and shelter services provided by RWOs, in particular, were often the only resources in rural communities for women in abuse situations. In addition, because RWOs were staffed primarily or only by women, they were able to provide services to women *by* women. In most rural areas, this type of gender-sensitive service is not otherwise available, and thus was highly valued by the study participants and rural women.

Women's Reasons for Consulting Rural Women's Organizations

The most urgent and immediate reason that women accessed RWOs was for physical health issues, such as help in escaping from domestic abuse and obtaining physical safety for themselves and their children. A participant explained, 'They access the RWO [because] it's an escape from ... really difficult and challenging situations that they live in on a daily basis.' Some women accessed RWOs because they needed someone to talk to, to help them through domestic or abuse situations so they did not have to leave their home and uproot their children. One participant noted that women in violent relationships will call the shelter and say, 'I'm not coming to the shelter ... [but] I ... need to touch base with somebody. [Women] are more reluctant to leave ... [they] don't [want] to risk losing ... money coming in.' Another participant also stated, 'We'll encourage them to keep calling us ... try to help them make a safety plan.'

Women also consulted RWOs for mental-health-related issues, such as drug and alcohol abuse, fetal alcohol syndrome, eating disorders, anxiety, and depression. Participants noted, '[Women] ... struggling with addiction, [this] has a huge impact on health,' and 'We have high incidence of fetal alcohol syndrome ... some people with severe brain damage are raising children with brain damage ... it's an area of concern for us.'

Another participant noted that addictions are one of the top health issues in rural communities and directly contribute to other issues, such as violence, sexual and physical abuse, and their sequelae. In addition, women accessed RWOs for reasons related to rural childcare and parenting, poverty, and farming. Women find it very costly and difficult to access childcare in rural areas. As one participant noted, 'We still have this problem ... ninety percent ... of women on farms are now working off the farm to subsidize ... put food on the table ... Paying for rural childcare ... is very expensive.' In addition, women in the 'sandwich generation' who are now faced with the task of caring for their elderly parents as well as their children often sought social and emotional support from RWOs. A participant explained, '[There is an] increase in the complexity of issues that women are bringing forward ... not only parenting ... [but also care] of an aging parent at home.' Participants stated that women tend to 'wear a lot of hats on the farm'; the personal impacts on women of these multiple roles include being overextended and burned out. RWOs helped women to deal with their multiple roles and overextensions. Women also consulted RWOs on issues relating to poverty and financial support. As one participant commented:

> Poverty is a serious issue ... that's one of the biggest determinants of health ... women who are struggling with poverty ... can barely afford to feed [themselves] ... how do [they] afford 20 bucks [of] gas it costs for getting from another rural community to meet with a worker?

Because of the lack of resources available in rural areas and the distances to travel to resources, women relied on RWOs to provide programs that addressed leadership training, finances, education, self-development, and mental health issues. As an example of the latter, one participant noted, 'We have horticulture therapy ... a lot of women ... with anxiety issues or depression ... this program helps them to go in and start something from a seed, nurture it, care for it and feel they're actually helping something grow and fix it.' Workshops related to women's role in farming were also provided, including 'training [for women] related to agriculture ... milking clinics ... proper sanitation ... bookkeeping ... computers ... accounting information to help them out in that role.'

Effects of Funding Cutbacks

Participants revealed that the main effects of funding cutbacks to RWOs related to staff issues, program and advocacy cutbacks, organization sustainability, the challenges of keeping up with changing community needs, and limitations to research projects and applying for funding. Funding cutbacks prevented or hindered RWOs from hiring qualified and experienced staff, maintaining existing long-term staff, keeping centres open with sufficient staff, meeting increasing service demands, and supporting staff with continuing education. More than one participant noted, 'Challenges [are] placed upon us by funding restrictions ... we aren't able to pay the staff at a reasonable rate, which affects retention.'

Women were reluctant to access services and discuss their problems with inexperienced, uneducated, and very young staff. One participant stated, '[Staffing] has an impact on ... women ... a woman who was admitted to our shelter recently ... didn't want to speak to the staff person ... because she was so young. She said "I can't burden her."' Several participants in the study reported that the hiring of inappropriate staff was occurring more frequently in rural women's organizations because of financial cutbacks; these cutbacks meant that RWOs did not have the funds to attract and retain suitably qualified staff. As a result, rural women were becoming more reluctant to access RWO resources, choosing instead to either accept or try to deal with issues on their own, even if they did not have the resources. As a consequence, it may seem that rural women do not need RWOs or are coping well without them when, in fact, decreased RWO support masks or hides problems in rural areas, which makes these problems more difficult to identify, more entrenched, and more challenging to address.

To cope with decreased funding, RWOs reduced or eliminated outreach programs, parenting and infant/tot programs, workshops, and transportation services. One participant noted, 'If we don't get funding ... that means we don't do outreach ... once you begin offering services and support to the community ... not being able to do that is not being fair.' The cutbacks to outreach and advocacy also meant that '[women's] voices aren't heard ... if organizations are not able to ... connect with [and advocate for] women.'

Funding cutbacks had a compounding effect on women and children, as one participant remarked: '[Loss of programs has] a profound effect on baby's health, mother's health and it has ripple effects into the community.' The effects included women having limited or no access to social support, education, and training, and the need to use their own limited resources to get what they needed, which resulted in lower socio-economic status and poorer physical and mental health.

As a consequence of cutbacks to RWO funding, women hesitated to build relationships with RWOs. A participant explained, 'It takes a long time to build trust relationships, especially with diverse communities, so you do it cautiously, carefully, because it's fragile. You don't want to be offering things that aren't sustainable, they must be sustainable.' Another participant explained, 'If somebody is sick or has to be on extended leave, we don't have the capacity to backfill ... [so] we can't deliver that service ... which means women don't get what they need.' Consequently, women were apprehensive about accessing services and trusting staff because they were unsure if the people would continue to be there and services would be continuously and consistently offered; they did not want to risk counting on resources that might not be there tomorrow.

Cutbacks to RWO funding made it difficult to keep up with the challenging and changing needs of rural communities, such as increasing homelessness and the need for housing and shelter, funding based on population size rather than needs, an increase in violence and addictions, and providing services to cultural populations. One participant summarized the perspectives of several others when she stated, 'Our [shelter] capacity is for ten ... we've had as many as twenty-three.' The increasing need for shelters stems from the increase in violent and abusive relationships, as well as an increase in homelessness because of limited affordable housing. As one participant explained, '[Homelessness] is ... an increasing issue ... people in our rural areas want to move in closer where the services are but ... homes that are available in the more central areas, the housing prices have gone through the roof.'

Without RWO services such as shelters, women are probably staying, or staying longer, in abusive or domestic violence relationships. As one participant noted, 'These cuts ... really impact further on women so that they're ... staying in their violent situation or ... giving up ... they're doing worse because of the multiple barriers these cuts have caused.' This is a very direct example of how the health, well-being, and safety of women's lives are being compromised as a consequence of limited RWO funding.

All the participants talked about how funding has not been increased to meet increasing needs. Funding is based on population rather than need. As one participant commented, 'Our money hasn't changed but our demand for services has tripled or quadrupled.' Because rural areas have low populations, they receive less funding than urban areas, even though rural needs may be equal to or even greater than in urban locations.

Because of funding cutbacks, RWOs also found it challenging to understand and meet the needs of diverse cultural groups. As one participant noted, 'I think becoming culturally aware and sensitive is ... key.' As a result of cutbacks, training for cultural safety and the provision of relevant services were curtailed or eliminated. This has the very real effect of creating barriers to services, as evidenced by the fact that some women chose not to access services because they felt there was a lack of sensitivity to their specific needs and a lack of cultural understanding and racism. A participant explained, 'There is a long history of ... racism by ... service providers ... willingness to trust is very weak, limited, and cautious ... [requiring] long-term building.'

Because of funding cutbacks, RWOs had limited staff to become involved in research projects and were apprehensive about applying for funding because they were uncertain of their organization's sustainability. As one participant explained, 'We've not gone after a lot of new grants because we haven't known if we would be around to finish them.' RWOs also reported difficulties with operating under short-term project-based funding that supported only specific research projects and not infrastructure or programmatic needs. Furthermore, instead of RWO directors being able to plan and support their organizations, because of cutbacks they were frequently faced with the need to engage in frontline service provision. These staffing issues created difficulties in sustaining the RWO organization, and in planning and meeting the evolving needs of rural women and their communities.

Participants' Recommendations

Longer-term rather than annual funding, more infrastructure funding, more core funding to pay for staff, funding for programs instead of pieces of programs, and funding based on community needs rather than population size were consistent recommendations. More funding would enable RWOs to hire, maintain, and retain qualified and experienced staff, provide education and training to existing staff, and increase effective service provision to communities. One participant stated:

> What we need are qualified individuals ... we don't have resources to ... deal with challenges we're experiencing ... we don't provide the kind of income that [staff require], the kind of background experience that [women] need ... people aren't going to apply for jobs ... just above minimum wage.

Other recommendations included the need for more advocacy and research on both prominent and under-considered issues, and more advocacy to advance women's perspectives and policies that address their needs. Participants suggested more focus on farm women's issues and rural childcare, research on targeted populations such as First Nations, issues relating to homelessness and mental health, and an increased focus on illness and injury prevention and health promotion for women, for example, through programs on gender sensitivity. Participants also recommended an increase in family violence services and in services that address addictions, violence, and physical and sexual assault. As a participant noted, '[They are] key problems. There's not ... many shelters [in rural areas] and where does a woman go ... [when she needs help]?'

In addition, participants recommended increasing multidisciplinary networking and service provision opportunities in rural communities, developing multi-issue centres that encompass a variety of services in one place, and creating wrap-around services, especially for abuse situations. As one participant remarked, 'All of the organizations and committees working together is essential ... we can no longer work as little islands ... we have to come together as a community to deal with the issues as an entire community.' Another participant advised, regarding shelters, '[We need wrap around services] ... [this] means that we want to have people who can begin ... working with women while they're in the shelter ... but can also move [their services] from the shelter into their homes.' Wrap-around services can provide consistent and informed care that is important for all rural women.

Implications and Conclusions

The numerous missions of the RWOs indicate their desire and the importance of these organizations to address diverse issues and to be relevant to the communities and women they serve. Many of the determinants of health, such as gender, culture, economics, and social support (Health Canada, 1996), form the basis of RWO missions and activities. Indeed, it seems that RWOs are attempting to be all things to all women, and it is true that in rural settings, RWOs may be a woman's only resource or the only resource that offers services provided by women. For example, physicians in rural communities, if they are available at all, are often male; and nurse practitioners and public health nurses, who are predominantly women, are not commonly available in most rural settings in Canada, and their work with women only as well as with women with families has often been minimized or eliminated. Rural women deal with sensitive and sometimes life-threatening issues, such as intimate partner violence, and they often prefer to deal with female health and social service providers (Leipert, 1999, 2006; Riddell, Ford-Gilboe, & Leipert, 2009). Because RWOS promote services for women and are generally staffed by women, their importance becomes clear.

Yet our study revealed that due to decreasing financial support from federal, provincial, and municipal governments, the presence and sustainability of RWOs are threatened, and the services and programs they can provide are becoming fewer and more limited in scope and depth. RWOs are less able to provide services to women in remote areas, and services are being provided by staff without the educational or experiential backgrounds or the maturity to adequately provide services. Because of understaffing, administrative staff are becoming frontline service providers, compromising the ability to engage in planning, support, advocacy, and research activities that advance women's health and well-being. If, as is often maintained, women are the backbone of rural communities, compromising RWOs and women also compromises the health and well-being of rural communities.

In spite of downsizing or eliminating programs due to funding cut-backs, RWOs refused to eliminate services that directly support women in abuse situations. However, these services, such as safe houses and transition housing, are definitely becoming less available and effective as less funding is provided to RWOs and the needs of rural communities increase. In addition, the quality of services related to counselling, outreach, and education is threatened as funds to attract and retain qualified staff diminish. As a consequence, women are more often forced to remain in abusive partner situations, not only at a serious cost to their health and well-being and that of their children, but also at the risk to their lives.

In accordance with several other studies (see Sutherns & Haworth-Brockman, chapter 1; Haworth-Brockman et al., chapter 2; Bushy, chapter 4; Coward et al., 2006; Leipert, 1999; Leipert et al., 2012; Sutherns et al., 2004), participants in our study highlighted the importance of providing more health promotion and illness and injury prevention services for women in rural settings. Health promotion services are essential in rural areas that have little or no resources to promote women's health (CIHI, 2006; Leipert, 1999, 2006; Leipert et al., 2011). However, participants revealed that many of these services have been minimized or discontinued due to lack of funding and changing government priorities. As a result, the advancement of changes that promote women's health and well-being is stalled, and changes in rural communities that would support women's health are not realized or are realized in much slower and less effective ways. The present situation is thus, as one participant commented, 'One step forward and two steps back.'

Study participants made several recommendations to strengthen RWOs and rural women's health: governments need to give priority to rural women's health and enrich funding to RWOs and rural women's health programs; RWOS need to enhance advocacy, health promotion, and research activities to address prominent as well as less obvious issues, provide multidisciplinary services in one location, and make available wrap-around services that follow the woman from service to home. Many of these recommendations have also been reflected in other research that has explored rural women's health issues from a social determinants perspective (CIHI, 2006; Leipert, 1999; Sutherns et al., 2004) as well as in recent government commissions (Romanow, 2002). Thus, the recommendations from this study reveal consistency in intent and purpose, as well as the ongoing nature of these issues.

Several of the organizations whose staff we interviewed for this study have now ceased to exist due to financial cutbacks and lack of support. We contend that these cuts have resulted from broader neoliberal ideas about reducing taxation and government interventions. Although these ideas have been adopted in Canada to a greater or lesser extent by all types and levels of government, they have arguably been more ideologically driven by Progressive Conservatives, as several participants in this study noted.

The major conclusion of this study is that rural women's organizations have played and where they can will continue to play a significant role in promoting, supporting, and serving the health and well-being needs of rural women. Nonetheless, governments at the federal and provincial levels seem reluctant to address the enduring and substantial rural health issues, and their continued cuts to rural women's organizations undermine much of the good – and fairly inexpensive – work that has been done. What will it take for governments, who represent rural as well as urban constituencies, to address rural women's health issues and effectively implement these recommendations?

Notes

1 The study was conducted as part of the Rural Women Making Change research alliance and funded by the Chair in Rural Women's Health Research at the University of Western Ontario and the Social Sciences and Humanities Research Council.

2 The Supreme Court of Canada ruled that on her divorce, despite twenty years of work on her husband's farm, Irene Murdoch was entitled only to support payments from her husband, not to a share in the value of the farm. Lobbying on this issue resulted in a change in the matrimonial property laws, and in 1976 Murdoch was awarded $65,000, representing about 24% of the value of the farm (Shortall, 1994, p. 281).

3 The Canadian Farm Women's Education Council, Canadian Farm Women's Network, Centres of Excellence for Women's Health, Farm Credit Canada, Manitoba Farm and Rural Stress Line, New Brunswick Farmer's Union and Partners in Agriculture, PEI Women in Agriculture, Provincial Association of Transition Houses, Saskatchewan Women's Agricultural Network (SWAN), Status of Women Canada, Women's Institutes, various rural women's resource centres and shelters, and a northern public health unit. SWAN, the Canadian Farm Women's

Network, the Canadian Farm Women's Education Council, and several of the rural resource centres closed just prior to or during the course of this study.

References

Brophy, J., Keith, M., Gorey, K., Luginaah, I., Laukkanen, E., Hellyer, D., Reinhartz, A., Watterson, A., Abu-Zahra, H., Maticka-Tyndale, E., Schneider, K., Beck, M., & Gilbertson, M. (2006). Occupation and breast cancer: A Canadian case-control study. *Annals of the New York Academy of Science, 1076*, 765–77.

Bruce, D. (2003). Housing needs of low-income people living in rural areas. Ottawa: Canada Mortgage and Housing Corporation.

Canadian Feminist Alliance for International Action (FAFIA). (2008). 'Women's inequality in Canada.' Submission of the Canadian Feminist Alliance for International Action to the UN Committee on the Elimination of Discrimination Against Women. Ottawa: FAFIA. Available at http://www.fafia-afai.org/files/FAFIA_Canada_CEDAW_2008.pdf.

Canadian Institute for Health Information (CIHI). (2006). How healthy are rural Canadians? An assessment of their health status and health determinants. Ottawa: CIHI.

Clark, K., & Leipert, B. (2007). Strengthening and sustaining social supports for rural elders. *Online Journal of Rural Nursing and Health Care, 7*(1), 13–26.

Corbett, M. (2007). *Learning to leave: The irony of schooling in a coastal community*. Black Point, NS: Fernwood.

Coward, R., Davis, L., Gold, C., Smiciklas-Wright, H., Thorndyke, L., & Vondracek, F. (Eds.). (2006). *Rural women's health: Mental, behavioural, and physical issues*. New York: Springer.

Dunkerley, C.M. (2004). Risky geographies: Teens, gender and rural landscape in North America. *Gender, Place and Culture, 11*(4), 559–79.

Fuller, T., & O'Leary, S. (2008). The impact of access to transportation on the lives of rural women. Guelph, ON: Rural Women Making Change. Available at http://www.rwmc.uoguelph.ca/document.php?d=181.

Gerrard, N., Thurston, W.E., Scott, C.M., & Meadows, L.M. (2005). Silencing women in Canada: The effects of the erosion of support programs for farm women. *Canadian Woman Studies, 24*(4), 59–66.

Gott, C. (1997). *Lessons learned, roads travelled: Mobilizing communities for rural child care*. Dundalk, ON: Bruce Gray United Way.

Halseth, G., & Ryser, L. (2006). Trends in service delivery: Examples from rural and small town Canada, 1998 to 2005. *Journal of Rural and Community Development, 1*, 69–90.

Health Canada. (1996). Towards a common understanding: Clarifying the core concepts of population health. Ottawa: Health Canada.

Heather, B., Skillen, L., Young, J., & Vladicka, T. (2005). Gendered identities and the restructuring of rural Alberta. *Sociologia Ruralis, 45*(1–2), 86–97.

Hornosty, J., & Doherty, D. (2003). Responding to wife abuse in farm and rural communities: Searching for solutions that work. In R. Blake and A. Nurse (Eds.), *The trajectories of rural life: New perspectives on rural Canada* (pp. 37–53). Regina: Saskatchewan Institute of Public Policy.

Kechnie, M. (2003). *Organizing rural women: The federated women's institutes of Ontario 1897-1919*. Montreal and Kingston: McGill-Queen's University Press.

Kubik, W., & Moore, R. (2003). Changing roles of Saskatchewan farm women: Qualitative and quantitative perspectives. In R. Blake & A. Nurse (Eds.), *The trajectories of rural life: New perspectives on rural Canada* (pp. 25–36). Regina: Saskatchewan Institute of Public Policy.

Leach, B. (1999). Transforming rural livelihoods: Gender, work and restructuring in three Ontario communities. In S. Neysmith (Ed.), *Restructuring caring labour: Discourse, state practice and everyday life* (pp. 209–25). Toronto: Oxford University Press

Leach, B. (2011). Jobs for women? Gender and class in Ontario's ruralized auto manufacturing industry. In B. Pini & B. Leach (Eds.), *Reshaping gender and class in rural spaces* (pp. 129–43). London: Ashgate.

Leach, B., Hawkins, L., & Pletsch, C. (2009). *What do rural women's organizations contribute to rural communities?* Unpublished manuscript.

Leipert, B. (1999). Women's health and the practice of public health nurses in northern British Columbia. *Public Health Nursing, 16*, 280–9.

Leipert, B. (2006). Rural women's health issues in Canada: An overview and implications for policy and research. In A. Medovarski & B. Cranney (Eds.), *Canadian woman studies: An introductory reader* (2nd ed., pp. 552–64). Toronto: Inanna Publications and Education.

Leipert, B. (2010). Rural and remote women and resilience: Grounded theory and photovoice variations on a theme. In C. Winters & H. Lee (Eds.), *Rural nursing: Concepts, theory, and practice* (pp. 105–129). New York: Springer.

Leipert, B., & George, J. (2008). The determinants of rural women's health: A case in southwest Ontario. *Journal of Rural Health, 24*(2), 210–18.

Leipert, B., Landry, T., McWilliam, C., Kelley, M., Forbes, D., Wakewich, P., & George, J. (2012). Rural women's health promotion needs and resources: A photovoice perspective. In J. Kulig and A. Williams (Eds.), *Health in rural Canada* (pp. 481–502). Vancouver: UBC Press.

Leipert, B., Plunkett, R., Meagher-Stewart, D., Scruby, L., Mair, H., & Wamsley, K. (2011). 'I can't imagine my life without it!' Curling and health promotion: A photovoice study. *Canadian Journal of Nursing Research, 43*(1), 61-78.

Machum, S. (2006). Commodity production and farm women's work. In B.B. Bock and S. Shortall (Eds.), *Rural gender relations: Issues and case studies* (pp.46–62). Wallingford, UK: CABI.

NVIVO. (1999). QRS NUD*IST VIVO. Melbourne, Australia: Qualitative Solutions and Research Pty. Ltd.

Raphael, D. (Ed.). (2008). *Social determinants of health: Canadian perspectives* (2nd ed.). Toronto: Canadian Scholars' Press.

Reinharz, S., & Kulick, R. (2007). Reading between the lines: Feminist content analysis into the second millenium. In S.N. Hesse-Biber (Ed.), *Handbook of feminist research: Theory and praxis* (pp. 257–75). London: Sage.

Riddell, T., Ford-Gilboe, M., & Leipert, B. (2009). Strategies used by rural women to stop, avoid, or escape from intimate partner violence. *Health Care for Women International, 30*(1), 134–59.

Riddell-Dixon, E. (2001). *Canada and the Beijing conference on women: Governmental politics and NGO participation.* Vancouver: UBC Press.

Romanow, R. (2002). *Building on values: The future of health care in Canada.* Ottawa: Commission of the Future of Health Care in Canada.

Shortall, S. (1994). Farm women's groups: Feminist or farming or community groups, or new social movements? *Sociology, 28*(1), 270–91.

Sutherns, R., McPhedran, M., & Haworth-Brockman, M. (2004). *Rural, remote, and northern women's health: Policy and research directions.* Winnipeg: Prairie Centre of Excellence for Women's Health.

World Health Organization. (2008). Commission on social determinants of health. Retrieved from http://www.who.int/social_determinants/en/.

4 Health Issues of Women in Rural United States: An Overview

Angeline Bushy

This chapter discusses the health concerns of rural women in the United States. It is important to emphasize that women cannot be viewed as isolated entities. Families, children, and significant others are an integral dimension of a woman's life, as are her health behaviours. In turn, a woman is integral to the health and well-being of her family and her community. The reader is reminded this is an infinitely broad topic and there is wide diversity among rural communities and the health status of women who live there. It is, therefore, with utmost caution that this author undertakes a discussion in a textbook chapter focusing on the health-related concerns of rural women in the United States.

Definitions of 'Rural'

Before we examine the health status and concerns of rural women, it is important to understand the meaning of the terms 'rural' and 'urban,' which can mean different things in different contexts. Imprecise definitions of 'rural' present concerns for policy makers, researchers, clinicians, and educators alike in that they hamper delineation and understanding of the epidemiology, health status, and care-seeking behaviours of women living in diverse rural contexts (Bushy, 2005, 2008; Satcher & Rubins, 2006). A range of official definitions exist, and most include geographic and population factors that differentiate rural from urban. For example, the given population residing within a circumscribed area is used to differentiate a Standard Metropolitan Statistical Area (SMSA) from a non-Standard Metropolitan Statistical Area (non-SMSA). An SMSA, defined as urban, refers to a city and/or its adjacent area having a population density of fifty thousand or more residents, while nonSMSAs, defined as rural, do not meet this level. SMSAs constitute about 80% of the total US population, nonSMSAs about 20% (approximately fifty-four million people), and the latter are dispersed across four-fifths (80%) of the US land mass (Rural Assistance Center [RAC], 2010a, 2010c; US Census Bureau, 2002). Other definitions differentiate 'urban,' 'suburban,' 'rural,' 'frontier,' and 'farm residency.' With this set of terms, 'rural' refers to a community having fewer than twenty thousand residents; a higher population density is considered urban. Of all rural residents, approximately 5% reside in towns of fewer than twenty-five hundred residents and less than 2% reside on a farm. Frontier areas have six or fewer residents per square mile (RAC, 2010a, 2010c). Other definitions take into consideration distance to services and/or time to access services; for example, 'rural' is defined as more than twenty miles or more than thirty minutes to access services. However, it must be noted that the delimiter of time to access services also is relevant to a woman living in the core of an inner city who must contend with transportation challenges to access services and health care (Coburn et al., 2007; RAC, 2010a).

Rural Socio-economic Considerations

Overall, rural areas have higher rates of poverty than urban, with more than 40% of families living below the poverty level. While children of minority background represent about 20% of the total rural population, minority children experience poverty to a greater degree than other rural and urban counterparts (Gamm, Hutchison, Dabney, & Dorsey, 2003a; RAC, 2010a). Impoverished rural families often must contend with substandard housing, poor sanitation, inadequate nutrition, and contaminated water, and lack public health services, in particular prenatal care for pregnant adolescents, immunizations, health screenings of various types, and health-promoting education (Kaiser Commission on Medicaid and the Uninsured, 2003; US Department of Health and Human Services–Office of Women's Health [USDHHS-OWH], 2008). Poverty dramatically affects access to health and social services. In rural or urban areas, racial and ethnic minorities and women in particular have a higher prevalence of poverty than other segments of the population (Gamm et al., 2003a; RAC, 2010a). Although the United States is highly industrialized, some rural regions reflect conditions found in low-income countries; this is especially true of those populated by racial minorities. Many of these households do not have such basic services as running water, electricity, indoor plumbing, and telephones. Life for low-income women who live in rural minority communities often is bleak, isolated, totally lacking in resources, and lived under dire economic hardships (Institute of Medicine [IOM], 2002; USDHHS-OWH, 2008).

Rural Demographic Trends

Demographic characteristics offer insights about the lifestyle and health problems of a given community. Overall, the demographic profile of rural communities reflects two ends of the lifespan continuum, that is, most rural residents are either under the age of seventeen or over the age of sixty-five (RAC, 2010a). Compared to urban populations, a greater proportion of rural people are married, did not complete high school, and have fewer years of formal education. Associated with higher fertility rates in rural areas, there are a corresponding greater proportion of children under eighteen years of age. Rural communities have a disproportionate population of older residents, with greater numbers of elderly women than elderly men (RAC, 2010a, 2010b). This trend is most dramatic in southern and midwest states. More rural older women live alone as widows or care for a disabled spouse or family member at home. Compared to urban counterparts, rural older women experience higher rates of poverty, chronic illnesses, and disability; have less education; and have limited access to transportation and health care providers (Gamm et al., 2003a; Gamm & Hutchison, 2004; Gamm, Hutchison, Dabney, & Dorsey, 2003b; RAC, 2010a).

Rural Social Structures

It is difficult to describe a 'typical' rural town, due to population and geographic diversity. A rural town in Alaska, for instance, is very different from one in Alabama, Colorado, or Tennessee, and there can be significant variations among communities in the same state. Rural communities with a population of twenty thousand residents have features that one expects to find in a large city, and residents in a community of two thousand people or less often perceive a community with a population of ten thousand to be a city. A person who lives in a geographically remote frontier region may not feel isolated because urban-based services are relatively easy for the family to access via telecommunication or dependable transportation. Yet, some features are common to small communities (Nelson, 2009; Winters & Lee, 2009). Compared to highly populated areas, small town social dynamics are conducive to familiarity among local residents. 'Rural' often connotes a high quality of life in non-material terms, with a limited range of industries and slower paced living. These and other contextual features of rural residency affect the lives and health of rural women and their families, sometimes for the better, sometimes for the worse.

Informal interpersonal exchanges can enhance a woman's support network; however, social support can be quickly diminished by the effects of the dynamic and active 'community grapevine.' In other words, familiarity presents challenges as well as benefits. On the one hand, rural residents often prefer to interact with others who hold similar perspectives, and some are reluctant to trust community outsiders (Bushy, 2005, 2008). On the other hand, familiarity poses threats to confidentiality, for instance, when a woman or someone in her family experiences a highly sensitive situation such as an unplanned pregnancy, sexually transmitted disease, domestic abuse or interpersonal violence, or emotional or behavioural health problems. It is also important to stress that rural communities possess resilience and resources that often are overlooked and not taken into consideration by outsiders. Historically, rural residents are known for their creativity and self-reliance in responding to the needs of the families in their midst (Bushy, 2005).

Rural Economic Infrastructures

Economic infrastructures can provide insights about a community's demographic profile and health status. While economies are widely diverse, rural infrastructures have some common features. The predominant employers in most rural communities are the education system (schools), the health care system (hospitals, public health centres, long-term-care facilities, medical practices, social service agencies), and public service utilities (road maintenance, water/sewage maintenance, etc.). Here, employee turnover tends to be very low. Other than these employers, rural communities have mostly small and/or family enterprises, such as grocery stores, service stations, banks, restaurants, and pharmacies, which support the predominant industry in the region. These enterprises usually offer part-time or seasonal employment opportunities to locals, generally without health insurance benefits. On the one hand, family enterprises can promote cohesiveness and autonomy for their members. Conversely, the business may cause excessive stress for the family, whose income may be directly dependent on local or regional industry (USDA, 2008, 2009). Sometimes one or two family members assume additional responsibilities to ensure success of the business or certain members subjugate personal goals for the sake of the family enterprise. During economic recessions, an individual may be expected or need to seek employment outside of the business to augment the family income (USDHHS-OWH, 2008).

Limited employment opportunities associated with rural economies are of particular concern for a woman with advanced education. It often is difficult, if not impossible, to find a job locally that is commensurate with her level of education or skill. Some commute great distances to work in an urban area. Others accept local employment even if it entails being underemployed for her level of education, for instance, a woman with a business degree accepts a secretarial position or a woman with a degree in education works as teacher's assistant in the local school system. In brief, rural economic infrastructures are a source of financial and emotional stress for many women, affecting their self-esteem and emotional well-being (Coward et al., 2004; Sawyer, Gale, & Lambert, 2006).

Rural Health Care

Access to quality health care and social services is of notable concern in rural regions, especially in remote and frontier areas. A continuum of health care services and providers either does not exist or is fragmented and difficult to navigate, especially for consumers who are more vulnerable. Specialty services are limited or non-existent. Recruiting and retaining qualified personnel in Health Professional Shortage Areas (HPSAs), that is, areas designated by USDHHS as having shortages of primary medical care, dental, or mental health providers, is of utmost concern to rural residents and policy makers (Bureau of Health Professions, 2010). Transportation barriers include extensive distances to medical specialists, poor travel conditions, and lack of a dependable vehicle or public transportation. For someone with a disability, transportation barriers often consist of physical obstacles. Language barriers are profound for a woman who cannot understand, speak, or read English. There are also barriers in the form of threats to confidentiality associated with small-town social networks (Nelson, 2009).

Rural Health Status

The objectives of the USDHHS's document *Healthy People 2020* target vulnerable and at-risk populations including, among others, pregnant women, children, older persons, and minorities (USDHHS, 2010). Rural women are less likely than urban counterparts to engage in preventive and health-promoting behaviours such as routine blood pressure checks, pap smears, and breast examinations (American College of Obstetricians and Gynecologists [ACOG]), 2009). Further, rural adults, both men and women, are more likely to engage in high-risk behaviours such as smoking, not wearing seat belts, and not engaging in regular exercise – all of which have implications for an individual's health status. Some speculate that the lifestyle behaviours of rural residents are associated with having limited access to health promotion education. Others propose that the health information that is disseminated may not be culturally appropriate for rural consumers. Still others suggest that the rural context is not conducive for health-promoting activities (e.g., they do not have access to biking and walking trails or fitness facilities for exercising). Suffice it to say, information is sparse and studies are needed that focus on the health beliefs and self-care practices of rural residents in order to develop culturally and linguistically attuned programs targeting age- and gender-specific aggregates.

Health Issues: Women

Regarding the health status of women, there are similarities and differences among rural and urban women (US Census Bureau, 2002; Gamm et al., 2003a, 2003b; Gamm & Hutchison, 2004). For both groups, birth rates have declined while death rates have remained the same. Both groups have experienced an increase in age at marriage and in divorce, while fertility rates and household size have declined. However, rural women are more likely to be married, have more children, live in larger families, and complete their families earlier in life. Rural households are larger in number, often comprised of several generations. Multigenerational living arrangements often emerge out of economic need and can enhance support to members of the family; however, extended family households have the potential for more familial conflicts. Rural women lag behind urban women in years of education. This may be attributable to the urban location of most institutions of higher learning. Lack of employment opportunities for college-educated women coupled with rural social dynamics tend to reinforce more traditional gender roles for women and men (Coward et al., 2004).

Morbidity and mortality data on rural populations focus on maternal, infant, and older populations (Gamm et al., 2003a, 2003b; Gamm & Hutchison, 2004). Information on those aggregates is more readily accessed and monitored when associated with funded initiatives targeting those communities, with the exception of Native Americans who receive care from the Indian Health Service (IHS, 2007, 2010) and African American communities benefitting from targeted health initiatives. However, there is a paucity of data focusing on other minority groups such as Asians and recent immigrants to the United States, and women of minority background in particular (Gamm et al., 2003a, 2003b; Gamm & Hutchison, 2004; RAC, 2010a). The deficit is partly attributable to very small numbers of rural residents in general, with even lower numbers of minority subgroups (Bushy, 2005). It is notable that regional variations are evident in health data for specific conditions even within a given community.

Health care utilization patterns indicate that the illnesses of rural women are similar to those of their urban counterparts (RAC, 2010b). Rural women, however, are reported to have higher rates of chronic conditions (especially hypertension), arthritis, back disorders, bursitis, hearing and visual impairments, heart disease, and cancer (RAC, 2010b). They tend to be diagnosed with breast and cervical cancer in later stages of the disease (Gamm et al., 2003a, 2003b; Gamm & Hutchison, 2004). For women with a diagnosis of diabetes, the risk of death is more common in those from forty-five to sixty-four years of age among rural as compared to urban residents. These disparities are associated with rural women being older, poorer, and less educated than urban populations, coupled with the lack of health care providers in more remote areas. In spite of the disparities, rural women have fewer doctor visits each year than urban women. However, when seeking care rural women tend to be sicker and are more likely to be hospitalized for a longer time period (Gamm et al., 2003a, 2003b; Gamm & Hutchison, 2004).

Gynecological and Obstetrical Services

Family planning and maternal, perinatal, and infant and child health care are lacking in rural areas (ACOG, 2009). Like the larger health system, maternal and infant health services in the United States are an ironic mixture of superb medical care for some segments of the population and inadequate care for many minorities and economically deprived groups. Associated with the rural context, rural women often must contend with extensive distances to access obstetrical, perinatal, and pediatric specialists. However, rural women who are also impoverished face even more barriers to access basic gynecological services for themselves and primary care services for children.

Although wide regional variations exist, generally there are higher rates of maternal and infant mortality and morbidity in rural areas than in urban areas (ACOG, 2009; Gamm et al., 2003a, 2003b; Gamm & Hutchison, 2004). Less than optimal pregnancy outcomes are more prevalent among rural minority women, specifically African Americans, Latinos, and Native Americans, with regional variations noted. The risks for less than optimal maternal/infant outcomes among rural minority groups include poverty, high fertility rates in younger women, exposure to toxic chemicals, physically demanding manual labour, and the lack of adequate medical insurance for many.

Pregnancy outcomes are directly associated with access to and availability of obstetrical and pediatric health professionals (ACOG, 2009). The escalating cost for medical malpractice insurance contributes to the inequitable rural distribution of health professionals, leaving an increasing number of communities without any obstetrical services. Provider shortages contribute to some women receiving no prenatal care or obtaining it late in pregnancy. In frontier regions, women sometimes must travel more than 150 miles one way to obtain care from an obstetrical provider. Cultural factors affect a pregnant woman's care-seeking behaviours and pregnancy outcomes, factors such as deciding whether or not to seek prenatal care from a physician, from an indigenous midwife, or from an elder female in the extended family. Rural women of minority background are less likely to initiate obstetrical care during their first trimester.

A woman living in an area with limited or no obstetrical providers is less likely to deliver in her local community hospital compared to one who lives in a community that has such providers. Women who are forced to seek obstetrical care elsewhere have higher rates of complicated and premature births, attributable in part to delays in seeking prenatal care early along with inadequate health-promoting education (Gamm et al., 2003a, 2003b; Gamm & Hutchison, 2004). Mothers and infants living in professionally underserved areas remain in the hospital longer after delivery; because of distance and unpredictable travel conditions coupled with a potential need for emergency services, these women are not discharged as quickly (Gamm et al., 2003a, 2003b; Gamm & Hutchison, 2004). For example, a new mother who lives many miles from an obstetrician, paediatrician, nurse practitioner, or public health nurse is less likely to be discharged with her new infant after twenty-four hours compared to one who lives where these providers are located (ACOG, 2009; Gamm et al., 2003a, 2003b; Gamm & Hutchison, 2004).

Recent closures of rural hospitals and obstetrical units have adversely affected access to care and pregnancy outcomes. These economically fragile health facilities are directly affected by local economies and reimbursement policies. Increasingly, large urban-based health care systems are purchasing rural hospitals and physician practices within and outside of their catchment area. Lacking an essential critical mass of consumers in the rural area, coupled with a greater proportion of children and older residents on fixed incomes, the urban-based purchasing entity often is unable to achieve a profit margin in that market area. Consequently, rural medical outreach services are reduced in frequency and sometimes eliminated. Such business-driven decisions leave an already underserved community with even less access to various types of health care providers, in particular obstetrical and paediatric services (IOM, 2005; USDHHS, 2009).

Occupational and Environmental Risks

Compared to rates within urban populations, there are rural disparities in accidents, trauma, disabilities, suicides, homicides, and use of alcohol and drugs. Rural populations suffer more injuries from lightning, farm machinery, and firearms, more drownings, and more accidents involving vehicles such as boats, snowmobiles, motorcycles, and all-terrain vehicles. However, separate rural morbidity and mortality data may not be available for these incidents (Gamm et al., 2003a, 2003b; Gamm & Hutchison, 2004).

Occupation-related injuries are of particular concern in rural communities. Of the four most dangerous industries (agriculture, fishing, mining, construction), agriculture has the highest morbidity and mortality rates, even though the number of people actively engaged in it is relatively small (OSHA, 2010). Not only is agricultural work inherently dangerous, it must be performed under adverse conditions such as snow, mud, and extreme heat or cold, and employees work extremely long hours.

The agricultural labour force is highly diverse in respect to age, work experience, education, and literacy levels. A typical agricultural enterprise is the 'family farm.' Here women, children, older persons, extended family members, and friends of all ages assist the owner with the work – usually without regard for an individual's competency level and without preliminary safety training. Women and children (whether family members or migrant workers) will often be operating machinery and performing repetitive heavy manual labour, work that can lead to musculoskeletal injuries, trauma, and sometimes death. For women who are more actively involved in work on the farm, automobile- and machinery-related injuries increase. Women and children suffer almost twice as many farm-related injuries as men, with 75% of their injuries being severe, permanent, or fatal (Gamm et al., 2003a, 2003b; Gamm & Hutchison, 2004). Clinicians practising in farming communities are likely to encounter women who have lost fingers or limbs or suffered back injuries, fractures, lacerations, or trauma to various body parts. Even when a woman is not the injured party, injury to a child or other family member can significantly affect her day-to-day life and ulti- mately her health status.

Agriculture is classified by OSHA as one of the highest-risk occupa- tions. As for the migrant work force in general, many are unable to understand or speak, much less read or write, English (NCFH, 2010; OSHA, 2010). Moreover, women and men of all ages work very long hours without the ability to read OSHA-mandated protective measures when working with agriculture chemicals used in crop production, or the ability to understand OSHA-safety briefs when operating farm machinery and equipment. However, morbidity and mortality data on migrant agricultural workers in general is sparse to nonexistent.

Chronic Health Problems

In general, rural residents are characterized by a relatively low mortal- ity rate but with high rates of chronic illness (Gamm et al., 2003a, 2003b; Gamm & Hutchison, 2004). The most critically needed services in rural areas are preventive services (e.g., health screening clinics, nutrition counselling, and wellness education) to prevent disabilities with chronic sequelae. There is an ever-present need in rural communities for home health services, adult daycare, respite services for family members, homemaker services, meal deliveries, and public transportation; these types of services support individuals with chronic conditions and allow them to remain at home rather than being placed in an assisted living or long-term care facility. Both urban- and rural-based programs must be- come more effective by decentralizing and providing in-home services via mobile units to reach those in need (Bushy, 2008; USDHHS, 2009).

Mental and Behavioural Health

Emotional and behavioural disorders affect approximately one-half of the US population over a lifetime and are among the most impairing conditions (Sawyer et al., 2006; USDHHS-OWH, 2008). Mental health disorders are widespread in rural as well as urban areas and affect approximately 20% of the total population in a given year. Emotional and behavioural health care is of particular concern in rural communities where there is a lack of all types of mental health professionals and services. More than 20% of non-SMSA counties lack mental health services, whereas only 5% of SMSA counties lack such services. Non-SMSA counties have on average less than two specialty mental health organizations; SMSA counties report an average in excess of thirteen such organizations (Sawyer et al., 2006).

The impact of mental illness and emotional and behavioural disorders on rural mortality and morbidity rates is evidenced on several fronts (Gamm et al., 2003a, 2003b; Gamm & Hutchison, 2004). For example, suicide rates, a standard indicator of mental illness, are higher in rural areas, particularly among adult males and children. Depression is an important cause and a frequent co-morbidity for other illness. More specifically, there is evidence that depression, anxiety, and other psychosocial factors contribute to progression and outcomes associated with chronic illnesses, such as heart disease (Coward et al., 2004). However, rural residents are less likely to report and seek treatment for serious mental illness than those residing in urban areas (Sawyer et al., 2006). More suicide attempts occur among depressed adults in rural areas than in urban areas. Rural primary care clinicians play a significant role in providing mental health services to their patients, due to the scarcity of mental health professionals as well as the stigma-associated reluctance to seek such services that may be increased for residents in rural areas. Threats to confidentiality and anonymity that characterize rural social dynamics, coupled with lack of knowledge about mental illness symptoms or treatments, are contributing factors to lower utilization of mental health services (Coward et al., 2004; Sawyer et al., 2006). Clinicians play an important role in educating the community to recognize self-destructive and risk-taking behaviours in family members and in providing specific details regarding resources (e.g., toll-free crisis hotlines) to facilitate early interventions and thus help to prevent tragic events. Following a tragic suicide event, the immediate family and loved ones as well as the entire community should be offered grief counselling; however, such counselling often is unavailable in rural settings.

Older Persons

The proportion of older women residing in rural communities is higher than that of both older women residing in urban areas and older men residing in rural communities (Gamm et al., 2003a, 2003b; Gamm & Hutchison, 2004). Of rural older women, most live in southern states (43%) and the Midwest (33%); the remainder (24%) are dispersed across the rest of the states. Rural older women's experiences and needs are often misunderstood and neglected, stemming from societal values in general and rural values in particular that emphasize productivity and a strong work ethic. These women have a high prevalence of chronic health problems but fewer resources to deal with these conditions. Rural women are more likely than urban women to self-treat with over-the-counter medications because they either cannot get to the doctor, cannot afford medical services, or both (Coward et al., 2004; Sawyer et al., 2006). Rural older persons are especially vulnerable to mental health issues because of a lack of mental health professionals, in particular gero-specialists. While as many as a quarter of older people suffer from a cognitive or emotional disorder, less than 5%of mental health professionals' practice time is spent with this age group (Coward et al., 2004).

Rural older women are more likely to enter an assisted living or long-term care facility at an earlier age and with fewer disabilities. Many rural communities do not have such facilities; thus, women may need to be placed in a facility located elsewhere. A contributing factor for this rural demographic phenomenon may be that young working-age adults, who historically provided care for family elders, are moving away from small towns to seek employment. Unfortunately, many small communities have not replaced these disintegrating informal helping networks with the formal services required to care for older individuals in a home setting.

Minorities

Blacks (African Americans)

More information about the health concerns of blacks living in rural areas has been gathered in the past two decades (Gamm et al., 2003a,

2003b; Gamm & Hutchison, 2004; RAC, 2010a). Of all rural blacks, 95% live in the south and almost all are poor (97%). Black women in the South work in the lowest-paying and least desirable jobs. Compared to urban and other rural counterparts, rural black women are reported to have a higher adolescent pregnancy rate with poor perinatal outcomes; higher rates of chronic illness and disability related to obesity, hypertension, and diabetes; and a higher breast cancer mortality rate. Human immunodeficiency virus (HIV) infection is an emerging problem in rural black women, but precise data are unavailable on the prevalence and incidence in this highly vulnerable group. Overall, these women experience any number of health disparities, most of which are associated with poverty and limited access to health care, along with cultural factors.

Latinos

Although they share a common language (Spanish), Latinos represent many nationalities, each having a distinct culture and, often, particular health problems. The majority of Latinos in the United States have Mexican origins, followed by immigrants from the Caribbean and Central and South America (RAC, 2010a). Precise data on Latinos living in the United States are unavailable since significant numbers are undocumented residents. Rural Latino families often live in substandard housing and lack access to potable water and toilet facilities. Women are at particular risk for the following: infectious diseases associated with poor sanitation, abuse, trauma, farm-machine accidents, exposure to toxic substances such as pesticides and herbicides, hepatitis, typhoid, and bladder and kidney infections (Gamm et al., 2003a, 2003b; Gamm & Hutchison, 2004). As with rural black women, HIV infection is on the increase for Latinos in rural environments but precise data are not available. Tracking use of health services by Latino migrants is problematic, as they travel from one state to another following the crop productions. There is a disparity for Latino migrant women in that they are less likely to receive prenatal care than other rural subgroups and low-income Latinos in urban areas (Gamm et al., 2003a, 2003b; Gamm & Hutchison, 2004). Urban residents are more likely to live near a federally qualified health clinic (FQHC). Such urban clinics are more likely to have bilingual staff than is a rural migrant health clinic. Availability of services and language both correlate positively with having prenatal care in the Latino population.

Native American Indians, Pacific Islanders, and Alaskan Natives

There is wide racial, ethnic, and cultural diversity among Native Americans (NA), which include American Indians, Hawaiian and Pacific Islanders, and Alaskan Natives (Gamm et al., 2003a, 2003b; Gamm & Hutchison, 2004). In general, NA as a group have the poorest overall health status of rural minorities on a number of indicators despite extensive federal and community-based initiatives. Demographically, the NA population has a higher percentage of females (51%) than males (49%). The population is a young one, with the median age of women being 25.3 years and of men 21.1 years. Early mortality and high birth rates influence the demographic profile of this population. The NA birth rate has been higher than all other races, but with some of the poorest perinatal outcomes and extremely high neonatal mortality rates. NA women have a lower life expectancy than other women, but live longer than NA men. More NA women are divorced, separated, or widowed than are NA men. About 25% of all American Indian and Alaskan Natives reside on reservations, located predominantly in isolated rural areas. Many, but not all, qualify for care from Indian Health Service (IHS), but distances to a community-based facility can be extensive. For many, time to access services can range from 30 to 150 minutes or more, depending on weather and road conditions and assuming the family has access to transportation.

Unemployment is rampant on reservations, ranging from 45% to 95%. Compared to other racial groups, both men and women have a very high prevalence of frostbite, tuberculosis, sexually transmitted diseases, diabetes, and cirrhosis of the liver, as well as vehicular and other types of accidents, violence, and suicide. NA women are employed in all salary levels except the highest. Women who live on reservations experience extreme poverty, illiteracy, cultural isolation, and discrimination. Many of these conditions could be prevented, in part, through improved socio-economic status, better education, and positive lifestyle change (Gamm et al., 2003a, 2003b; Gamm & Hutchison, 2004).

Women and Interpersonal Violence

Violence against women and children is an important issue for US residents, urban and rural alike (Gamm et al., 2003a, 2003b; Gamm & Hutchison, 2004; USDHHS-OWH, 2008). Prevalence estimates vary, and reported cases probably are only the tip of the iceberg. Under-reporting of abuse events is probably even higher in rural than in urban settings. Factors complicating safe and appropriate resolution for rural women experiencing violence include geographic and social isolation, more readily available hunting weapons in the home environment, the lack of safe residential shelters, and informal rural social structures that threaten confidentiality and anonymity. Economic stressors and seasonal unemployment that accompany rural industries contribute to increased alcohol consumption by males and increased incidents of domestic violence. Increasingly, rural communities are acknowledging that domestic violence exists, yet for the most part services to support local women in these situations are still inadequate or nonexistent.

Women with Alternate Sexual Orientation

Women with alternate sexual orientation who live and work in rural settings are another group about which little has been written (USDHHS-OWH, 2008). Anecdotal reports indicate that homophobia, both within the local community and especially among rural health professionals, is one of the major concerns of this group of women. Likewise, anecdotal comments seem to reflect that some suicides among adolescents may be related to unresolved sexual orientation issues. Some speculate that traditional attitudes regarding women's roles, a preponderance of male physicians, and threats to confidentiality contribute to inadequate care and lack of support systems for rural women of all ages who have a sexual orientation other than heterosexual. For women with alternative sexual orientations, access to health care is usually limited to crisis care, while health promotion services are virtually nonexistent.

Conclusion

Rural and urban women confront many similar concerns, yet as other chapters in this book have found (see, for example, the previous three chapters), economic, social, geographic, environmental, and cultural factors create some unusual barriers to health for rural women. There is a great need for further empirical data substantiating the health status and health care needs of the various subgroups of women in diverse rural contexts.

References

American College of Obstetricians and Gynecologists (ACOG). (2009). Committee Opinion no. 429: Health disparities for rural women. *Obstetrics and Gynecology, 113*(3), 762–5.

Bureau of Health Professions. (2010). *Shortage areas: HPSA by state & county* (Data file). Available from Health Resources and Services Administration website, http://hpsafind.hrsa.gov.

Bushy, A. (2005). Needed: A more inclusive research paradigm to learn about the health needs of rural women. *Women's Health Issues, 15*(5), 204–8.Bushy, A. (2008). Community health nursing in rural areas. In C. Smith & F. Maurer, *Community health nursing: Theory and practice* (3rd ed.). Philadelphia: W.B. Saunders.

Coburn, A.F., MacKinney, A.C., McBride, T.D., Mueller, K.J., Slifkin, R.T., & Wakefield, M.K. (2007). *Choosing rural definitions: Implications for health policy* (Rural Policy Research Institute Health Panel Issue Brief no. 2). Retrieved from http://www.cdktest.com/rupri/Forms/RuralDefinitionsBrief.pdf.

Coward, R., Davis, L., Gold, C., Smiciklas-Wright, H., Throndyke, L., & Vondracek, F. (2004). *Rural women's health: Mental, behavioral, and physical issues.* New York: Springer.

Gamm, L.D., & Hutchison, L.L. (Eds.). (2004). *Rural healthy people 2010: A companion document to Healthy People 2010 (Vol. 3).* College Station, TX: Texas A&M University System Health Science Center, School of Rural Public Health, Southwest Rural Health Research Center. Retrieved from http://www.srph.tamhsc.edu/centers/rhp2010/Volume_3/Vol3rhp2010.pdf.

Gamm, L.D., Hutchison, L.L., Dabney, B.J., & Dorsey, A.M. (Eds.). (2003a). *Rural healthy people 2010: A companion document to Healthy People 2010 (Vol. 1).* College Station, TX: Texas A&M University System Health Science Center, School of Rural Public Health, Southwest Rural Health Research Center. Retrieved from http://www.srph.tamhsc.edu/centers/rhp2010/Volume1.pdf.

Gamm, L.D., Hutchison, L.L., Dabney, B.J., & Dorsey, A.M. (Eds.). (2003b). *Rural healthy people 2010: A companion document to Healthy People 2010 (Vol. 2).* College Station, TX: Texas A&M University System Health Science Center, School of Rural Public Health, Southwest Rural Health Research Center. Retrieved from http://www.srph.tamhsc.edu/centers/rhp2010/Volume2.pdf.

Indian Health Service (IHS). (2007). *Facts on Indian health disparities.* Retrieved from http://info.ihs.gov/Files/DisparitiesFacts-Jan2007.doc.

Indian Health Service (IHS). (2010). *IHS fact sheets*. Retrieved from http://info. ihs.gov.

Institute of Medicine (IOM). (2002). *Unequal treatment: What health care providers need to know about racial and ethnic disparities in health care* (Report Brief). Retrieved from http://www.iom.edu/Reports/2002/Unequal-Treatment-Confronting-Racial-and-Ethnic-Disparities-in-Health-Care.aspx.

Institute of Medicine (IOM). (2005). *Quality through collaboration: The future of rural health*. Retrieved from http://www.iom.edu/Reports/2004/Quality-Through-Collaboration-The-Future-of-Rural-Health.aspx.

Kaiser Commission on Medicaid and the Uninsured. (2003). *The uninsured in rural America*. Retrieved from http://www.kff.org/uninsured/upload/The-Uninsured-in-Rural-America-Update-PDF.pdf.

National Center for Farmworkers Health (NCFH). (2010). *Fact sheets about farmworkers*. Retrieved from http://www.ncfh.org/?pid=5.

Nelson, W.A. (Ed.). (2009). *Handbook for rural health care ethics: A practical guide for professionals*. Hanover, NH: Dartmouth College. Retrieved from http://dms.dartmouth.edu/cfm/resources/ethics.

Occupational Safety & Health Administration (OSHA). (2010). *Safety and health topics: Agricultural operations*. Retrieved from http://www.osha.gov/SLTC/agriculturaloperations/index.html.

Rural Assistance Center (RAC). (2010 a). *Rural demographic maps*. Retrieved from http://www.raconline.org/maps/.

Rural Assistance Center (RAC). (2010 b). *Rural women*. Retrieved http://www.raconline.org/info_guides/public_health/womenshealth.php.

Rural Assistance Center (RAC). (2010c). *What is rural*. Retrieved from http://www.raconline.org/info_guides/ruraldef/.

Satcher, D., & Rubins, P. (2006). *Multicultural medicine and health disparities*. New York: McGraw-Hill.

Sawyer, D., Gale, J., & Lambert, D. (2006). *Rural and frontier mental and behavioral health care: Barriers, effective policy strategies, best practices*. Waite Park, MN: National Association for Rural Mental Health. Retrieved from http://www.narmh.org/publications/archives/rural_frontier.pdf.

US Census Bureau. (2002; rev. December 2009). *Census 2000 urban and rural classification*. Retrieved from http://www.census.gov/dmd/www/glossary.html.

US Citizenship and Immigration Services (USCIS). (2010). *Working in the US*. Retrieved from http://www.uscis.gov/portal/site/uscis.

US Department of Agriculture (USDA). (2008). *Briefing rooms – Measuring rurality*. Retrieved from http://www.ers.usda.gov/Briefing/Rurality.

US Department of Agriculture (USDA). (2009). *Browse by subject – Rural economy*. Retrieved from http://www.ers.usda.gov/Browse/view.aspx?subject= RuralEconomy.

US Department of Health and Human Services (USDHHS). (2009). *The 2009 report to the Secretary: Rural health and human services issues*. Annual report by the National Advisory Committee on Rural Health and Human Services to the Secretary of the US Department of Health and Human Services. Retrieved from http://ruralhealth.hrsa.gov/reports/2009_NAC.pdf.

US Department of Health and Human Services (USDHHS). (2010). *Healthy people 2020: The road ahead*. Retrieved from http://www.healthypeople.gov/hp2020/default.asp.

US Department of Health and Human Services – Office on Women's Health (USDHHS-OWH). (2008). *Charting New Frontiers in Rural Women's Health Conference: Summary report*. Proceedings of the conference held in Washington, DC, 13–15 August 2007. Retrieved from http://www .womenshealth.gov/archive/rwhc/conference.cfm.

Winters, C., & Lee, H. (Eds.). (2009). Rural nursing: Concepts, theory and practice (3rd ed.). New York: Springer.

PART TWO

Health and Environment

Beverly D. Leipert

The environment is increasingly being seen as a significant determinant of rural women's health, globally and nationally. Brophy, Keith, Watterson, Gilbertson, and Beck discovered, in their work in occupations and health, that farm life has had significant effects on the health of women who grew up there, and specifically a higher incidence of breast cancer in these women as a result of their early farm years. Clearly more research is needed to fully understand and prevent these serious long-term environmental impacts on the health of rural girls and women.

McIntyre and Rondeau discuss the beliefs, obligations, and actions of farm women regarding the provision of healthy food for their families within the context of their daily food provisioning practices. These authors' unique focus on the daily food practices of rural women provides important knowledge about not only food provisioning and its effect on family health, cohesion, and support, but also about the effect on rural women's health of environmental issues related to the changing nature, demands, and stresses of farming.

In the following chapter, Kubik and Fletcher explore issues of climate change, commercialized agriculture, food production, and farm women's health in order to examine how each is linked to the overarching concern about health. The stress for farm women of sustainable agriculture is clearly an important consequence of the rural environment.

In their chapter about Old Order Mennonite women, Dabrowska and Wismer examine several determinants of rural women's health to reveal important environmental, cultural, and social forces that shape the health of this population of rural women. Interestingly, these authors reveal that the health of Old Order Mennonite women is influenced in a different way than would be predicted by prevailing assumptions concerning socio-economic factors such as limited education, low income, patriarchal relations, and lifestyle.

The chapters in this section significantly enrich our understanding of how the changing rural and farming environments affect the health of rural women. This new and vital information can substantially enrich the development of policies and practices that advance the health of rural women – fundamental figures in rural families and communities – and also enrich understanding of women's experience of farming and living in rural environments.

5 Farm Work in Ontario and Breast Cancer Risk

James T. Brophy, Margaret M. Keith,
Andrew Watterson, Michael Gilbertson,
and Matthias Beck

Does farming in Ontario increase breast cancer risk? Our research suggests there may be a causal link. We have learned that farm women, through their residential and work environments, have been exposed to an array of agricultural chemicals – often beginning at childhood. These early exposures may be of particular concern because immature breast tissue is especially vulnerable to genetic damage that might result in cancer later in life (Brody et al., 2007).

There is limited research on the effects of farming on women's health (Zahm & Blair, 2003). As Kubik and Fletcher note in chapter 7, farm women do not often self-identify occupationally as farmers. Likewise, researchers have historically viewed women as not directly occupationally engaged in farming, and therefore have either not examined their exposures or have excluded them due to small numbers (McDuffie, 1994). Because women and men differ biologically and often have somewhat different occupational roles, this research gap raises concerns about possible unidentified health vulnerabilities.

Several pesticides have been shown to be mammary carcinogens in animal bioassays (Rudel, Attfield, Schifano, & Brody, 2007). Many are endocrine disrupters and interfere with normal hormone metabolism and functioning (Diamanti-Kandarakis et al., 2009). However, epidemiological research has not been consistent in its findings of an association between pesticide exposures and breast cancer. Epidemiological studies in this area tend to be limited in number, and many lack the methodological design features that would enable them to accurately assess the effects of specific exposures (Brody et al., 2007).

Background

Breast cancer, the primary focus of our research, is the most prevalent cancer among women in Canada, where 'rates are amongst the highest in the world' (Canadian Cancer Society, 2007, p. 71). In Ontario alone, it was projected that there would be nine thousand new diagnoses in 2011 (Canadian Cancer Society, 2011). Less than half of these cases can be explained by known or suspected risk factors, such as age, reproductive history, hormone replacement therapy, family history, and other factors (Gray, Evans, Taylor, Rizzo, & Walker, 2009).

Our interest in the possible association between farming and breast cancer first arose with findings from our initial exploratory case-control study, which we launched in partnership with the Windsor Regional Cancer Centre in 1995. The study was designed to collect the occupational histories of male and female cancer patients in order to explore possible associations between *any* occupation and the risk for *any* type of cancer. After four years of data collection, we found that the largest group in our completed dataset was women with breast cancer. The work histories for the 299 cases were compared to the histories of another 237 women who had been diagnosed with cancers other than breast or ovary. Our findings, while not statistically strong due to the relatively small number of subjects, indicated a nine-fold increase in risk for breast cancer among women who had ever farmed, particularly among those aged fifty-five and younger (OR = 9.05 [95% CI, 1.06–7.43]). This hypothesis-generating study was limited in that broad occupational groups were used as surrogates for exposure, it did not account for most of the other recognized risk factors, and the control group was not randomly selected from the community (Brophy et al., 2002).

With an expanded research team, we undertook a subsequent case-control study in 2000 to test the farming–breast cancer hypothesis. Our methods were improved. The controls were randomly selected from the community. The questionnaire was enhanced to control for the generally accepted breast cancer risk factors such as reproductive history and included more detailed questions about the subjects' occupational histories. The dataset, compiled over two and a half years, included 564 cases and 599 controls. Analysis revealed an almost tripling of breast cancer risk among women with an occupational history of farming (OR = 2.8 [95% CI, 1.6–4.8]). The risk also appeared to be elevated for women who worked in farming and were subsequently employed in health care (OR = 2.3 [95% CI, 1.1–4.6]) or auto-related industries

(OR = 4.1 [95% CI, 1.7–9.9]). We observed that farming tended to be among the earlier jobs worked, often in the teen years. As Brophy and colleagues (2006) noted, 'Because many women who worked in farming began during adolescence, it is plausible that the timing of exposure is of significance in terms of risk' (p. 774). While this second study indicated an elevated risk for breast cancer among women who had farmed, it was somewhat limited by its relatively small number of subjects and the lack of specific exposure information (Brophy et al., 2006).

We were concerned about these findings and their potential ramifications for women in farming communities. We knew, however, that we had to identify *specific* exposures in order to contribute in a meaningful way to the formulation of prevention strategies. This would also require us to overcome some of the methodological limitations of standard epidemiological approaches. With that goal, we launched two integrated follow-up studies in south-western Ontario. The Lifetime Histories Breast Cancer Research Study was a more comprehensive case-control study than the previous two. The Exposure Exploration Study was a qualitative study designed to provide us with a deeper understanding of the historic working conditions experienced by women employed in a few key occupations, including farming.

The Lifetime Histories Breast Cancer Research Study

Data collection began in 2003. The interviewer-administered questionnaire gathered information about the subjects' socio-economic status, lifestyle, reproductive history, family history, parental occupations, residency, and work history. It also included many open-ended questions about working conditions and occupational exposures.

During the five years of data collection, 1,006 women with breast cancer and 1,146 randomly selected women from the community were interviewed. Together our cases and controls identified 466 subjects as having worked in agriculture at some point in their lives, and all together they held a total of 576 different farming jobs. We assessed and coded each job for age at time of employment, duration, and types of exposures.

The Exposure Exploration Study

We undertook the qualitative exposure study in 2007 to gather data to enhance the exposure information provided by subjects in the case-control study, which had inherent limitations due to its methodological design

(Teschke, Smith, & Olshan, 2000). For example, some of the subjects were unable to accurately recall details of their past work or lacked precise knowledge regarding specific chemicals used, their particular application, or their concentrations.

We utilized an ethnographic research methodology for the qualitative study. Because cancer has a long latency period between exposure and identification of the disease, it was essential for us to know what agricultural chemicals farmwomen were exposed to and how these were employed over a period of thirty or more years. ·

Unlike the modern industrial workplace, many farming operations are living environments for workers and their families. These operations also vary in size and crop production mix. We sought the participation of men and women from a wide range of age groups and types of farming. Because of the exploratory nature of the study, inclusion criteria were broad; that is, we included adult males and females who had lived and/or worked on a farm in Essex or Kent counties. Recruitment was conducted by word-of-mouth invitation with the help of contacts within the rural community. Both individual and collective interviews were conducted. The total number of participants was forty-four women and thirty-one men. Their ages ranged between twenty-five and ninety years.

As one data-gathering technique, we had participants draw on large pieces of paper to show their farming work and residential settings as they existed in decades past as well as the present. We asked them to include the farm layout, work processes, and chemicals used. Such graphic representations seemed to help participants recall details and more clearly describe the conditions to us – even those existing in the more distant past (Keith et al., 2001). Interviews were audiotaped and transcribed.

Two complementary techniques were used to analyse the data: (1) a thematic qualitative approach providing insight into individual experiences and the contextual environment; and (2) a network analysis approach of structures found within the data related to chemical exposures (Tashakkori & Teddlie, 1998). Systematic coding procedures were developed to facilitate a structured code book in which a negotiated list of themes emerged from the analysis of the transcripts by three team members working both independently and as a team.

The information we gathered resulted in a breadth of experiential recollections that painted a vivid picture not only of life on the farm but also of the timing, degree, and types of exposures borne by women in farming work or residential settings at various periods in their lives. Often several informants would tell similar stories, which served to bolster our confidence in the accuracy of the various recollections. It emerged that women's exposures on the farm differed from men's and that young girls often played an active role in farm work.

We have selected a number of the narratives that best reflect important themes for inclusion in this chapter. These excerpts provide snapshots of individual personal experiences of agricultural practices and types of exposures. We have supplemented the information provided by participants with a review of reports regarding the use of various agricultural chemicals on Ontario crops over the past three decades and a review of relevant scientific literature.

Unravelling the Mystery

Historically, agricultural communities in North America, not to be confused with rural, non-agricultural communities (Leipert, 1999), were viewed as healthier in some respects than their urban counterparts due to lower smoking rates, better diet, and increased physical activity (Alavanja et al., 1996). Despite these comparative lifestyle advantages, several epidemiological studies have shown that farming populations have an elevated risk of some types of cancers.

Among women engaged in farming, excess risks have been observed for non-Hodgkin's lymphoma, leukaemia, multiple myeloma, soft tissue sarcoma, and cancers of the breast, ovary, lung, bladder, cervix, and sinonasal cavities (McDuffie, 1994). The excess cancers may be related to farming exposures, either singularly or in combination. Possible causative agents include pesticides, solvents, engine exhaust, viruses, and others (Coble et al., 2002). It is notable that while there is a broad range of potential exposures, the bulk of the research that has been done on the occupational health hazards of farming (excluding traumatic injuries) is mainly in the area of agricultural chemical pesticides. This is true of our research as well.

In 1993, the US National Cancer Institute launched a large Agricultural Health Study that involved tens of thousands of agricultural workers (Alavanja et al., 1996). The study was designed to determine whether particular exposures increase cancer risk. A nested case-control study of pesticide applicators and their spouses was conducted using data from the large cohort that included 89,000 subjects. Analysis revealed that herbicides, and in particular pendimethalin and s-ethyl dipropylthiocarbamate (EPTC), appeared to be associated with an increased risk for pancreatic cancer (Andreotti et al., 2009).

Animal bioassays have found that over 216 chemicals, including 10 pesticides, induced tumours in the mammary glands of laboratory animals (Rudel et al., 2007). Many of these substances are particularly persistent and bioaccumulate in the adipose tissue, which can include breast tissue. Several of the pesticides shown to be animal mammary carcinogens have been used or are still being used in Ontario. Rudel and colleagues (2007) state that the list is not complete, as many chemicals have not been fully tested. The International Agency for Research on Cancer (IARC) has classified a number of other pesticides as carcinogens, although they are not identified specifically as mammary carcinogens (IARC, 1991).

The Setting for Our Research

Essex and Kent, Ontario's southernmost counties, make up the geographic setting for our case-control and qualitative studies. These counties are home to field crops, orchards, vineyards, animal husbandry, and an enormous greenhouse industry. In Essex County, agriculture involves over 325,000 acres and produces as much as any one of the Atlantic provinces (Brophy et al., 2002). Furthermore, 'greenhouse vegetable production in Essex County is the most intensive in all of Canada' (Corporation of the County of Essex, 2009, para. 3). Agriculture in the neighbouring Kent County also plays a significant economic role (Ontario Ministry of Natural Resources, 2009).

Emergence of Concern Regarding Pesticide Use

Pesticide use in Ontario appears to have begun in 1885 when acetoarsenite and copper sulphate were applied as insecticides to apple orchards (Grabusky, Martin, & Struger, 2004). Grabusky and colleagues state: 'Since then, pesticides have gone through several transitions: from primarily inorganic and organometallic formulations to organochlorine insecticides, triazine herbicides, organophosphorous, carbamate, and later, pyrethroid insecticides; and, more recently, to sulfonylurea and imidazolinone herbicides' (p. 4).

These pest and weed control innovations were seen as both labour saving and a boon to production. An Essex County farmer recalled the days before insecticides were widely available:

I can remember when that corn borer first started. I was just a little guy ... we had to cut our corn – took the fodder and all into the field and, when it turned cold, we'd take a railroad iron and break all the stalks off, break them all up and burn them. And there was an inspector that would come around and check.

Another farmer remembered: 'The way of controlling the weeds in the old days was to manually hoe them. Their kids were out there hoeing ... It takes a long time to hoe thirty acres one chop at a time.' A woman who had personally experienced the hardship of manual hoeing explained why pesticides were so welcomed: 'That's why people turned to chemicals. Because it is brutally hard work farming if you don't have the chemicals.'

In 1962 Rachel Carson published her seminal book *Silent Spring*, which warned of the public health and environmental risks associated with pesticides, especially DDT (Carson, 2002). The predominant evidence of harm Carson presented focused on declines in populations of peregrine falcons and bald eagles contaminated by exposure to pesticide residues, but she also voiced concern about the possible risk of cancer for the human population. It was not until years later that the agricultural community was informed about the risks, thus substantiating Carson's contention about the eerie 'silence' of government regulators. Although DDT is now banned in Canada, it was widely used throughout Essex and Kent counties in the 1950s, 1960s, and early 1970s along with numerous other pesticides. A former food inspector recalled the results of soil and food tissue sampling:

We did find through the process that some of the residuals ... from lindane, aldrin, dieldrin, and DDT ... were staying in the soils for years. Because some of the chemicals, which were no longer available to farmers, were showing up in the food tissue tests, that's what tipped us off [to their persistence].

More scientific evidence of the risks of pesticides began to emerge through the 1970s and 1980s. The Great Lakes Basin became a focal point for this forensic research, which contributed to the development of a new field of scientific enquiry into the potential harm of hormone-mimicking chemicals called endocrine disrupters (Fox, 2001). Reproductive and developmental damage has been discovered in the turtles, frogs, fish, and birds in agricultural areas in the Great Lakes watershed. For example, 42% of the male leopard frogs examined in areas in Kent

County that are heavily contaminated with pesticides, especially those with a combination of atrazine and nitrate, showed evidence of feminization, that is, the occurrence of testicular ovarian follicles (McDaniel et al., 2008).

Colborn, Dumanoski, & Myers (1996) have articulated this scientific phenomenon in their groundbreaking book *Our Stolen Future*. Their findings about the impact of endocrine-disrupting substances challenged age-old assumptions in toxicology. The adage that the 'dose makes the poison' was now understood to have limitations in relation to chemicals that mimic hormones. The timing of the exposure to endocrine disrupters, particularly for developing fetuses and children, appears to have more relevance than the amount (van Larebeke et al., 2008). Further, it would seem that lower-level exposures might be more damaging than higher levels, again depending on the timing. These new hypotheses have implications for agricultural populations, especially for men and women of reproductive age and for children and young adults who are often directly or indirectly exposed to hormone-disrupting pesticides through farming activities or household contamination (Clark & Snedeker, 2006).

Pesticides and Breast Cancer Hypothesis

The European Commission's Endocrine Disrupter Research has found evidence of hormone mimicking from a number of pesticides (some of which are now banned): insecticides such as DDT, endosulfan, dieldrin, methoxychlor, dicofol, and toxaphene; herbicides such as alachlor, atrazine, and nitrofen; fungicides such as mancozeb and tributyltin; and nematocides such as aldicarb and dibromochloropropane (Pesticide Action Network UK, 2009). Depending on the nature of the endocrine disrupters, they can exert their effects in many different ways and on various body systems. Chemicals that mimic estrogens are of particular concern in relation to the development of breast cancer (Davis et al., 1993). Estrogen (i.e., estradiol) is a known human breast carcinogen. Women naturally produce estrogen, particularly between menarche and menopause. Late menarche and early menopause, in addition to multiple pregnancies and lactation, reduce the lifetime body burden of naturally occurring estrogen, thereby providing some protection. An increased load of estradiol, whether naturally occurring or through pharmaceutical supplementation, may increase breast cancer risk (Birnbaum & Fenton, 2003).

Some epidemiological studies have found an association between farming and breast cancer while others have not. In several large cohort studies no elevated risk was observed among women who farmed compared to the general population (Brody et al., 2007). These studies, however, did not control for specific exposures or timing of exposures. The Agricultural Health Study, while inconclusive, found 'risk was elevated among post-menopausal women whose husbands used aldrin, chlordane, dieldrin, heptachlor, chlorpyrifos, diazinon, malathion, 2,4,5-TP and captan' (Clapp, Jacobs, & Loechler, 2008, p. 7).

There have also been several studies exploring the possible link between DDT and breast cancer, with equivocal results (Snedeker, 2001). However, a recent study found that young women exposed to DDT before the age of fourteen had a five-fold excess breast cancer risk before age fifty (Cohn, Wolff, Cirillo, & Sholtz, 2007).

In a case-control study of British Columbia breast cancer patients, Band and colleagues (2000) found a three-fold elevated breast cancer risk among women who had ever been employed in fruit and other vegetable farming. This study did not control for specific exposures.

Another case-control study, which controlled for both traditional breast cancer risk factors and farming exposures, resulted in complex findings (Duell et al., 2000). When the data were analysed without controlling for pesticide exposure or the use of protective equipment, breast cancer risk was found to be below the expected. However, women who reported having been present in the fields during or shortly after pesticide application had an 80% increased risk of developing breast cancer. Among those who reported using pesticides without protective clothing, there was a two-fold excess breast cancer risk, while women with protective clothing had a lower than expected risk, albeit not statistically significant. The researchers concluded that while farming may not present an elevated risk per se, farming women exposed to pesticides might have an elevated breast cancer risk.

These studies demonstrate the weakness in using occupation as a surrogate for exposure, since misclassification occurs when subjects with less exposure are aggregated with the more highly exposed. Such non-differential misclassification decreases the probability of detecting associations and tends to underestimate the risks (Blair et al., 1993). Although epidemiology remains the gold standard in determining causal links between exposures and disease in human populations, it is difficult to study the effects of specific exposures using epidemiological methods because, in the real world, multiple exposures and mixtures can confound results (Jaga & Dharmani, 2007).

The Use of Suspected Carcinogenic and Endocrine-Disrupting Pesticides

Regular surveys of pesticide use have been conducted by the Ontario government beginning in the 1970s, and these provide summaries of pesticides used on various crops and comparisons for different time periods. Unfortunately, the surveys do not include information about greenhouses where suspected carcinogens and endocrine disrupters are used and exposures may be more concentrated. These surveys indicate that, in general, pesticide use in Ontario 'increased by 46% from 1973 to 1983' (Gallivan, Surgeoner, & Kovach, 2001, p. 798). In the twenty-year period between 1983 and 2003, there was 'a 52 percent reduction in total pesticide usage ... Atrazine use in field corn was maintained at 80 percent of the 1998 usage, at 499,000 kg ... Total usage [of glyphosate] was 1,171,000 kg, which has increased by 58 percent since 1998' (McGee, 2004, p. 5).

Atrazine is a triazine herbicide and is considered to be an endocrine disruptor and suspected human carcinogen (Nudelman et al., 2009). In animal studies, in utero atrazine exposure delayed breast gland development and was suspected of conferring 'an extended window of sensitivity to potential carcinogens after sexual maturity' (Birnbaum & Fenton, 2003, p. 393). Recent animal studies have confirmed that exposure to atrazine at critical moments, such as prenatally, predisposes the animal to breast cancer later in life (Birnbaum & Fenton, 2003). It should be noted that while it is still being used in Canada and the United States, atrazine is banned in the European Union (Sass & Colangelo, 2006).

Glyphosate is now the most widely used weed control chemical in the world. It has been largely regarded as safe, yet very recently it has come under more careful scrutiny. Although it is not listed by the European Commission's Endocrine Disrupter Research as an endocrine disrupter, a recent study in France found it to have both endocrine-disrupting and carcinogenic effects on human cell lines (Gasnier et al., 2009).

There is still debate regarding potential carcinogenic and endocrine-disrupting effects of 2,4-D, another heavily used herbicide in Canada (Sierra Club of Canada, 2005). In a Canadian case-control study exploring occupational risk factors for non-Hodgkins lymphoma, a 30% increased risk was found among men exposed to 2,4-D (McDuffie et al., 2001).

Scientists have recently identified that the fungicide vinclozolin may pose human health risks that have the potential to continue into following generations. Studies of pregnant rats exposed to vinclozolin found increased risks for breast cancer that affected up to three subsequent generations of offspring, none of which had any exposure (Anway, Memon, Uzumcu, & Skinner, 2006). Vinclozolin is banned in some European countries due to its carcinogenic and endocrine-disrupting properties (Pesticide Action Network Europe, 2006). In 2003, 899 kilograms of vinclozolin were used in Ontario (McGee, 2004).

Exposure Pathways

Farm family members and rural residents in close proximity to active farms may be at risk for exposure to pesticides through numerous pathways. Pesticides have been detected in ambient air, drinking water, garden soils, household carpeting, and foods (Clark & Snedeker, 2006). Studies of human exposures in farming communities in the United States have found residual pesticides in the blood and urine of family members (Arcury et al., 2007; Gladen et al., 1998). A study of the families of agricultural pesticide applicators in the United States found that there were ample opportunities for exposure: '51% of wives of applicators worked in the fields in the last growing season, 40% of wives have ever mixed or applied pesticides, and over half of children aged 11 or more do farm chores' (Gladen et al., 1998, p. 581).

Drinking Water

A rural resident now living on what had been a family farm in Essex County described the issue of contaminated well water:

> They did a study here back in the late eighties and they found a tremendous amount of the wells out here were contaminated with atrazine. Atrazine was used a lot in corn and they didn't realize the build-up of it in the fields and it wasn't that common to rotate your herbicides. So if atrazine was good this year then let's keep on and let's use it next year, and next year.

Well water sampling from 596 wells was conducted in southern Ontario between 1969 and 1984. The sampling revealed that 293 wells had pesticide concentrations above the detection level. Atrazine, found in 18% of the samples, and 2,4-D, found in 16.3% of the samples, were the most commonly detected, while several others were also present in a small percentage of samples (Frank, Braun, Clegg, Ripley, & Johnson, 1990). There were similar findings from well water sampling carried out in subsequent years (Agriculture Canada, 1992).

While drawing the layout of the farm on which she grew up, a young woman pointed out the vulnerability of their drinking water: 'This is all corn, this is cucumbers, there's your cows, there's our house, and there's our little well, and [my dad] would spray all the way around here ... He died of cancer at 56.'

Household and Chore-Related Exposures

Agricultural chemicals tend to drift from the intended targets and can contaminate households in surrounding areas. Pesticides can also be tracked into homes on footwear, clothing, and pets. Pesticides have been measured in carpeting in homes near farm fields and orchards (Lu, Fenske, Simcox, & Kalman, 2000). For example, in a study of house dust in agricultural areas in Iowa positive results were found for a range of pesticides including 2,4-D, atrazine, and others. Concentrations were significantly associated with the size of the treated acreage (Ward et al., 2006).

Such bystander exposure may have implications for farm women's breast cancer risk. For example, in the large US Agricultural Health Study breast cancer was found to be elevated in women whose homes were nearest to areas of pesticide application (Engel et al., 2005). In addition, farm women often handle chemically contaminated clothing when they wash clothes, and they may wash them with other family members' clothing, thereby exposing not only themselves but their whole family to contaminants.

According to a farmer in Essex County, family-owned and -operated farms were commonplace in the early and middle years of the past century. It was typical of a farm family to live in a house surrounded by gardens, fields, orchards, livestock, storage, and equipment facilities. The farmer drew a large diagram for us and described the typical farm layout as follows:

The orchards surrounded the house, and the tomato fields and the onion fields ... The farmer himself typically was the person that would have been doing any [pesticide] applications. But the family was living in that environment that whole time period. I remember when they first started to introduce the wine grapes to this area ... there were serious numbers of farmhouses directly around these spraying sites.

A woman who had grown up on a farm described the setting of her childhood home: 'You'd look out down the fields and the spray would be going over and the laundry had just been hung out so obviously it was getting all over what we would consider clean clothing – towels, dishtowels ... everything.'

We were told that, on a typical family farm, mixed crops and orchards surrounding the farmhouse were sprayed at regular intervals, often with kitchen or bedroom windows open. A woman whose childhood family farm was primarily devoted to raising livestock recalled:

Neighbouring our farm was a fruit and vegetable farm ... and they would spray. There were cucumbers, raspberries, strawberries ... sweet corn, and all of those things were sprayed at various times to try to control the pests and yet that spray would also float over. I mean it's hard to spray and have a day when there's absolutely no wind.

Another woman remembered:

We'd be in the house at night when [my uncle] would go and spray. We wouldn't shut any windows and we knew exactly where he was and what was going on. You'd smell it. And of course that whole area, if it wasn't him that was spraying, it was somebody else. It was all just a cloud.

We were informed that it was sometimes the job of the farm women or children to mix powdered fertilizers or herbicides into a solution prior to application. Having been directed to ensure 'no undissolved powder remained to clog the sprayer nozzles,' they would 'mix the solution with their bare arms.' An informant recalled that, as a child, she helped her mother mix pharmaceuticals into poultry feed:

I can remember we had a small kitchen and the powder would be in the air. [My mother] tried to come up with different methods so that it would sort of dampen it and then mix it and add a bit more to keep it from floating so much in the air in the kitchen. And we did that four times a year every year for two weeks at a time, every time you got a crop of turkeys. And I kind of remember there was always the 'well if a little bit's good, double it and it's better.'

In interviews with dairy farmers, we learned that in the 1950s and 1960s it was sometimes the responsibility of the women or children to spray the dairy cows with DDT fly spray in the barn prior to milking. As one woman told us: 'We always sprayed the cows in the summertime. Because otherwise, they'd kill you with their tails if you would have sat there and milked by hand.' Another woman who grew up on a dairy farm remembered:

> When dad would bring the cows in to milk them, they would just be covered in flies. So we had a pump can and you just sprayed ... so, here you are as a little seven year old ... the air would just be like a fog after you're finished.

As noted by McIntyre and Rondeau in chapter 6, historically food provisioning for the family fell to the farm women and children. This role included tending the family garden plot:

> All of the farms that I'm aware of had large gardens to feed their family or extended family ... spraying was done at different times ... You dust for various pests on broccoli and cauliflower ... no one wore masks, no one wore gloves, you washed when you came up to the house but often you were snacking out of the garden.

A young mother from Kent County who developed breast cancer in her thirties recalled: 'I remember as a little kid ... being in the field and dad spraying while we're hoeing the cucumbers.'

What We Have Learned

The health and environmental effects of many chemical pesticides are being debated by scientists and regulators, and as a result farmers receive many mixed messages. As one woman put it: 'What they say is acceptable now, 20 years from now you find out is a big mistake.' Driven by the need to produce bountiful crops in order to survive the economic pressures of the changing farming industry, farmers have relied on the recommendations provided by government agencies and have heard assurances by pesticide suppliers that their products could be used safely. As revealed by the increasing size and complexity of the publications guiding farmers in the use of pesticides, farmers have much more information available to them today than in the past and some working practices seem to have improved. A recently retired farmer observed:

> I have noticed since probably the early nineties, the farmers are becoming very, very aware of the danger of the chemicals they're handling. And they are handling them differently ... their children aren't out there doing the things that I did as a kid ... But those are the things we didn't know at the time.

While our research is ongoing, and to date our current case-control study data have not been fully analysed, our work has revealed that in Ontario there was, and continues to be, widespread use of agricultural chemicals known or suspected of causing cancer or hormone disruption. Our research has consistently shown an elevated breast cancer risk among women who have worked in agriculture. We have learned that while there is an increasing body of scientific research literature showing a link between pesticides and diseases, including breast cancer (Clapp et al., 2008), scientists do not hold an unequivocal view regarding the human health risks of exposure to pesticides, nor do they have a uniform understanding of the biological mechanisms at play. Recent reviews, however, have established that the weight of the evidence strongly supports a causal link between breast cancer and other adverse health endpoints, and endocrine-disrupting chemicals. (Kortenkamp et al., 2012; Vandenberg et al., 2012).

It is clear to us from our interviews with farming men and women that agricultural farming practices were, and continue to be, such that farmers, their families, farm workers, and neighbouring residents are exposed to pesticides to varying degrees and of varying concentrations and levels of toxicity, and more research is urgently needed. It is our hope that our research will contribute to the understanding of possible cancer risks from pesticide exposures and that the information we are bringing to light through these studies will provide the agricultural community with evidence with which to demand regulatory protection and economic supports for any related transitions. There has been inadequate public health attention paid to the well-being of agricultural communities. Effective prevention policies and practices must be based on the precautionary principle, which asserts, 'when an activity raises threats of harm to human health or the environment, precautionary measures should be taken even if some cause and effect relationships are not fully established scientifically' (Kriebel et al., 2001, p. 871).

Acknowledgments

The authors acknowledge the contributions to this research made by the co-investigators for the Lifetime Histories Breast Cancer Research case-control study, by research assistants Jane McArthur, Kathy Mayville, and Daniel Holland, by Kandy Flood who facilitated many of the contacts with members of the farming community, and by Dale DeMatteo, Sean Griffin, Robert Park, and Robert DeMatteo who reviewed the chapter.

The Canadian Breast Cancer Foundation – Ontario Region provided funding for the case-control study and related qualitative research. The Breast Cancer Society of Canada and the Windsor Essex County Cancer Centre Foundation provided additional funding for the case-control study. The Ontario Trillium Foundation provided project funding for interviews with members of the farming community, the information from which supplemented the data gathered in the qualitative research study. The University of Windsor hosted and provided ethical approval for the research. The case-control study was conducted in partnership with the Windsor Regional Cancer Centre (Windsor Regional Hospital), which provided additional ethical approval. The Occupational Health Clinics for Ontario Workers (OHCOW) co-sponsored the studies.

References

Agriculture Canada. (1992). *Ontario Farm Groundwater Quality Survey Winter 1991/92*. Retrieved from http://gis.lrs.uoguelph.ca/AgriEnvArchives/esi/esiprog.html.

Alavanja, M.C., Sandler, D.P., McMaster, S.B., Zahm, S.H., McDonnell, C.J., Lynch, C.F., Pennybacker, M., Rothman, N., Dosemeci, M., Bond, A.E., & Blair, A. (1996). The Agricultural Health Study. *Environmental Health Perspectives, 104*(4), 362–9.

Andreotti, G., Beane Freeman, L.E., Hou, L., Coble, J., Rusiecki, J., Hoppin, J.A., Silverman, D.T., & Alavanja, M. (2009). Agricultural pesticide use and pancreatic cancer risk in the Agricultural Health Study cohort. *International Journal of Cancer, 124*, 2495–2500.

Anway, M.D., Memon, M.A., Uzumcu, M., & Skinner, M.K. (2006). Transgenerational effect of the endocrine disruptor vinclozolin on male spermatogenesis. *Journal of Andrology, 27*, 868–79.

Arcury, T.A., Grzywacz, J.G., Barr, D.B., Tapia, J., Chen, H., & Quandt, S.A. (2007). Pesticide urinary metabolite levels of children in eastern North Carolina farmworker households. *Environmental Health Perspectives, 115*(8), 1254–60.

Band, P.R., Le, N.D., Fang, R., Deschamps, M., Gallagher, R.P., & Yang, P. (2000). Identification of occupational cancer risks in British Columbia. *Journal of Occupational and Environmental Medicine, 42*(3), 284–310.

Birnbaum, L.S., & Fenton, S.E. (2003). Cancer and developmental exposure to endocrine disrupters. *Environmental Health Perspectives, 111*(4), 389–94.

Blair, A., Linos, A., Stewart, P.A., Burmeister, L.F., Gibson, R., Everett, G., Schuman, L., & Cantor, K.P. (1993). Evaluation of risks for non-Hodgkin's lymphoma by occupation and industry exposures from a case-control study. *American Journal of Industrial Medicine, 23*(2), 301–12.

Brody, J.G., Moysich, K.B., Humblet, O., Attfield, K.R., Beehler, G.P., & Rudel, R.A. (2007). Environmental pollutants and breast cancer: Epidemiologic studies. *Cancer, 109*, 2667–2711.

Brophy, J.T., Keith, M.M., Gorey, K.M., Laukkanen, E., Hellyer, D., Watterson, A., Reinhartz, A.D., & Gilbertson, M. (2002). Occupational histories of cancer patients in a Canadian cancer treatment centre and the generated hypothesis regarding breast cancer and farming. *International Journal of Occupational and Environmental Health, 8*, 346–53.

Brophy, J.T., Keith, M.M., Gorey, K.M., Luginaah, I., Laukkanen, E., Hellyer, D., Reinhartz, A., Watterson, A., Abu-Zahra, H., Maticka-Tyndale, E., Schneider, K., Beck, M., & Gilbertson, M. (2006). Occupation and breast cancer: A Canadian case-control study. *Annals of the New York Academy of Sciences, 1076*, 765–77.

Canadian Cancer Society. (2007). *Canadian cancer statistics.* Retrieved from http://www.cancer.ca/ontario/About cancer/Cancer statistics.aspx?sc_lang=en.

Canadian Cancer Society. (2011). *Ontario cancer statistics.* Retrieved 22 March 2012 from http://www.cancer.ca/canada-wide/about%20cancer/cancer%20statistics.aspx).

Carson, R. (2002). *Silent spring* (40th anniversary ed.). New York: Houghton Mifflin.

Clapp, R., Jacobs, M., & Loechler, E. (2008). Environmental and occupational causes of cancer: New evidence 2005–2007. *Review of Environmental Health, 23*, 1–37.

Clark, H., & Snedeker, S. (2006). *Farm family pesticide exposure: New pathways for understanding risk.* Ithaca, NY: Program on Breast Cancer and Environmental Risk Factors. Cornell University. Retrieved from http://envirocancer .cornell.edu/FactSheet/Pesticide/fs54.farmexposure.cfm.

Coble, J., Hoppin, J.A., Engel, L., Elci, O.C., Dosemeci, M., Lynch, C.F., & Alavanja, M. (2002). Prevalence of exposure to solvents, metals, grain dust, and other hazards among farmers in the Agricultural Health Study. *Journal of Exposure Analysis and Environmental Epidemiology, 12,* 418–26.

Cohn, B.A., Wolff, M.A., Cirillo, P.M., & Sholtz, R.I. (2007). DDT and breast cancer in young women: New data on the significance of age at exposure. *Environmental Health Perspectives, 115,* 1406–14.

Colborn, T., Dumanoski, D., & Myers, J.P. (1996). *Our stolen future.* Toronto: Dutton.

Corporation of the County of Essex. (2009). *County of Essex.* Retrieved from http://www.countyofessex.on.ca/general/home.asp.

Davis, D.L., Bradlow, H.L., Wolff, M., Woodruff, T., Hoel, D.G., & H Anton-Culver, H. (1993). Medical hypothesis: Xenoestrogens as preventable causes of breast cancer. *Environmental Health Perspectives, 101*(5), 372–7.

Diamanti-Kandarakis, E., Bourguignon, J.P., Giudice, L.C., Hauser, R., Prins, G.S., Soto, A.M., Zoeller, R.T., & Gore, A.C. (2009). Endocrine-disrupting chemicals: An Endocrine Society scientific statement. *Endocrine Reviews, 30*(4), 293–342.

Duell, E.J., Millikan, R.C., Savitz, D.A., Newman, B., Smith, J.C., Schell, M.J., & Sandler, D.P. (2000). A population-based case-control study of farming and breast cancer in North Carolina. *Epidemiology, 11*(5), 523–31.

Engel, L.S., Hill, D.A., Hoppin, J.A., Lubin, J.H., Lynch, C.F., Pierce, J., Samanic, C., Sandler, D.P., Blair, A., & Alavanja, M.C. (2005). Pesticide use and breast cancer risk among farmers' wives in the Agricultural Health Study. *American Journal of Epidemiology, 161,* 121–35.

Fox, G. (2001). Wildlife as sentinels of human health effects in the Great Lakes–St. Lawrence Basin. *Environmental Health Perspectives, 109*(Suppl. 6), 853–61.

Frank, R., Braun, H.E., Clegg, B.S., Ripley, B.D., & Johnson, R. (1990). Survey of farm wells for pesticides, Ontario, Canada, 1986 and 1987. *Bulletin of Environmental Contamination and Toxicology, 44,* 410–19.

Gallivan, G.J., Surgeoner, G.A., & Kovach, J. (2001). Ecological risk assessment: Pesticide risk reduction in the province of Ontario. *Journal of Environmental Quality, 30,* 798–813.

Gasnier, C., Dumont, C., Benachour, N., Clair, E., Chagnon, M.C., & Séralini, G.E. (2009). Glyphosate-based herbicides are toxic and endocrine disruptors in human cell lines. *Toxicology, 262*(3), 184–91.

Gladen, B.C., Sandler, D.P., Zahm, S.H., Kamel, F., Rowland, A.S., & Alavanja, M.C. (1998). Exposure opportunities of families of farmer pesticide applicators. *American Journal of Industrial Medicine, 34*, 581–7.

Grabusky, J., Martin, P.A., & Struger, J. (2004). *Pesticides in Ontario: A critical assessment of potential toxicity of urban use products to wildlife, with consideration for endocrine disruption* (Technical Report Series 410). Ottawa: Canadian Wildlife Service, Environment Canada.

Gray, J., Evans, N., Taylor, B., Rizzo, J., & Walker, M. (2009). State of the evidence: The connection between breast cancer and the environment. *International Journal of Occupational and Environmental Health, 15*, 43–78.

International Agency for Research on Cancer (IARC). (1991). *Occupational exposures in insecticide application and some pesticides* (IARC Monographs on the Evaluation of the Carcinogenic Risk of Chemicals to Humans, Vol. 53). Lyon, France: World Health Organization.

Jaga, K., & Dharmani, C. (2007). Pesticide exposure and breast cancer. In A.P. Yao (Ed.), *New developments in breast cancer research* (pp. 45–78). New York: Nova Science.

Keith, M., Cann, B., Brophy, J., Hellyer, D., Day, M., Egan, S., Mayville, K., & Watterson, A. (2001). Identifying and prioritizing gaming workers' health and safety concerns using mapping for data collection. *American Journal of Industrial Medicine, 39*, 42–51.

Kortenkamp, A., Evans, R., Martin, O., McKinlay, R., Orton, F., & Rosivatz, E. (2012). *State of the art assessment of endocrine disrupters – Final report* (Project contract no. 070307/2009/550687/SER/D3). Retrieved 27 March 2012 from http://ec.europa.eu/environment/endocrine/documents/studies_en.htm.

Kriebel, D., Tickner, J., Epstein, P., Lemons, J., Levins, R., Loechler, E.L., Quinn, M., Rudel, R., Schettler, T., & Stoto, M. (2001). The precautionary principle in environmental science. *Environmental Health Perspectives, 109*(9), 871–6.

Leipert, B. (1999). Rural women's health issues in Canada: An overview and implications for policy and research. In A. Medovarski & B. Cranney (Eds.). *Canadian woman studies* (pp. 552–64). Toronto: Inanna.

Lu, C., Fenske, R.A., Simcox, N.J., & Kalman, D. (2000). Pesticide exposure of children in an agricultural community: Evidence of household proximity to farmland and take-home exposure pathways. *Environmental Research, 84*, 290–302.

McDaniel, T.V., Martin, P.A., Struger, J., Sherry, J., Marvin, C.H., McMaster, M.E., Clarence, S., & Tetreault, G. (2008). Potential endocrine disruption of sexual development in free ranging male northern leopard frogs (*Rana pipiens*) and green frogs (*Rana clamitans*) from areas of intensive row crop agriculture. *Aquatic Toxicology, 88*(4), 230–42.

McDuffie, H. (1994). Women at work: Agriculture and pesticides. *Journal of Occupational Medicine, 36*(11), 1240–46.

McDuffie, H.H., Pahwa, P., McLaughlin, J.R., Spinelli, J.J., Fincham, S., Dosman, J.A., Robson, D., Skinnider, F.L., & Choi, N.W. (2001). Non-Hodgkin's lymphoma and specific pesticide exposures in men: Cross-Canada study of pesticides and health. *Cancer Epidemiology, Biomarkers & Prevention, 10*(11), 1153–63.

McGee, B. (2004). *Survey of pesticide use in Ontario, 2003.* Toronto: Ontario Ministry of Agriculture and Food, Economics and Policy Coordination Branch.

Nudelman, J., Taylor, B., Evans, N., Rizzo, J., Gray, J., Engel, C., & Walker, M. (2009). Policy and research recommendations emerging from the scientific evidence connecting environmental factors and breast cancer. *International Journal of Occupational and Environmental Health, 15*, 79–101.

Ontario Ministry of Natural Resources. (2009). *Stewardship Kent – People and the economy.* Retrieved from http://www.ontariostewardship.org/councils/kent.

Pesticide Action Network Europe. (2006). *Eight hazardous pesticides banned or restricted in the EU Market* (Newsletter 29). Retrieved from http://www.pan-europe.info/Resources/Newsletter/Archive/news29.htm.

Pesticide Action Network UK (2009). *A catalogue of lists of pesticides identifying those associated with particularly harmful health or environmental impacts* (3rd ed.). Retrieved from http://www.pan-uk.org/List%20of%20Lists.html.

Rudel, R., Attfield, K., Schifano, J., & Brody, J. (2007). Chemicals causing mammary gland tumors in animals signal new directions for epidemiology, chemicals testing, and risk assessment for breast cancer prevention. *American Cancer Society, 109*(12), 2635–66.

Sass, J.B., & Colangelo, J.D. (2006). European Union bans atrazine, while the United States negotiates continued use. *International Journal of Occupational and Environmental Health, 12*, 260–7.

Sierra Club of Canada. (2005). *2,4-D pesticide fact sheet.* Retrieved 23 March 2012 from www.sierraclub.ca/national/programs/health-environment/pesticides/2-4-D-fact-sheet.shtml.

Snedeker, S. (2001). Pesticides and breast cancer risk: A review of DDT, DDE, and dieldrin. *Environmental Health Perspectives, 109*(Suppl 11), 35–47.

Statistics Canada (2008). *Section 5 Rural and urban populations by sex and age for the total population and the farm population.* Retrieved from http://www.statcan.gc.ca/pub/95-633-x/2007000/t/6500022-eng.htm#35.

Tashakkori, A., & Teddlie, C. (1998). *Mixed methodology: Combining qualitative and quantitative approaches.* Thousand Oaks, CA: Sage.

Teschke, K., Smith, J.C., & Olshan, A.F. (2000). Evidence of recall bias in volunteered vs. prompted responses about occupational exposures. *American Journal of Industrial Medicine, 38,* 385–8.

Vandenberg, L.N., Colborn, T., Hayes, T.B., Heindel, J.J., Jacobs, D.R., Lee, D.-H., Shioda, T., Soto, A.M., vom Saal, F.S., Welshons, W.V., Zoeller, R.T., & Myers, J.P. (2012). Hormones and endocrine-disrupting chemicals: Low-dose effects and nonmonotonic dose responses. *Endocrine Reviews, 33*(3), 378–455. doi:10.1210/er.2011-1050.

van Larebeke, N., Sasco, A.J., Brophy, J.T., Keith, M.M., Gilbertson, M., & Watterson, A. (2008). Sex ratio changes as sentinel health events of endocrine disruption. *International Journal of Occupational and Environmental Health, 14,* 138–43.

Ward, M.H., Lubin, J., Giglierano, J., Colt, J.S., Wolter, C., Bekiroglu, N., Camann, D., Hartge, P., & Nuckols, J.R. (2006). Proximity to crops and residential exposure to agricultural herbicides in Iowa. *Environmental Health Perspectives, 114*(6), 893–7.

Zahm, S.H., & Blair, A. (2003). Occupational cancer among women: Where have we been and where are we going? *American Journal of Industrial Medicine, 44,* 565–75.

6 An Exploration of Canadian Farm Women's Food Provisioning Practices

Lynn McIntyre and Krista Rondeau

Given the inextricable link between food and health (World Health Organization, 2012), much research has been dedicated to understanding the determinants of food choices and food consumption patterns in order to improve the health and nutritional status of individuals and populations. Why people eat what they eat is a complex process that is influenced by historical, physical, social, cultural, environmental, and economic conditions, in addition to individual factors (DeVault, 1991; Furst, Bisogni, Sobal, & Falk, 1996; Mead, 2008; Schubert, 2008). This chapter focuses on the relationship between food and health by exploring the experience of a unique rural population – farm families who are adapting to agricultural transition – from the viewpoint of the primary food provider: farm women.[1] We describe the food provisioning construct as a tool for the study of farm women's experiences as food provider, and then discuss the evolving nature of farm families and farm women in Canada. We present an overview of the food provisioning framework that arose from interviews with twenty-two farm women in Alberta, Ontario, and Nova Scotia. We conclude with a discussion of the beliefs, obligations, and actions of farm women regarding the provision of healthy food for their families within the context of their daily food provisioning practices.

Background

Food Provisioning

The study of food provisioning is a way to understand the underlying factors that influence the daily food routine and the eventual relationship between food choices and consumption patterns and health. Food provisioning is a construct that informs everyday food consumption in a specific social setting – the household – by making visible the socio-cultural and environmental factors that shape these activities (DeVault, 1991; Schubert, 2008; Whitehead, 1984). Far from being mundane, food provisioning involves a breadth of complex activities (acquisition, preparation, production, consumption, and disposal of food) where technical skills (e.g., growing food, shopping, meal planning, preserving, cooking) and resources must be tacitly coordinated, often by a primary food provider within the social context and demands of household members as well as within the broader environment in which the household lives (Bava, Jaeger, & Park, 2008; Charles & Kerr, 1988; DeVault, 1991; Marshall, 1995; Schubert, 2008; Whitehead, 1984). Thus, food provisioning practices are the enactment of complex processes and mechanisms that link socio-cultural and environmental factors to both household and individual dietary practices (Schubert, 2008). As such, they illuminate the lived experience of both farm women and their households.

Farm Families and Farm Women in Canada

Although often studied in conjunction with rural populations, farm families are distinct from the general rural population because their agricultural occupation base is also their home (Meares, 1997). The farm population in Canada is in decline: in 1931, 31.7% of Canadians lived on farms, but in 2006, those living on farms accounted for only 2.2% of all Canadians (Statistics Canada, 2008). Across Canada, the proportion of the farm population ranges from 0.4% in Newfoundland and Labrador to 31.0% in Saskatchewan (Statistics Canada, 2008). The number and size of farm families living on single unincorporated farms is also declining: in 2006 there were 175,810 family farms, a 9.5% decrease from 2001, with an average household size of 3.1 (Statistics Canada, 2008). At the same time, farms are getting larger, and farmers are increasingly directing their commodities towards large urban areas and export markets and away from local markets and home use (Statistics Canada, 2008).

Since Canada began counting its farm population in 1931, Canadian farm families have had to adapt to changing market conditions, environmental stresses, and new technologies (Statistics Canada, 2008). More recently, the discovery of bovine spongiform encephalopathy

(BSE), or mad cow disease, in Canada in 2003 had significant impact on the economic health of farm commodities (Samarajeewa, Weerahewa, Bredahl, & Wigle, 2006). Concurrently, farm families are seeking employment off the farm; agriculture-population linkage data from the 2006 census revealed that the largest source of income for farm families was wages and salaries (62.2% of total income), while net farm income represented 6.3% of their total household income (Statistics Canada, 2008).

Empirical research has shown that farm women in Canada play a significant role in the successful operation and management of the family farm. They work on the farm while maintaining traditional responsibilities in the home, including primary responsibility for household food provisioning activities, and often have off-farm employment in addition (e.g., Kubik & Moore, 2005; Martz & Brueckner, 2003). As a result, farm women are likely to reveal a range of factors that influence their food provisioning practices (DeVault, 1991). How farm women discuss their daily activities may inform not only an understanding of the modern lives of farm families but also how they cope and adapt during times of farm stress (Bailey, Convery, Mort, & Baxter, 2006).

Methods

For this study, we recruited twenty-two farm women (six in Alberta, six in Ontario, and ten in Nova Scotia) with at least two children under the age of eighteen years who lived on farms of varying commodities. Semi-structured in-person interviews were conducted with participants in their homes between the months of June and November 2007, which allowed us to observe any food provisioning supports that they may have discussed (e.g., garden, cold storage, animals for home consumption, etc.). Farm women were asked to discuss what they did in an average day to manage food and meals for themselves and their families, with a particular focus on food acquisition strategies, sources of food, meal planning and preparation, and consumption. Farm women were also asked to comment on the impact of rurality, various agricultural crises (e.g., drought, grasshopper infestations, BSE), and social movements (e.g., local food movements such as the 100-mile diet, organic foods) on their food provisioning practices. Socio-demographic information on their household and farm operations as well as the household's food security status (i.e., whether the household was worried about obtaining or unable to obtain sufficient, nutritious foods through socially acceptable means due to a lack of income [Davis & Tarasuk, 1994]) was collected. Table 6.1 presents the socio-demographic profile of participants. Table 6.2 provides farm location and commodity for each of the participants, who are listed by pseudonym.[2] Analysis was conducted using conventional qualitative content analysis techniques (Hsieh & Shannon, 2005), as well as techniques such as immersion/crystallization (Borkan, 1999), memoing (Bryman, 2004), visual displays (Miles & Huberman, 1994), peer debriefing, and member-checking (Lincoln & Guba, 1985).

Socio-demographic Profile of Participants

The mean age of participants was forty-two years, and their farms represented a variety of commodities, with an emphasis on cattle. Women were generally well educated, and 40.9% ($n = 9$) reported off-farm employment. Two households were identified as food insecure based on their response to the household food security questionnaire, and a third volunteered after the interview that she had withheld this information because her husband was in the room during the interview.

Food Provisioning Framework

This section examines the foremost aims of the food provisioning process that influenced farm women in their role as primary food provider, followed by a review of factors that led to manifest food provisioning practices. This framework is outlined in Figure 6.1.

Aims of Food Provisioning Practices

CREATE AND SUPPORT A STRONG FAMILY ENVIRONMENT
Farm women's food provisioning practices reflected a desire to create and support a strong family environment. Food provisioning activities such as gardening, raising animals, going to the farmer's market, making maple syrup, or catching fish were occasions that allowed the family to spend time together. Often, children accompanied participants during grocery shopping trips and assisted with meal preparation; however, as children grew older and became more independent, the opportunities to engage in family food provisioning activities decreased. Gwen recalled how her daughters, as they approached adulthood, avoided activities that once brought the family together:

Table 6.1 Selected Socio-demographic Variables of Participants (*n* = 22)*

Variable	Description
Province	*n*
Nova Scotia	10
Ontario	6
Alberta	6
Type of farm	*n*
Beef / bison	7
Dairy	7
Mixed, with beef	4
Other	4
Age of women**	*Years*
Average age	41.7
Range	25–50
Education	*n*
Less than high school	0
Graduated high school	3
Some post-secondary	2
Graduated post-secondary	14
Unknown	3
Children living in household < 18 years	
Average age of children	10.0 years
Average number	*n* = 2.4
Range	0–5
Farms with off-farm income	*n (%)*
	14 (63)
Farms reporting food insecurity	*n (%)*
	2 (9)

*   McIntyre & Rondeau (2009); McIntyre et al. (2009); Rondeau & McIntyre (2010).
** The age of four participants is missing.

They never really came out and said it but you could see them kind of shrinking away … it would be like, 'Can you guys help me weed the garden?' 'Ah, I got a date' (laughter) and they'd be gone, so you accept those kinds of things.

A common feature of all participants' food provisioning practices was commensality, which refers to eating with others, with the family being the most fundamental commensal unit (Sobal & Nelson, 2003). Although current trends are towards fewer home-prepared meals (Canadian Council of Food and Nutrition [CCFN], 2008), farm women

Table 6.2 Participant Profile

Pseudonym	Farm location	Farm commodity*
Mary	Alberta	Beef
Kelly	Alberta	Mixed, with beef
Carol	Alberta	Beef
Tammy	Alberta	Mixed, with beef
Barbara	Alberta	Other
Olivia	Alberta	Beef
Denise	Ontario	Beef
Eleanor	Ontario	Other
Gwen	Ontario	Beef
Holly	Ontario	Dairy
Iris	Ontario	Dairy
Natalie	Ontario	Mixed, with beef
Rose	Nova Scotia	Dairy
Sally	Nova Scotia	Dairy
Tenille	Nova Scotia	Other
Valerie	Nova Scotia	Dairy
Julie	Nova Scotia	Mixed, with beef
Leanne	Nova Scotia	Dairy
Jennifer	Nova Scotia	Dairy
Amanda	Nova Scotia	Other
Carrie	Nova Scotia	Beef
Joan	Nova Scotia	Mixed, no beef

* Unique commodities were masked to protect the identity of the participant.

reported that the majority of meals were consumed at home. Dinner was consistently reported to be a family event, and many families also ate breakfast and lunch together. While the content and elaborateness of the meal varied, the sole requirement was 'everybody will be sitting at the table having something together' (Barbara), and many women specifically stated that meals were not to be consumed in front of the television. Participants reported that shared family meals were opportunities for family bonding and sharing stories about the day, as well as opportunities to model habits and behaviours for children and discuss troublesome behaviour. While the shared family meal was the ideal, there were often factors that influenced whether or not this actually occurred, as is discussed later.

Figure 6.1 Farm Women's Food Provisioning Framework

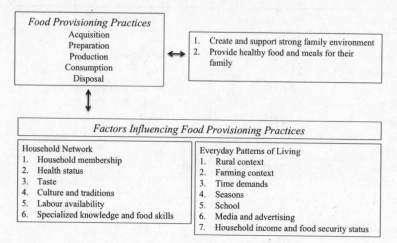

PROVIDE HEALTHY FOOD AND MEALS

A second aim of farm women's food provisioning practices centred on providing food and meals that they believed to be healthy (McIntyre, Thille, & Rondeau, 2009). Farm women spontaneously drew on healthy eating guidelines such as *Canada's Food Guide* (Health Canada, 2007) to describe their food provisioning practices, with specific mention of choosing minimally processed foods (i.e., minimal added sodium, sugar, fat, and preservatives), whole grains, healthy fats (e.g., grass-fed saturated fat, cod liver oil), and 100% juice.[3] In their discussion of their food provisioning practices, farm women articulated principles of balance, variety, and moderation. For example, Iris contended: 'I think they eat well. [T]hey eat a fairly broad spectrum of, you know, Canada's Food Guide. They, you know, maybe there's some days where Canada's Food Guide gets thrown out the window, and I think everybody is the same.'

While these guidelines helped farm women provide foods that they deemed healthy, they also relied on food provisioning practices that enabled them to 'know what had gone into their food,' as they believed this would yield safe, healthy, and wholesome food (Rondeau & McIntyre, 2010), that is, trusted foods. Farm women explicitly referred to food production methods that allowed them to know what had gone into their food, such as growing and raising their own food, obtaining food from trusted farmers, family, or friends, and otherwise acquiring foods that had been produced according to Canadian food safety regulations (Rondeau & McIntyre, 2010). In addition, advanced food processing and preservation techniques, such as freezing, canning, and making preserves, allowed farm women to prepare and consume trusted foods beyond the typical growing season. Processing and preservation tended to be done in the home, although some would rely on their neighbours for specialized equipment (e.g., grist mill, wine press). Making food and meals from scratch was also a common way to provide trusted foods because it allowed farm women to eliminate ingredients that were unwanted, such as preservatives, allergens, or contaminants, or those that were perceived to be unhealthy.

In turn, farm women reported that the foods and meals they provided for their family came to be preferred by family members. Joan, who raised chickens for her family's consumption, recalled her family's reaction when she served chicken she had purchased:

> I bought chicken one year 'cause we ran out of chickens and I cooked it and put it on the table and my oldest one looked at me and she said, 'You really don't expect us to eat that, now do you?' (Laughter) ... It took me days to get rid of that chicken. (Laughter). I had one more [chicken] left. I made soup and gave it to the neighbours.

Farm women expressed satisfaction that the work they did to provide food for their families was appreciated by both their children and husbands, who would, on occasion, convey appreciation for their efforts: 'I do think they appreciate the work I do in the kitchen. Like they'll often say, "Oh, that was a really good meal, Mom" or "thank you"' (Carol). Farm women subsequently gauged their success at providing appropriate food for their families by reporting that their children were 'good eaters.' Most children did not have food restrictions due to allergies or dislikes, and they were expected to eat what was served.

Factors Influencing Food Provisioning Practices

Although farm women's food provisioning practices were driven by the desire to provide healthy and trusted foods for their families while also creating and supporting a strong family environment, there were a number of factors that influenced the types of foods and meals that they acquired, prepared, and ultimately consumed.

HOUSEHOLD NETWORK

Farm women's household network included their immediate household, such as their family and extended family, and, to a lesser extent, neighbours, friends, and other farmers in their vicinity. These social relationships drove their food provisioning practices and are described below.

Household membership. Farm women's household membership, especially children, had a strong impact on their food provisioning practices. Many reported paying more attention to the quality of their diet once they became pregnant or when their children were born. Rose, who lives on a dairy farm, began purchasing and consuming pasteurized milk for the family once she became pregnant: 'We did drink unpasteurized milk ... But once I was pregnant I knew you weren't supposed to, so I started drinking pasteurized and we've never changed.' As families grew with the birth of additional children, and subsequently shrank when children grew up and left the home, food provisioning practices changed as well. Elaborate food provisioning activities like gardening and preservation were no longer appropriate once children left home: 'I used to do the canning of beans and all those good things, and make jams and everything, but as the kids grew up and started leaving home and they didn't eat those things, I quit doing that' (Denise).

Health status. The health status of family members also had an impact on farm women's food provisioning practices. Farm women modified their food provisioning practices in an effort to ensure optimal growth and development, maintain good health, and prevent disease or cope with new or pre-existing conditions, such as allergies, migraines, elevated blood sugar levels, ulcers, or cancer. Some women reported a desire to lose weight themselves or prevent excessive weight gain in children, and this led to food provisioning activities such as purchasing low-fat dairy, avoiding starchy foods (e.g., potatoes, bread), minimizing desserts, or preparing and consuming more fruits and vegetables.

Taste. Taste preferences of family members were a strong factor in determining the food provisioning activities of farm women. Many women revealed their family's preference for fresh or homemade products and consequently reported acquiring fresh foods from their own garden or their agricultural exchange network and making and preparing foods and meals from scratch. While farm women were unwilling to prepare multiple meals for family members to meet food and taste preferences, they were also unwilling to spend the time, money, and energy to buy, grow, and prepare foods that their family members would not consume because they did not like them: 'I find that they eat better if they have a say into it so I'd just rather it be that way' (Tenille).

Culture and traditions. Cultural foods and traditions also played a strong role in the food provisioning practices of farm women. For some, cultural traditions were only enacted during holidays; for others, cultural traditions influenced the daily food routine (e.g., green salad accompanying dinner [Holly]). Farm women also spoke of 'family foods' and traditions, that is, eating patterns that they experienced as children that were incorporated into their food provisioning practices: 'Suppertime was always important [when I was a child] and [my mother] always made sure we had a good meal at suppertime, so I guess that's why [we do the same]' (Leanne).

Labour availability. Many farm women relied on their children and extended family to help out with food provisioning activities, such as grocery shopping, gardening, food preservation, and meal preparation. Children most often assisted with grocery shopping, gardening, setting the table, cooking, and baking, roles that could become more complex as they grew older. The family garden was a good example of the need for assistance; many women once had a large and thriving garden, but they now lacked the assistance from children and relatives to maintain it. In addition, advanced food production and preparation techniques, such as butchering and freezing animals, were often done with the assistance of extended family members; once they were no longer available to help out, these activities were likely to be abandoned.

Specialized knowledge and food skills. Farm women's specialized knowledge and food skills, and that of their extended family, played a role in the food provisioning activities. Many farm women reported learning how to grow, process, preserve, and prepare food from their parents, most often their mother or mother-in-law. Others reported learning how to do these activities through self-directed learning, trial and error, and home economics classes. In addition, the preparation of cultural foods was often taught and assisted by the farm women's extended family.

EVERYDAY PATTERNS OF LIVING

While farm women described ideal food provisioning practices that responded to those in their local social network, there were many other
external everyday factors that influenced the daily food routine.

Rural context. The rural location in which farm women lived influenced
their food provisioning practices. Although some farm women reported good access to fresh produce, ironically, other farm women reported
higher prices and decreased availability and variety of fresh, quality
produce in small, rural grocery stores. Being in a rural setting meant
that farm women generally had better access to land, equipment, and
resources required to produce and process food (e.g., garden, pasture,
water [fish], land [hunting], dugout water for watering the garden,
slaughtering facilities) and to store food (e.g., freezer space, cold storage) than would be available in a non-farm or urban setting. However,
farm women had to contend with the particular geography and climate
of the region in which they lived and its impact on food production; for
example, drought was common in Alberta, while poor-quality, rocky
soil was a problem in some Ontario communities, and seasonal storms
were a threat in Nova Scotia. Participants tended to have fewer opportunities to purchase prepared meals outside the home, as rural locations generally have poor access to restaurants and fast food outlets.

Farming context. Farm life played a key role in farm women's food provisioning practices. During high seasons (i.e., seeding, calving, harvest-
ing), meals tended to be less elaborate and mealtimes could be sporadic.
While farm women reportedly fed their children at regular mealtimes,
their husbands, who were working on the farm, would come in for a
meal when they had a break in their schedule. Some farm women prepared meals for the farm workers employed during high season in addition to feeding their own family members. Denise, who also helped
with farm work, said:

> In the wintertime when we're just feeding the cows, we'll have supper
> probably around six o'clock and it's pretty much fixed. Come calving, I try
> to have [supper] fixed but you know if [you] gotta go and be a midwife for
> a little bit, then you know, supper might be delayed or pushed forward or
> something, but it's during springs and summer that mealtimes are all over.

Some farm women indicated that farm animals had priority over certain foodstuffs and resources. For example, the pigs and veal calves that

Natalie raised had priority over the household for the milk produced on the farm, which resulted in the family's inability to produce cheese from home-produced milk.

Time demands. Farm women would tailor their food provisioning practices to the schedules of family members. In particular, children's school schedules and extra-curricular activities demanded specific mealtime requirements and also influenced farm women's ability to plan and prepare a meal, since they were often responsible for driving children to and from activities. Mealtimes could be delayed and preparation was often less elaborate (e.g., leftovers, easily prepared casseroles) on these days. On the other hand, farm women would plan trips to the grocery store around their children's schedules as it often brought them into town during the day.

The daily farm schedule was also a strong determinant of mealtimes: 'we just kind of live around my husband's schedule' (Denise). Chores had to be done at specific times, and meals would be planned around these requirements. In addition, participants' farm work had implications for the food provisioning activities they were able to perform:

> Normally when the potatoes need to be dug and the beans and that kind of stuff needs to be picked, I'm ... either running around like a mad hatter trying to get equipment ready or bins ready [for] harvest. Like it coincides with both. (Barbara)

For farm women who had off-farm employment, food provisioning practices had to be balanced against time availability. Some activities, such as gardening, meal planning, and preparing foods from scratch, became increasingly difficult when women worked off the farm:

> When I stopped [working] to have kids, when I had more time, I would do [a lot of preparation from scratch]. I'd bake bread every week. I even had sourdough bread ... Since I started work, too much part time, I just hadn't had the time for it. (Kelly)

For some, work schedules limited their ability to shop at farmer's markets, which typically have limited hours of operation. While some women preferred to work outside the home and subsequently buy foods rather than grow food, others had to abandon gardening as a preferred practice due to time constraints.

Farm women expressed the need to balance food provisioning activities with family time. Activities like gardening and advanced food production are time consuming, and some women expressed concern that engaging in these activities would take time away from being with their children:

> [If] I'm doing all this stuff in the [house and in the garden], then basically all they're going to do is see me work. They don't see anything else (chuckle) you know. They're only young once so you kinda have to make a compromise I find. (Holly)

Seasons. Not surprisingly, farm women reported that their food provisioning practices were affected by the seasons. For example, barbecuing was preferred over stews and roasts during the summer months; fresh vegetables and fruits were eaten in greater quantity and variety during the summer and early fall, whereas frozen or canned goods were more readily consumed in the winter. Certain foods were only purchased, prepared, and consumed when they were in season, and bumper crops were reflected in the composition of meals.

School. For many farm women, the types of foods that could be included in their children's lunch were partially determined by the school's food and nutrition guidelines. In addition, many schools had breakfast clubs, hot lunch programs, or a cafeteria or concession where children could purchase lunch, subsequently influencing the foods and meals that needed to be provided.

Media and advertising. On occasion, farm women discussed the role of media and advertising in their food provisioning practices. Many women referred to weekly flyers for ideas on foods to purchase that week and subsequent meals to prepare. For some, reports on the health and safety implications of certain foods could influence the foods they acquired. For example, Natalie, who raised a variety of animals for home consumption, discussed how her family had watched a documentary on the ethical treatment of animals and subsequently refused to consume commercially produced meats.

Household income and food security status. While most women expressed an awareness of cost when purchasing and preparing food (e.g., they stocked up on items on sale, minimized waste through leftovers, bought certain items in bulk) and expressed concerns over the rising costs of food and fuel, they were unwilling to compromise on the quality of foods purchased: 'If I decide I want to buy mangoes or avocados or anything, if it's a bit expensive, or grapes or any fruit, I don't worry about it. I just buy it' (Carol).

The influence of household income on the food provisioning practices of farm women was most evident in food-insecure households. Farm women in food-insecure households reported coping strategies that included purchasing food on credit, skipping other bill payments, using coupons, shopping on discount days (e.g., 10% off grocery bill on the first Tuesday of every month), purchasing items on sale or items that had been reduced (e.g., day-old bread), comparison shopping, and borrowing food from friends and neighbours. In the situation of more severe food insecurity, Barbara sacrificed her food intake for her children:

> I'll take like a sandwich with me or some fruit or something with me. If there's nothing like fruit left, then I'll just make a sandwich like a piece of bread or something like that. As long as I've got water (chuckle), I'm good.

The unpredictability of farm income due to variations in the cost of inputs and commodity market prices, in addition to significant operating costs, made budgeting adequately for food a difficult task for food-insecure families.

Discussion and Conclusion

In our study, we began with a simple request: 'tell me what you do in an average day to manage food and meals for yourself and your family.' As Silverman (2006) has suggested about qualitative study, our inquiry about the family food provisioning experience served as an entry point for a larger conversation on farm women's lived experience. What farm women shared was a comprehensive assessment of their role as primary food provider; their beliefs, obligations, and actions regarding the provision of safe, healthy, and wholesome foods (Rondeau & McIntyre, 2010); and the myriad of factors both within and external to their household that influenced their everyday actions of managing the family's food resources, health, and well-being in the context of farm life. These results are notable, as there are relatively few examples in the literature where this strategy has been used to understand the daily food practices of households (e.g., Bava et al., 2008; Jabs et al., 2007; Whitehead, 1984), and of farm families and farm women in particular.

The findings of this study suggest that farm women's food provisioning experiences reflect a traditional farming lifestyle and heritage. Consistent with traditional gender roles that place women at the helm of feeding work (Cummins, 2005; Heather, Skillen, Young, & Vladicka, 2005; Meares, 1997; O'Sullivan, Hocking, & Wright-St. Clair, 2008; Van Esterik, 1999), farm women are the primary food provisioning agent, engaging in complex activities to provide desired and trusted food and meals while nurturing family life. Unique features of farm life, including ancillary work on the farm, the farm cycle, and unpredictable farm income, place real constraints on farm women's food provisioning activities. At the same time, farm women must also navigate modern stressors that are typical in all households, such as time constraints deriving from employment and children's school and extracurricular schedules.

Food preparation from scratch appears to be the most durable aspect of farm women's food provisioning practices, even amongst farm women who experienced food insecurity. While many women typically have less time to spend in the kitchen because they are working outside the home and thus rely more on convenience foods (Bava et al., 2008; Blake et al., 2009; Jabs et al., 2007; O'Sullivan et al., 2008), it seems that farm women are better able than non-farm women to manage these constraints. In fact, farm women's food provisioning practices are more typical of those of older women who 'take pride in their ability to provide a meal from scratch using ingredients at hand, believing home-made food to be the basis of good health and an important aspect of caring for their family' (O'Sullivan et al., 2008, p. 65). Furthermore, contrary to current trends to consume meals away from home (CCFN, 2008) or in social isolation (Sobal & Nelson, 2003), we found that farm families routinely engage in communal eating, with family meals in the home serving as social events for its members (DeVault, 1991). The salience of communal eating patterns can likely also be attributed to the remote geographical location of farms as well as the need to remain in close proximity to the field or the barn throughout the day, factors that limit opportunities to leave the farm and eat at food outlets.

Nonetheless, while we have provided an initial examination of farm women's ability to adapt to modern stresses, this is an area of inquiry that would benefit from further investigation. In addition, farm women's ability as primary food provider to influence the consumption and subsequent nutritional well-being of household members requires further exploration given recent interest in the concept of the household's nutritional gatekeeper (e.g., Rosenkranz & Dzewaltowski, 2008; Wansink, 2006). It also remains unclear how the experiences of farm women and farm families are distinct from those of the rural population as a whole, of whom only 10.3% live and work on farms (Statistics Canada, 2008). The framework that we have described in this chapter is an important foundation for examining these issues in a larger sample, an expanded sample, and with more direct questioning.

Ultimately, these results can be applied to understanding the relationship between food provisioning practices, food consumption, and the health of farm families. Public health and nutrition policy initiatives can often focus on an individualistic health promotion model that fails to recognize how consumption and dietary patterns occur within households (Schubert, 2008). For example, both Charles and Kerr (1988) and DeVault (1991) reveal that efforts to improve the healthfulness of family diets by targeting nutrition education efforts at women would likely increase their burden of guilt because healthy eating concepts may not be congruent with the responsibility of feeding their families a 'proper' meal. Understanding and making visible the ecological picture underlying daily food practices could enable future efforts to influence the health and nutritional status of groups and populations, such as farm families, to be more targeted and more effective, and unintended consequences could be reduced (Charles & Kerr, 1988; DeVault, 1991; Jabs et al., 2007; Mead, 2008; Schubert, 2008; Whitehead, 1984).

The health risks for farm women and their families are further explored in chapter 5 by Brophy and colleagues, who investigate exposure to pesticides through its application and subsequent contamination of groundwater, soil, and air. In chapter 7, Kubik and Fletcher move beyond household-level analysis to explore commercial food production practices and their possible relationship to the health of farm women and the viability of family farming practices. Evidently, the factors that influence the nutritional health and well-being of farm women are broad and complex and require elaboration in future research.

Acknowledgments

We thank the women who shared their insights with us during interviewing, and acknowledge Bonnie Anderson, interviewer for Nova

Scotia. Partial financial support was received from PrioNet Canada, the Alberta Prion Research Institute, and the faculties of Medicine and Veterinary Medicine and the Vice-President Research at the University of Calgary.

Notes

1 We chose to use the term *farm women* as they are not necessarily farm operators, but nor are they simply *farm wives* (Sachs, 1996). We use the term *farm families* to refer to families who live on unincorporated farms where at least one family member is a farm operator.

2 Note that the pseudonyms will be cited as the source of quotes from the data used in this chapter.

3 In Canada, nutrition and health professionals typically describe healthy eating as consumption patterns that are outlined in *Canada's Food Guide*. Eating patterns based on these recommendations, built on principles of balance, variety, and moderation, help to ensure that adequate micro- and macronutrients are consumed, some chronic disease risk is reduced (e.g., obesity, type 2 diabetes, heart disease, osteoporosis, certain types of cancer), and overall health and vitality are encouraged (Health Canada, 2007).

References

Bailey, C., Convery, I., Mort, M., & Baxter, J. (2006). Different public health geographies of the 2001 foot and mouth disease epidemic: 'Citizen' versus 'professional' epidemiology. *Health and Place, 12*, 157–66.

Bava, C.M., Jaeger, S.R., & Park, J. (2008). Constraints on food provisioning practices in 'busy' women's lives: Trade-offs which demand convenience. *Appetite, 50*, 486–98.

Blake, C.E., Devine, C.M., Wethington, E., Jastran, M., Farrell, T.J., & Bisogni, C.A. (2009). Employed parents' satisfaction with food-choice coping strategies: Influence of gender and structure. *Appetite, 52*, 711–19.

Borkan, J. (1999). Immersion/crystallization. In B.F. Crabtree & W.L. Miller (Eds.), *Doing qualitative research* (2nd ed., pp. 179–94). Thousand Oaks, CA: Sage.

Bryman, A. (2004). *Social research methods* (2nd ed.). Oxford: Oxford University Press.

Canadian Council of Food and Nutrition (CCFN). (2008). *Tracking nutrition trends VII*. Retrieved from http://www.ccfn.ca/events/agm.asp.

Charles, N., & Kerr, M. (1988). *Women, food and families*. Manchester: Manchester University Press.

Cummins, H.A. (2005). Unraveling the voices and identity of farm women. *Identity, 5*, 287–302.

Davis, B., & Tarasuk, V. (1994). Hunger in Canada. *Agriculture and Human Values, 11*, 50–7.

DeVault, M.L. (1991). *Feeding the family*. Chicago: University of Chicago Press.

Furst, T., Connors, M., Bisogni, C.A., Sobal, J., & Falk, L.W. (1996). Food choice: A conceptual model of the process. *Appetite, 26*, 247–66.

Health Canada. (2007). *Eating well with Canada's food guide*. Retrieved from http://www.hc-sc.gc.ca/fn-an/food-guide-aliment/index-eng.php.

Heather, B., Skillen, L., Young, J., & Vladicka, R. (2005). Women's gendered identities and restructuring of rural Alberta. *Sociologia Ruralis, 45*, 86–97.

Hsieh, H., & Shannon, S.E. (2005). Three approaches to qualitative content analysis. *Qualitative Health Research, 15*, 1277–88.

Jabs, J., Devine, C.M., Bisogni, C.A., Farrell, T.J., Janstran, M., & Wethington, E. (2007). Trying to find the quickest way: Employed mothers' constructions of time for food. *Journal of Nutrition Education and Behaviour, 39*, 18–25.

Kubik, W., & Moore, R.J. (2005). Health and well-being of farm women: Contradictory roles in the contemporary economy. *Journal of Agricultural Safety and Health, 11*, 249–56.

Lincoln, Y.S., & Guba, E.G. (1985). *Naturalistic inquiry*. Beverly Hills, CA: Sage.

Marshall, D. (1995). *Food choice and the consumer*. Glasgow: Blackie.

Martz, D.J.F., & Brueckner, I.S. (2003). *The Canadian farm family at work: Exploring gender and generation*. Retrieved from the National Farmers Union website http://www.nfu.ca/women.html.

McIntyre, L., & Rondeau, K. (2009). Surviving bovine spongiform encephalopathy (BSE): Farm women's discussion of the effects of BSE on food provisioning practices. *Journal of Toxicology and Environmental Health, 72*, 1083–5.

McIntyre, L., Thille, P., & Rondeau, K. (2009). Farmwomen's discourses on family food provisioning: Gender, health, and risk avoidance. *Food and Foodways, 17*, 80–103.

Mead, M. (2008). The problem of changing food habits. In C. Counihan & P. Van Esterik (Eds.), *Food and culture: A reader* (2nd ed., pp. 17–27). New York: Routledge.

Meares, A.C. (1997). Making the transition from conventional to sustainable agriculture: Gender, social movement participation, and quality of life on the family farm. *Rural Sociology, 62*, 21–47.

Miles, M.B., & Huberman, M. (1994). *Qualitative data analysis: An expanded sourcebook*. Thousand Oaks, CA: Sage.

O'Sullivan, G., Hocking, C., & Wright-St. Clair, V. (2008). History in the making: Older Canadian women's food-related practices. *Food and Foodways, 16*, 63–87.

Rondeau, K., & McIntyre, L. (2010). 'I know what's gone into it': Canadian farmwomen's conceptualisation of food safety. *Health, Risk, and Society, 12*, 211–29.

Rosenkranz, R.R., & Dzewaltowski, D.D. (2008). Model of the home food environment pertaining to childhood obesity. *Nutrition Reviews, 66*, 123–40.

Sachs, C.E. (1996). *Gendered fields: Rural women, agriculture, and environment.* Boulder, CO: Westview Press.

Samarajeewa, S., Weerahewa, J., Bredahl, M., & Wigle, R. (2006). Impacts of BSE crisis on the Canadian economy: An input-output analysis. Retrieved from the University of Minnesota Department of Applied Economics website http://purl.umn.edu/34179.

Schubert, L. (2008). Household food strategies and the reframing of ways of understanding dietary practices. *Ecology of Food and Nutrition, 47*, 254–79.

Silverman, D. (2006). *Interpreting qualitative data.* London: Sage.

Sobal, J., & Nelson, M.K. (2003). Commensal eating patterns: A community study. *Appetite, 41*, 181–90.

Statistics Canada. (2008, 2 December). *Agriculture-population linkage data for the 2006 census.* Retrieved from http://www.statcan.gc.ca/ca-ra2006/agpop/article-eng.htm.

Van Esterik, P. (1999). Gender and sustainable food systems: A feminist critique. In M. Koc (Ed.), *For hunger-proof cities: Sustainable urban food systems* (pp. 157–61). Ottawa: IDRC Books.

Wansink, B. (2006). Nutritional gatekeepers and the 72% solution. *Journal of the American Dietetic Association, 106*, 1324–7.

Whitehead, T.L. (1984). Food habits in a southern community. In M. Douglas (Ed.), *Food in the social order* (pp. 97–142). New York: Russell Sage Foundation.

World Health Organization. (2012). *Nutrition.* Retrieved from http://www.who.int/topics/nutrition/en/.

7 The Multiple Dimensions of Health: Weaving Together Food Sustainability and Farm Women's Health

Wendee Kubik and Amber Fletcher

The long-term sustainability of wholesome food, along with its clear links to health, are becoming issues of global concern. In the current context of increasingly commercial agriculture and rapid climate change, food sustainability and food security issues are putting Canadians at a strategic crossroads in their food production decisions. In Canada, farm women hold the key to a healthier and more sustainable food system; however, their livelihoods and health are being jeopardized by the very system that threatens food sustainability and food security around the world. With the dire predictions about the effects of climate change and the resulting consequences for food security[1] and sustainability, there is a need to expand our vision towards the production of food, taking into consideration the human side of agriculture.

This chapter weaves together the seemingly diverse issues of climate change, commercialized agriculture, food production, and farm women's health in order to examine how each is linked to the overarching concern about health. We argue that large-scale commercial agriculture poses a threat to environmental stability and thus to long-term food sustainability and security, while the family farm holds the key to a more secure and environmentally accountable system of food production; and we examine how commercial agriculture affects the livelihood of family farmers on the Canadian prairies.

Close examination of the family farm dynamic reveals that farm women are now ensuring the farm's survival with their labour, both on and off the farm. This means that the survival of the family farm – which, we argue, is the key to a healthier, more sustainable and secure food supply – is dependent on the increasing flexibility of farm women's labour capacity. However, the situation has dire consequences for

Canadian farm women's health. As a result of this increased pressure, farm women experience high levels of stress and long-term health problems, as well as facing issues of health care access and balance between work and home life.

Working at a broad theoretical level, this chapter posits the possibility of a linkage between the family farm crisis and the increased presence of large-scale commercial agriculture on the Canadian prairies. Furthermore, we point to the family farm as a more environmentally sustainable and secure system of food production. The focus on health is twofold: at the macro level, concern over food security and sustainability, particularly in the face of impending climate change, suggests a looming global health threat; at the micro level, the survival of the family farm – as a more sustainable provider of healthy food – assumes the infinite elasticity of farm women's work, leading to high levels of stress-related illness in farm women. The most sustainable method of food production hinges on the contributions of farm women; therefore, we promote measures to enable farm women to stay on the farm without the continued exploitation of their labour.

The Changing Context of Food Production

Climate Change and Agriculture

Rapid changes in the Canadian climate are becoming increasingly evident, with higher overall temperatures and weather extremes becoming more common. Temperature records show a consistent upward trend in temperature across the Prairies, with an overall temperature increase of 1.6 degrees Celsius since 1895, and particularly dramatic increases since the 1970s (Sauchyn & Kulshreshtha, 2008). These heightened temperatures have led to climate-change projection scenarios that emphasize the risk of moisture deficit and drought on the Prairies (Sauchyn & Kulshreshtha, 2008; Watson, Zinyowera, & Moss, 1997). Importantly, such changes can have dramatic effects on soil quality. The Intergovernmental Panel on Climate Change (IPCC) definitively stated that 'loss of organic soil matter, leaching of soil nutrients, salinization, and erosion are likely consequences of climate change' (Watson et al., 1997, 8.3.4). Such changes can dramatically affect agricultural output in the short term as well as agricultural sustainability in the long term.

Along with these scenarios, a rise in global extreme precipitation events has been predicted (Kharin & Zwiers, 2000), suggesting an increased possibility of flooding and other precipitation-related threats to agricultural production (Sauchyn & Kulshreshtha, 2008). For agriculture, additional consequences of climate change include 'variations in conditions such as length of growing season, timing of frosts, [and] heat accumulation' (Wall, Smit, & Wandel, 2004, p. 1). Such changes to temperature and growing season allow for increased survival and reproductive rates of pests and insects, and increases in associated diseases in livestock. Diseases previously considered rare (e.g., West Nile virus) are becoming increasingly common.

Since the Prairies contain more than 80% of the agricultural land in Canada (Sauchyn & Kulshreshtha, 2008), the potential risks of climate change to the Prairies could pose a significant challenge to the country's food production system. Mitigation and adaptation have been promoted as complementary strategies to cope with climate change (Lemmen, Warren, Bush, & Lacroix, 2008). Increases to a system's adaptive capacity, or its ability to cope with climate change, can play a key role in the process of adaptation (IPCC, 2008).

Although the building of adaptive capacity involves technological and infrastructural investments, experts have recognized the importance of social elements of adaptive capacity, such as equity and community networks (Adger, 2003; Sauchyn & Kulshreshtha, 2008; Warren & Egginton, 2008). Wolfgang Sachs (1999) also emphasized the necessity of a shift in human thinking and values in the face of impending climate change; indeed, Lemmen and colleagues (2008) argued that 'adaptation involves making adjustments in our decisions, activities and thinking because of observed or expected changes in climate' (p. 4).

The Cost of Large-Scale Commercial Farming

It can be argued that large-scale commercial agriculture works against the mitigation of, and adaptation to, climate change. Thus, it poses a risk to the long-term sustainability and security of our food supply. Commercial farms are often defined in opposition to the family farm, because in a commercial farm 'the operator is engaged in less of the ownership, management, risk and/or reward of the farming operation even though farm operators and their families continue to provide the labour to the agricultural production operation' (Furtan, 2006, p. 10). This is because, in commercial farming, integrator companies often contract the labour of farmers and direct the process of production (Furtan, 2006).

Factory farms, also known as Intensive Livestock Operations (ILOs), are a product of the commercial agricultural presence. Industrial-scale hog barns have become a familiar scene – as well as a cause of controversy – in many Prairie communities. Large-scale commercial facilities have been linked to a number of environmental problems, from air pollution and odour issues (Paton, 2003), to the build-up of manure cesspools (Norberg-Hodge, Merrifield, & Gorelick, 2002). Slurry from industrial hog facilities is typically disposed of by spreading it upon the land; however, due to the total amounts of slurry and its high concentrations of methane and nitrogen, it can negatively affect soil fertility (Ervin, Holtslander, Qualman, & Sawa, 2003). Furthermore, off-gassing from manure pools emits high levels of these gases into the air, which then act as agents of global warming (Ervin et al., 2003). For these reasons commercial farming has been criticized for its negative environmental impacts. Indeed, in their analysis of climate change, Sauchyn and Kulshreshtha (2008) suggested that human impacts on soil quality are affected by the rising influence of multinational corporations in the agricultural production sector (p. 295).

The increased presence of vertically integrated commercial operations has been enabled by neoliberal trade policies (Barry, 1995; Desmarais, 2007). Global trade liberalization, enabled by such agreements as the World Trade Organization (WTO) Agreement on Agriculture and the North American Free Trade Agreement (NAFTA), has meant that domestic producers are increasingly unable to compete with low-cost imported products – some of which are produced, processed, and marketed by a single multinational corporation. Family farmers are often unable to compete with integrated corporations because the 'balance of market power determines the distribution of profits within the agri-food production chain' (National Farmers Union, as cited in Desmarais, 2007, p. 63). Corporate dominance of the global food system means that family farmers must exponentially increase the size of their operations just to compete, or else they are forced to leave agriculture altogether (Desmarais, 2007).

The driving out of local producers has negative consequences for food security. Many countries no longer produce enough food domestically to ensure their own food security (Barry, 1995). Paradoxically, farmers are being forced to stop producing when, for six of the past seven years, we as a global society have consumed more grain than was produced (Qualman, 2007). Despite the demand, agricultural commodity prices have remained low, a fact that is reflected in farmers' financial statements. In Canada, only 55.8% of all farms reported gross farm receipts greater than, or equal to, their total operating expenses, while 44.2% fell into debt (Statistics Canada, 2009a). Of those farms experiencing the greatest financial instability, the majority are small- to medium-sized family farms. Indeed, in 2006, approximately 70% of small farms reported that their total expenses were greater than their total income (Statistics Canada, 2009a). Meanwhile, the largest commercial farms – those with over one million dollars in annual revenue – continue to thrive.

In his analysis of the prairie hog sector, Qualman (2001) offered an explanation for continued low commodity prices, attributing them to the increased presence of vertically integrated agricultural corporations. He explained that such corporations are less dependent than family farms on earning a rate of profit from the production sector. Rather, low commodity prices can, in fact, be beneficial for integrated corporations. Qualman argued that 'low prices allow [corporations] to take their profits in their packing plants and to secure additional hog supplies from independent producers at low cost' (p. 26). The immense size and market power of corporate operations, as well as their ability to undercut family operations, explains why large-scale farms currently receive 40% of total farm income in Canada, despite comprising only 2.6% of all farms in the country (Statistics Canada, 2009a).

Because commercial farming poses a threat to the survival of family farms, it can be argued that commercial farms also harm the social structure of rural communities (Lobao & Stofferahn, 2008). Indeed, Lind (1995) argued that there is a 'strong connection' between 'the sustainability of farm families and the sustainability of rural communities,' and that the problems faced by family farms have implications for the survival of nearby communities (p. 25). This can be seen in the fact that family farmers tend to support their local businesses, whereas corporate operations can often obtain low-cost inputs as part of an integrated corporation or from other corporate affiliations. When local businesses close for lack of patronage, the economy of rural communities is damaged, and the remaining family farmers are forced to travel farther for the products they require. When rural economies are thus diminished, small communities are no longer able to sustain themselves – residents leave, hospitals are closed, and schools shut down. Such changes make rural and agricultural life an impossibility, with fewer people wanting to live in or around rural communities. To cite just one example, in the following chapter Dabrowska and Wismer note the importance that strong community support has for the well-being of the Old Order of Mennonite Women.

Sustaining the Family Farm: Labour and the Farm Family

The continued presence of small- and medium-sized family farms, despite the challenges they face, suggests an important question: why do many family farmers continue farming when faced with such an uncertain future, stress, ongoing crises, low returns and high input costs, and eroding rural infrastructures (among other considerations)? In a qualitative and quantitative Canadian study of farm women conducted in 2002, numerous farm women talked about why they wanted to remain in farming despite the many difficulties they were facing (Kubik, 2004). Several women mentioned that, in spite of the stress, they loved the lifestyle of farming. They cherished the close-knit community support and believed it was one of the best places to raise children.

When discussing viability, however, one farm woman expressed her concern:

> I've come to look at farming as a great lifestyle but an impossible way to make a living. I'm thankful that we could raise our children on the farm. The values and work ethics they have learned are invaluable to them no matter what their future lives hold. However, had we kept trying to make our living by farming alone, I think the stress would far outweigh any benefits...It's been one 'crisis' after another from the time we started – 25 years ago – so we decided we would farm because we love to farm but we would work elsewhere to support our family and our lifestyle. (interview with W. Kubik, 2004).

Considering that the number of farm families has been steadily declining over the decades, the farmers who remain are economically able to finance their businesses, or they are farmers because they want to be and they supplement their farm production by other means.

One of the major ways farmers stay on the land is by supporting the farm and supplementing their agricultural income with off-farm work. Women make a major contribution to this off-farm work. Statistics Canada (2009b) reported that more farmers were working off the farm in 2006 than five years ago; nearly half (48.4%) of all farm operators reported an off-farm job or business, compared with 44.5% in 2001. Furthermore, in 2006, for the first time, the percentage of female operators who had off-farm work reached one-half (50.4%), in comparison to the 47.6% of male operators who had off-farm work (Statistics Canada 2009b).

Over the past twenty-five years, the many contributions farm women make to their farms and farming communities has begun to be analysed. Martz and Brueckner (2003) noted that 'the number of women who engage in farm field work tasks on a regular basis has increased by an average of 12 percent while the number engaged in farm management tasks on a regular basis has increased by 22 per cent from 1982 to 2001–2002' (p. 30). Farm women often perform the majority of bookkeeping for the farming operation (Alston, 2006; interview with A. Fletcher, 2011).The majority of household and care-giving work is still done by farm women (Kubik, 2005, p. 87; Morris & Little, 2005, p. 24; Roppel, Desmarais, & Martz, 2006, p. 24), even when they hold off-farm jobs. Because of the work done by these 'super women' (Kemp, 1999), they play a pivotal role in sustaining farm production and may hold the long-term key to healthy, secure, and sustainable food production in Canada.

The question of whether family farming provides a more progressive and sustainable approach to agriculture and food production than does corporate farming requires further systematic research and analysis. Although the discourse of 'farming as a business' is in the ascendancy in many quarters, the family farm is a business like no other. Harriet Friedmann (1978, 1986) is among the scholars who have noted distinct differences. She suggested that family farmers, unlike capitalist enterprises, do not have to make a profit to stay in business, nor do they consistently make production decisions based on necessity to earn average rate of profit. The decision to remain farming, despite profit shortages, is largely a product of lifestyle choices and a preference for farm life (Kubik, 2004).

Among the survival tactics farmers employ to stay in business is the reduction of household consumption rates to subsistence levels, in order to sustain the farm business. Friedmann (1978) also noted the capacity for self-exploitation through longer working hours and the participation of more and more family members in farm production. This tendency is particularly pertinent considering the recent pressure for farmers to expand their operations in order to compete with large-scale agri-business. As noted, many stay in business by supplementing farm income with off-farm income. In addition, family farmers seem prepared not just to forgo making a profit, but to accumulate debts beyond normal definitions of business viability. Very few if any other businesses continue to operate with ever-increasing debt loads in order to continue the business, a business that is clearly more like a vocation.

Family Farmers and Environmental Sustainability

This unique commitment to farming is part of a commitment to the larger community in which the farming activity occurs and to which family members belong. Because family farmers are also members of their local and regional community, they generally have a vested interest in the local environment and the processes via which that community responds and adapts to climate change. Environmental stewardship and a focus on sustainability are more likely to be significant values for those less driven by the bottom line.

For example, in Lind's (1995) study, most farmers expressed concern about climate change. Many had incorporated some form of environmental strategy into their operation, such as tree planting. Although family farmers felt that they had high stakes in environmental farming practices, many have found themselves forced to engage in environmentally damaging practices (e.g., using large amounts of chemicals to reduce tillage and increase production) in order to 'compete' in the corporate-dominated marketplace. Lind aptly argued that farmers must be able to afford to engage in conservation measures, which is clearly made difficult by the current system of agricultural economics. It is important to note, then, that the family farm is not an inherently unsustainable form of food production. Farmers possess the awareness of, and desire to participate in, sustainable practices. Brophy, Keith, Watterson, Gilbertson, and Beck in chapter 5 document the harmful consequences that exposure to pesticides has had, particularly for farm women. In addition, from a gendered perspective, Carolyn Sachs (2006) noted that women farmers are more likely than other producers to use sustainable agricultural practices and are less likely to use pesticides, chemical fertilizers, genetically modified seeds, and animal growth hormones.

Another factor that drives family farmers' environmental awareness is the emphasis on intergenerational transmittance of land. However unrealistic it may be, considering the recent exodus of young people from rural areas (Diaz, 2003), many farmers want to bequeath their land to their heirs. To such farmers, ensuring the long-term environmental sustainability of the land is of central importance. For other family farmers, the long-term profitability of the land is a consideration in planning for for resale value upon retirement. Because environmental stewardship can require 'practices that are sustainable in the long-run but not profitable in the short-run,' family farmers are more likely than corporate farm operators to undertake such environmental practices, as the profits will be captured in the price of the land (Furtan, 2006, p. 13). Overall, then, the family farm is at the centre of a 'triple bottom-line' that ranks community and environment as motivations alongside profits.

The many challenges that farm families face today are not individual producer problems; they are linked to the economic, environmental, social, and political structures that we as a society have created. This means that as a society and political force we can change and restructure our food system. Indeed, as already noted, climate change experts predict that the key to survival is adaptation. Farmers want to be able to produce healthy food, and they want to make a viable living doing so. For the past number of years the only way they can do so is by working long hours, both on and off the farm, in order to subsidize their farms. Most farm women and men want to stay on the farm because they enjoy the satisfaction of producing healthy food, enjoy the lifestyle, and believe it is a good place to raise children (Kubik, 2004).

The Contributions and Roles of Farm Women in Canadian Agriculture

Farm women's labour is structured by a particular gender ideology, which shapes their forms of self-identification, their labour roles, and also the social and political recognition of their labour. Lynn McIntyre and Krista Rondeau in chapter 6 note that farmwomen are primarily responsible for the complex activities of food provision. Farm women remain overwhelmingly responsible for childcare and household tasks (Kubik, 2005; Roppel et al., 2006; Shaver, 1996; Statistics Canada, 1999), yet they also perform a substantial portion of the on-farm work.

Added to this is a discourse of family farming that overshadows the increased workloads that burden farm women (Brandth, 2002). Work roles are delineated along traditional gender lines, but gendered expectations have expanded for farm women, adding on-farm and off-farm work to existing expectations in the home and community. Women are increasingly called upon as a source of family farm labour, and their off-farm labour provides the income necessary for many families to remain in farming (Kubik & Moore, 2005). Farm women often do not get credit or even acknowledgment for their work on the farm (Prince Edward Island Advisory Council on the Status of Women, 2003; Shortall, 1999).

This invisibility of work that farm women do, and the lack of recognition for their many contributions, ultimately enables the representation of farm women as second-class citizens in the countryside. This has consequences for the way women view themselves and their contributions. Lack of recognition has costs in terms of stress for the women themselves and in the larger political arena, for example, through the lack of public policy and government services focused on farm women. Farm women's labour is essential for the survival of the family farm and, by connection, for long-term sustainable food production; however, their contributions to food production systems often remain overlooked and unacknowledged.

Acknowledging farm women's contributions means understanding how their lives differ from those of urban women and farm men. In terms of work, farm women often face the triple responsibility of farm labour, off-farm waged labour, and domestic labour and caregiving work. Women's on-farm work is often invisible due to conservative attitudes about men's and women's work (e.g., ideology of farming as men's work despite women's increasing participation). Stress can be exacerbated by a lack of social support in rural areas; many rural areas lack childcare and sufficient eldercare services (Kubik, 1996). In addition, farm women's stress often results from a lack of agency and control over resources (i.e., financial and environmental). They also face differential susceptibility and exposure to gendered risks such as sexual or domestic violence, due to their increased isolation. In rural areas, women often have little or no access to resources such as women's shelters.

Despite these specific concerns, Canada currently has very few policies or programs specifically geared towards farm women. A spate of federal agriculture programs that focused on farm women were created throughout the 1980s: the Farm Women's Information Initiative in 1985, the Canadian Farm Women's Education Council in 1987, and the Farm Women's Advancement Program in 1988. In 1981 the Farm Women's Bureau – whose mandate included consultations with farm women's organizations as part of the policy-making process – was established as a unit within the federal Department of Agriculture. Unfortunately, these programs were eliminated throughout the 1990s, with 2003 marking the elimination of the Farm Women's Bureau as a distinct entity within the Department of Agriculture. Policy makers' lack of attention to farm women's health means continued consequences for the health and well-being of those women, particularly given the increased pressure on farm women's labour capacity in an increasingly corporate-dominated agricultural environment.

Farm Women, Stress, and Health

For Canadian farm families it is increasingly difficult to achieve a quality of life and health comparable to those enjoyed by urban residents (Romanow, 2002). In some provinces, hospital closures and health care cutbacks in agricultural communities have meant that women often engage in increased care-giving work to compensate for these cutbacks. Indeed, Luxton (2007) noted that neoliberal policy decisions often have gendered consequences, as when governmental responsibility for caring services is offloaded.

In rural areas, the presence of a strong gender ideology that emphasizes women's primary responsibility for care-giving and domestic labour means that women are more likely to assume care-giving responsibilities in the face of this offloading (Alston, 2006; Kubik & Moore, 2003). Because the rural population is, on average, older than the general Canadian population (Crosato & Leipert, 2006), health care restructuring has placed added responsibility for eldercare squarely on the shoulders of rural women (Jaffe & Blakley, 2000). The lack of formal support systems for caregivers in rural areas can contribute to poor health in rural caregivers, particularly in terms of caregiver stress and burnout (Jaffe & Blakley, 2000; Crosato & Leipert, 2006).

For farm women, this care-giving work is increasingly undertaken in combination with paid labour to support the family farm. A 1996 study illustrated that 60% of rural caregivers also engaged in paid labour away from home (Keefe, 1997). Bedard, Koivuranta, and Stuckey (2004) found that 35% of rural caregivers were employed full time, as opposed to 6% of their urban counterparts. These trends allow us to postulate a *triple day* for farm women specifically. In addition to increasing care-giving responsibilities (which usually require time-consuming and expensive travel away from the farm), farm women are also working both on- and off-farm at significantly higher rates. As mentioned above, this increased on- and off-farm labour is often the key to sustaining the family farm in an atmosphere that is increasingly dominated by agribusiness corporations. However, sustaining the farm often comes at a cost to farm women's health and well-being.

In a similar vein, yet another major source of stress for farm women lies in coping with their families' stress. Alston's (2006) research on drought and farm women in Australia exposed the specifically gendered effects of agricultural stress on the health of farm women. Alston noted:

> Women...tend to focus on their roles on and off the farm, and report a constant monitoring of the health of family members. They are deeply affected by their inability to change the deteriorating circumstances around them. As a consequence of this monitoring, they tend to prioritize their own needs and health as a very low priority. A constant theme in their conversations is the need to keep going for everyone else's sake. (p. 175)

In their study of 657 farm women, Carruth and Logan (2002) argue that a multitude of responsibilities, environmental and social influences, and stressors place farm women at high risk for depressive symptoms. A great deal of stress for farm women comes from balancing farm and home responsibilities, increased off-farm work, and concern for family members (Gerrard & Russell, 2000; Kubik & Moore, 2005). An increase in the availability of public supports – such as investments in rural childcare, eldercare, and health care services – could ameliorate some of this stress; furthermore, it would enable, and indeed encourage, more women to see farming as a viable opportunity.

Conclusion: Refocusing on Sustainability and Health

In this chapter, we have illustrated several key linkages between seemingly disparate phenomena: climate change, food sustainability, family farming, and the health of farm women in Canada. These phenomena exist at various scales of analysis, from the macro-level threat of global climate change to the health of farm women at the micro level of lived experience. Climate change projections indicate future challenges for the agricultural sector, such as increased drought and other extreme weather events, and it is thus necessary to refocus on the most sustainable systems of food production. Such systems are not found in large-scale commercial production, which have negative implications for both environmental and rural sustainability. Corporate farms are responsible to their shareholders when faced with unprofitable scenarios, and are able to leave such circumstances with relative ease.

In contrast, family farmers hold a long-term interest in the sustainability of their land, and are often willing to engage in environmental practices if they are empowered to do so (Lind, 1995). Currently, farm women experience high levels of stress and associated health consequences as they attempt to support their farms, families, and communities. It is necessary to establish supports that enable families to remain in farming, particularly during times of drought and extreme weather. Such supports must be designed with the full inclusion of farm women, who are currently overlooked in agricultural policy-making processes (Roppel et al., 2006). In addition, attention must be paid to gender-specific support services, such as childcare and eldercare programming in rural areas (Jaffe & Blakley, 2000). Adaptation to climate change involves more than simply physical infrastructure. It involves changes to our ways of thinking about, and interacting with, the physical environment (Lemmen et al., 2008; Sachs, 1999). Adaptation requires a shift in focus towards more sustainable food systems and, indeed, towards sustaining those who will continue to produce our food in the future.

Notes

1   The definition of food security put forth by the Food and Agriculture Organization (FAO) of the United Nations states, 'Food security exists when all people, at all times, have physical and economic access to sufficient, safe and nutritious food that meets their dietary needs and food preferences for an active and healthy life' (World Food Summit, 1996, as cited in FAO, 2006).There are four elements of food security:food availability, food access, utilization, and stability. For the purposes of this paper, we draw attention to the element of stability, which emphasizes that 'to be food secure, a population, household or individual must have access to adequate food at all times. They should not risk losing access to food as a consequence of sudden shocks (e.g. an economic or climatic crisis) or cyclical events (e.g. seasonal food insecurity) (FAO, 2006). We argue that increased corporatization of agriculture, and the associated decline of local family farm systems, increase the risk of food insecurity over the long term through their degenerative effects on environmental and social sustainability.

References

Adger, W.N. (2003). Social aspects of adaptive capacity. In J. Smith, R. Klein, & S. Huq (Eds.), *Climate change, adaptive capacity and development* (pp. 29–49). London: Imperial College Press.

Alston, M. (2006). The gendered impact of drought in rural gender relations. In B. Bock &Shortall, S. (Eds.), *Rural gender relations: Issues and case studies* (pp. 165–80). Wallingford, UK: CABI.

Barry, T. (1995). *Zapata's revenge: Free trade and the farm crisis in Mexico.* Boston: South End Press.

Bedard, M., Koivuranta A., & Stuckey, A. (2004). Health impact on caregivers of providing informal care to a cognitively impaired older adult: Rural versus urban settings. *Canadian Journal of Rural Medicine, 9*(1),15–23.

Brandth, B. (2002). On the relationship between feminism and farm women. *Agriculture and Human Values, 19*(2), 107–17.

Carruth, A., & Logan, C. (2002). Depressive symptoms in farm women: Effects of health status and farming lifestyle characteristics, behaviours and beliefs. *Journal of Community Health, 27*(3), 213–28.

Crosato, K.E., & Leipert, B. (2006). Rural women caregivers in Canada. *Rural and Remote Health, 6,* 520. Retrieved from http://www.rrh.org.au/articles/showarticlenew.asp?ArticleID=520.

Desmarais, A., (2007). *La Via Campesina: Globalization and the power of peasants.* Halifax: Fernwood.

Diaz, H.P. (2003). School, knowledge and skills in the farm community. In H.P. Diaz, J. Jaffe, & R. Stirling (Eds.), *Farm communities at the crossroads: Challenge and resistance* (pp. 91–106). Regina: Canadian Plains Research Center.

Ervin, A.M., Holtslander, C., Qualman, D., & Sawa, R. (Eds.). (2003). *Beyond factory farming: Corporate hog barns and the threat to public health, the environment, and rural communities. Proceedings of the 2ⁿᵈ Annual National Conference on Intensive Livestock Operations, Saskatoon, 9 November 2002.* Saskatoon: Canadian Centre for Policy Alternatives.

Food and Agriculture Organization (FAO) of the United Nations. (2006). *Food security.* Retrieved from ftp://ftp.fao.org/es/ESA/policybriefs/pb_02.pdf.

Friedmann, H. (1978). Simple commodity production and wage labour in the American plains. *Journal of Peasant Studies, 6*(1), 71–100.

Friedmann, H. (1986). Patriarchy and property: A reply to Goodman & Redclift. *Sociologa Ruralis, 26*(2), 186–93.

Furtan, H. (2006). *The need for direction: The Canadian grains sector at a crossroads.* Saskatoon: Knowledge Impact in Society Publications.

Gerrard, N., & Russell, G. (2000). *An exploration of health-related impacts of the erosion of agriculturally focused support programs for farm women in Saskatchewan.* Regina: Prairie Women's Health Centre of Excellence.

Intergovernmental Panel on Climate Change (IPCC). (2008). Summary for policy makers. In M.L. Parry, O.F. Canziani, J.P. Palutikof, P.J. van der Linden, & C.E. Hanson (Eds.), *Climate change 2007: Impacts, adaptation and vulnerability. Contribution of Working Group 11 to the Fourth Assessment Report of the Intergovernmental Panel on Climate Change* (pp. 7–22). Cambridge: Cambridge University Press. Retrieved from http://www.ipcc .ch/pdf/assessment-report/ar4/wg2/ar4-wg2-spm.pdf.

Jaffe, J., & Blakley, B. (2000). *Coping as a rural caregiver: The impact of health care reforms on rural women informal caregivers.* Regina: Prairie Women's Health Centre of Excellence.

Keefe, J. (1997). The likelihood of combining employment and helping elderly kin in rural and urban areas among Canadian regions. *Canadian Journal of Regional Science, 20,* 367–87.

Kemp, L. (1999). For farm women, agriculture is just the beginning. *Canadian Agriculture at a Glance 1999.* Ottawa: Statistics Canada. Retrieved from http://www.statcan.ca/bsolc/english/bsolc?catno=96-325-X19960014840.

Kharin, V., & Zwiers, F. (2000). Changes in the extremes in an ensemble of transient climate simulations with a coupled-atmosphere-ocean CGM. *Journal of Climate, 13,* 3760–88.

Kubik, W. (1996). The study of farm stress and coping: A critical evaluation. Master's thesis, University of Regina.

Kubik, W. (2004). The changing roles of farm women and the consequences for their health, well being, and quality of life. Doctoral diss., University of Regina.

Kubik, W. (2005). Farm women: The hidden subsidy in our food. *Canadian Woman Studies, 24*(4), 85–90.

Kubik, W., & Moore, R. (2003). Changing roles of Saskatchewan farm women: Qualitative and quantitative perspectives. In R. Blake & A. Nurse (Eds.),*The trajectories of rural life: New perspectives on rural Canada* (pp. 25–36). Regina: Canadian Plains Research Center.

Kubik, W., & Moore, R. (2005). Health and well-being of farm women: Contradictory roles in the contemporary economy. *Journal of Agricultural Safety and Health, 11*(2), 249–56.

Lemmen, D., Warren, F., Bush, E., & Lacroix, J. (Eds.). (2008). *From impacts to adaptation: Canada in a changing climate 2007.* Ottawa: Government of Canada. Retrieved from http://adaptation.nrcan.gc.ca/assess/2007/ index_e.php.

Lind, C. (1995). *Something's wrong somewhere: Globalization, community and the moral economy of the farm crisis*. Halifax: Fernwood.

Lobao, L., & Stofferahn, C.W. (2008). The community effects of industrialized farming: Social science research and challenges to corporate farming laws. *Agriculture and Human Values, 25,* 219–40.

Luxton, M. (2007). Family responsibilities: The politics of love and care. In L. Lucas (Ed.), *Unpacking globalization: Markets, gender, and work* (pp.131–44). Lanham, MD: Lexington.

Martz, D., & Brueckner, I. (2003). *The Canadian farm family at work: Exploring gender and generation.* Muenster, SK: Centre for Rural Studies and Enrichment. Retrieved from http://www.nfu.ca/epff/documents/The_ Canadian_Farm_Family_at_Work.pdf.

Morris, C., & Little, J. (2005).Rural work: An overview of women's experiences. In J. Little & C. Morris (Eds.), *Critical studies in rural gender issues* (pp. 9–26). Aldershot, UK: Athenaeum Press.

Norberg-Hodge, H., Merrifield, T., & Gorelick, S. (2002). *Bringing the food economy home: Local alternatives to global agribusiness.* Halifax: Fernwood.

Paton, B. (2003). The smell of intensive pig production on the Canadian prairies. In A.M. Ervin, C. Holtslander, D. Qualman, & R. Sawa (Eds.), *Beyond factory farming: Corporate hog barns and the threat to public health, the environment, and rural communities. Proceedings of the 2nd Annual National Conference on Intensive Livestock Operations, Saskatoon, 9 November 2002* (pp. 79–109). Saskatoon: Canadian Centre for Policy Alternatives.

Prince Edward Island Advisory Council on the Status of Women. (2003). *Policy guide: Women and unpaid work.* Charlottetown: Author.

Qualman, D. (2007). Peak food: The growing challenge of feeding civilization. *Briarpatch, 31*(1), 16–19.

Qualman, D. (2001). Corporate hog farming: The view from the family farm. In R. Epp & D. Whitson (Eds.), *Writing off the rural West: Globalization, governments, and the transformation of rural communities* (pp. 21–38). Edmonton: University of Alberta Press.

Romanow, R. (2002). *Building on values: The future of health care in Canada.* Ottawa: Government of Canada.

Roppel, C., Desmarais, A., & Martz, D. (2006). *Farm women and Canadian agricultural policy.* Ottawa: Status of Women Canada.

Sachs, C. (2006). Rural women and the environment. In B. Bock & S. Shortall (Eds.), *Rural gender relations: Issues and case studies* (pp. 288–302). Cambridge, MA: CABI.

Sachs, W. (1999). *Planet dialectics: Explorations in environment and development.* London: Zed Books.

Sauchyn, D., & Kulshreshtha, S. (2008). Prairies. In D. Lemmen, F. Warren, E. Bush, & J. Lacroix (Eds.), *From impacts to adaptation: Canada in a changing climate 2007* (pp. 275–328). Ottawa: Government of Canada.

Shaver, F. (Ed.). (1996). *Women in agriculture*. Canadian Rural Restructuring Foundation, ARRG Working Papers Series, no. 8. Brandon, MB: Brandon University.

Shortall, S. (1999). *Women and farming: Property and power*. Houndmills, UK: Palgrave Macmillan.

Statistics Canada. (1999). *National population health survey (Cycle 3)*. Ottawa: Statistics Canada, Health Statistics Division.

Statistics Canada. (2009a). *The financial picture of farms in Canada*. 2006 Census of Agriculture Highlights and Analyses. Ottawa: Statistics Canada. Retrieved from http://www.statcan.gc.ca/ca-ra2006/articles/finpicture-portrait-eng.htm.

Statistics Canada. (2009b). *Snapshot of Canadian agriculture*. 2006 Census of Agriculture Highlights and Analyses. Ottawa: Statistics Canada. Retrieved from http://www.statcan.gc.ca/ca-ra2006/articles/snapshot-portrait-eng.htm.

Wall, E., Smit, B., & Wandel, J. (2004). *Canadian agri-food sector adaptation to risks and opportunities from climate change*. A position paper. Guelph, ON: C-CIARN Agriculture, University of Guelph.

Warren, F.J., & Egginton, P. (2008). Chapter 2: Background information: Concepts, overviews and approaches. In D. Lemmen, F. Warren, E. Bush, & J. Lacroix (Eds.), *From impacts to adaptation: Canada in a changing climate 2007* (pp. 27–56). Ottawa: Government of Canada.

Watson, R.T., Zinyowera, M.C., & Moss, R.H. (1997). *The regional impacts of climate change: An assessment of vulnerability*. A special report of IPCC Working Group II. Paris: WMO/UNEP.

8 Outside Assumptions: Research with the Old Order Mennonite Women in Ontario – An Exploratory Study

Ewa M. Dabrowska and Susan K. Wismer

Romantic visions of the healthy pastoral life have more recently had to take into account the reality that many rural communities face serious problems related to air, soil, and groundwater contamination (see Brophy et al., chapter 5). This chapter examines how Old Order Mennonite (OOM) women in one Ontario community see environmental risk in the context of their orthodox religious beliefs, their agricultural way of life, and the health of their families. Our exploratory research demonstrates that health effects related to environmental risks are experienced and understood contextually and are not clear cut. Results of our study call for varied understanding of health and of health promotion, taking into account diverse realities. This chapter also raises some interesting questions regarding feminist research. Engaging respectfully and effectively with our participants required us to set aside a number of assumptions about method and about what it means to create opportunities for the voices of women to be heard and valued.

Background

Our study site, surrounding the town of Elmira in the Ontario Township of Woolwich, is one where local aquifers have been heavily polluted with contaminants, including cancer-causing N-nitroso-dimethlamine (NDMA), such that in 1989 the Ontario Ministry of Environment permanently shut down the town's wells (Conestoga-Rovers & Associates, 2003). Elmira's industrial history includes manufacture of highly toxic pesticides and herbicides. Hazardous wastes from the industrial site percolated into the soil and aquifers as well as into the surface water of Canagagigue Creek, the town's main body of water. High concentrations of dioxin, DDT, and other toxic carcinogenic compounds have been found in sediments along the Canagagigue Creek. Farming families living along the creek have been exposed to chemical waste products for more than half a century. In 2003, the potential health effects of contamination of the Canagagigue Creek flood plain were analysed in a Human Health Risk Assessment; findings indicated that residents downstream from the plant faced a much greater risk of developing cancer than other Canadians (Conestoga-Rovers & Associates, 2003).

The primary focus of remediation work along the creek since then has been to cut off sources of contamination and prevent soil erosion in order to decrease dioxin concentrations on the farms located downstream from the chemical plant (S. Bryant, personal communication, 15 October 2004). In 2005, residents along the creek were advised to fence off the flood plain and creek to reduce exposure to accumulated toxins. Residents included OOM farm families living very close to the polluted creek. This research project was the first study to examine health effects in the Elmira area as experienced and reported by OOM women.

Determinants of Rural Women's Health

In a recent study, Leipert and George (2008) analysed determinants of rural women's health in southwestern Ontario. That study describes the three key determinants of rural change, rural culture, and rural pride that have provided a useful general analytical frame for the research reported here. In that context, we have extended the definitions of the Leipert and George study to address the diverse perspective of a culturally distinct rural minority group, the conservative Anabaptist community of OOM women and their families farming along the Canagagigue Creek.

Rural change relates primarily to impacts of technological change, which may be positive or negative. In our study, for example, the relatively recent introduction of the household telephone has had a significant and largely positive impact on women's lives. In rural communities more generally, the costs of technological changes have significantly increased pressures on rural women to find off-farm employment, adversely affecting their families and increasing their reported stress levels. *Rural culture* refers to the enforcement of gendered roles of women. At least one previous study has noted that discrimination against women who do not adhere to wider rural community norms may adversely affect their health (Little, 2002). This was an issue of particular concern for this research, since we engaged OOM women in speaking for the first time to outside researchers, and was one reason for a two-year period of preparation for the study. *Rural pride* addresses women's pride in their capacity to raise their families with limited material resources and their strength in creating healthy local communities. Social networks and social support are essential to their well-being in rural communities (Leipert & George, 2008). In our study, rural pride, based on OOM beliefs and faith-based cultural values, was a key theme found in our interviews.

Other previously identified determinants affecting Canadian rural women's health include limited employment options and limited power; limited access to resources, education, and health care; negative attitudes towards rural women's roles; and lower social status expressed in the undervaluing of women's opinions and the silencing of their voices (Leipert & Reutter, 2005).

In Canada, health field studies of conservative Anabaptist communities are rare. Kulig and her colleagues completed research with Kanadier (Mexican) Mennonite women on the Canadian prairies (Kulig, Babcock, Wall, & Hill, 2006). They found for this non-homogeneous conservative Mennonite group that women's health-related behaviours varied with religious affiliation, differences in interpretation of the Bible, community rules, and personal preferences. Their study suggests that health programs based on assessments of health determinants need to take into account epistemic differences among researchers and participants in order to arrive at nuanced and respectful understandings of cultural difference.

Bennett (2003), who worked collaboratively with the conservative Anabaptist community in Ontario for several years, argues that 'the policy of the state to treat everyone the same has been oppressive to the Old Order Amish' (p. 158). From this perspective, the OOM community is a population vulnerable to adverse health effects because government and industrial decisions do not take into account OOM priorities regarding preserving their ethno-religious identity and maintaining separation from the multicultural rural society (Bennett, 2003). Analysis of issues of power in rural places is complex (Philo, 1992), and research concerning women's health among ethno-religious minority groups from already 'marginalized' rural places clearly requires a careful analysis of assumptions.

Old Order Mennonites

The OOM group has about fifty-eight hundred members divided into eighteen churches in northern Waterloo County (Peters, 2003). European ancestors of this Mennonite group fled religious persecution, migrating through Germany, Switzerland, Austria, and France and arriving in Pennsylvania in the 1700s. After the American Revolution, and in order to avoid military service, some Mennonites moved to new settlements in Upper Canada (Ontario), coming to the Waterloo area in the early 1800s. The Old Order Mennonite Church in Ontario was established as a distinct group in 1889 (Horst, 2000).

Each denomination of conservative Mennonite congregations has its own *Ordnung*, a book of rules, which functions to foster a God-pleasing life. Old Order Mennonites speak a High German dialect called Pennsylvania Deutsch (Peters, 2003). Their language helps them to maintain separation from the secular, largely English-speaking society that surrounds them. Horse and buggy transportation (see Figure 8.1), traditional clothing, and a legacy of Mennonite quilt-making and woodworking are some outward symbols of cultural identity.

Farming is integral to OOM values and traditions. Moral codes (*Gemeinschaft*) prioritize the needs of the community: 'Its members are prepared to give up individual rights and freedoms in favour of the collective good and the preservation of a faithful lifestyle' (Gingrich & Lightman, 2006, p. 186). Self-sufficiency is highly valued. They support their own schools and have negotiated with the Canadian and Ontario governments to be exempt from social insurance numbers, driver licensing, and registration with the Ontario Federation of Agriculture. OOMs do not use the Ontario Health Insurance Plan (OHIP), and they accept neither Canada Child Tax Benefits nor Old Age Security payments (Peters, 2003). These practices make them responsible for paying 100% of the cost of health care and other government-funded services.

Old Order Mennonites place stringent limits on the use of electricity and avoid use of technologies such as radio, TV, or the Internet. Telephones are permitted, but often are not used by church and community leaders (Gingrich & Lightman, 2006). OOMs communicate mainly through personal interactions and by traditional mail.

The OOM traditional patriarchal social order permeates every aspect of community life, dictating acceptable roles and behaviour for males and females of every age (Horst, 2000). OOM women have a religious

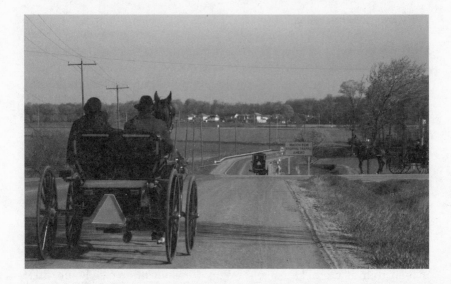

Figure 8.1 Old Order Mennonites travelling to the town of Elmira.
© Eva Dabrowska

obligation to be subordinate to their husbands, fathers, and brothers. This has a significant effect on their lives; for example, women are expected to be mostly silent in public settings (Epp, 2008). They do not read newspapers and they do not attend school beyond grade 8.

Methodology

Our study took place within this highly specific geographic and socio-cultural context in Ontario. After a two-year period of preparation and networking, access to the OOM community was granted with the help of two non-Mennonite women who had worked as community leaders in Elmira for more than fifteen years. These women introduced the primary researcher to an OOM 'cultural broker,' a man who had previously engaged with the outside world. The man's wife offered to serve as a gatekeeper and introduced the researcher to members of her community, arranging for the researcher to interview women living within close proximity to the Canagagigue Creek. As OOM women usually do not meet alone with outsiders, in all cases the wives followed a formal procedure of confirming arrangements for interviews with their spouses.

Interviews took place over a three-month period in 2005 and 2006. The study sample included fifteen OOM women, each living in the Township of Woolwich for all their lives. The women were 23 to 64 years of age, with the average age 49.7 years. Twelve women were married and three were single (never married). All women but one shared ownership of homes and family farms with husbands or sisters, and all had grade 8 education.

Participants were assured of anonymity and confidentiality throughout the research. Direct quotations used to illustrate key interview themes were chosen based on understandability to readers and maintaining anonymity, which was especially important because of the small sample size and the small number of farms located along the Canagagigue Creek. Questions, focusing on perceptions of health and environmental concerns, were prepared with the help of an OOM woman who assessed their appropriateness for her community. All participants completed a brief questionnaire providing demographic information and a history of major health episodes in their families. The survey also allowed women to express their opinions in writing, as one part of our research effort to address cultural constraints on open verbal expression for women.

Based on the three rural determinants of women's health (Leipert & George, 2008) that provided the theoretical framework for our study, our analysis explored understandings of health and health-environment relationships in the lives of the OOM women in our study.

Rural Culture

OOM women presented a theologically based understanding of health: 'Health is a gift from God.' Three women referred to the Bible as the primary source of knowledge. A younger woman explained that she has no worries about her health and health of her children: 'Our health is in the hands of God. I am not afraid for the health of new generations.'

All the women in our study stated that following their religion and traditions was an important aspect of taking responsibility for maintaining the health that is God's gift. One woman explained that taking care of her own health is her ongoing obligation: 'This is our responsibility to care about our health. We should eat healthy food and avoid obesity. We should care about our spiritual well-being.' One woman who has a chronic and disabling illness spent her days reading the

Bible, despite her problems with vision: 'I use this glass to read the Bible every day [She pointed to a large magnifying glass on string which was placed next to the Bible at the table]. My eyes are very bad. I always had very bad eyes.'

OOM women are educated in parochial schools. Teachers (single women only) are members of their community and also have just a grade 8 education. The curriculum in their parochial schools exclude secular and scientific knowledge, and OOM women do not learn much of what is taught about environmental issues in elementary schools in the rest of Canada. One woman explained that she did not understand issues of environmental pollution and the possibility of danger to her health: 'I do not know. I realize that I have never, ever studied it. I have to sort of look at things as they are.' Thus, the knowledge base of OOM women differs considerably from that of many other members of Canadian society.

The gender roles of women in this patriarchal community can be identified as a factor contributing to their vulnerability (Leipert & Reutter, 2005). A husband's evaluation of his wife's predetermined role in society influences her sense of well-being: 'My husband should an-swer the question how my health is. I had one kidney removed because of cancer five years ago. Now, I am fine.' One husband remarked: 'My wife is in good health, she works hard.'

OOM women reflected on their obligation to be obedient, accepting God's will. Two women explained how they accept God's will when children die, trusting that 'it will be better for them to be in heaven.' Three women, who reported multiple spontaneous abortions, did not question the reasons. Their obedience to God's will means that they do not need to search for scientific explanation or blame environmental impacts for their health concerns: 'Not everybody can have everything. I will have other children.' A mother of eight emphasized that her faith helps her in taking care of her children: 'Some of our children have dis-abilities, some are healthy. Health is a gift from God. We must accept it. We are providing for all our children's needs.'

Women are primary care givers for their families, caring for children, parents, and grandparents. Often a 'grandfather' house is built for ag-ing relatives, adjacent to the main farm house. It keeps the family to-gether, facilitating provision of care and support. OOM women in our study viewed births as making them 'a good member of the commu-nity.' We noticed that younger generations typically had fewer children (an average family in our sample had seven children, with a range from four to ten). All reported on their mothers' health by analysing health experiences with reference to identified roles:

My mother's health was quite good. She had fifteen of us and she is eighty-five now ... She had not time to teach us gardening, so we needed to learn ourselves ... She has now arthritis and rheumatic fewer.

My mother's health was not good. My mother had twelve of us ... They say that after each child it takes about three years for a women's body to recover from the previous pregnancy. She had diabetes, kidney failure, a hysterectomy and gall bladder problems.

Good health is understood as a lack of physical illness and capacity to carry out roles at home and in the community:

Interviewer: Why do women say when I ask about their mother's health, 'I have seen her nothing but working'?
OOM woman: If they did not see her mother lying in bed, this means she was healthy. This is why they answer that. This is what I would answer you.

Work for the family and community is an essential part of well-being. If women are able to do what is expected of them they consider themselves to be healthy. One chronically sick OOM woman explains: 'I do not know how my health is. Some people say that I do nothing. Some people say that they will not be able to do so much as I do every day.'

Importance of community was another key theme. Networks of social relations connect OOM women's lives, creating meaningful links among church members, neighbours, and extended families. 'Selflessness' is highly respected, as needs of others should always be considered before one's own. One woman describes her obligation to service:

A woman from Mount Forest was asking if I have any work and can I help sell her quilting because she needs money to pay for gas [for the stove]. Isn't it our role to help other people, when they need help? I will not sell my quilting but I will sell hers.

Another woman explains: 'The other women come to quilt together in my house. They know that my son is getting married and my health does not let me to quilt on my own. My son will get five quilts.'

Community members know about their neighbours' problems and challenges. Because they value mutual aid, knowing about others is important: 'There are no secrets in our community.'

Rural Change

Conservative Mennonites struggle with the dilemmas of preserving their culture and religion in a constantly changing world. Of the fifteen women, ten responded that we should talk to their husband about environmental concerns, but all confirmed that they knew that their spouses include pesticides in their current farming practices. Farmers without electric- or diesel-powered cooling systems cannot sell milk, so many OOMs have begun to use electricity. One woman commented that electricity helps her in preparing healthy meals: 'Not too long ago, without having a fridge, we were eating food at the age of getting spoiled.' Recently, community leaders have granted permission to use the telephone, and such access has improved health and safety: 'Now we can call for help when we need it.' However, not all families have installed telephones.

Several important changes were observed in recent farming practices (Bennett, 2003). The OOM use horses and buggies for their private transportation needs, but many now use tractors on the farm or hire the services of farmers with modern mechanical equipment. OOM women support their husband's decisions in these areas: 'This is my husband's department. He does what he needs to do.'

Despite well-known concerns about the environmental situation in Elmira, our OOM participants provided polite answers to our questions, expressing lack of interest in exploring health-environmental connections: 'I would say I have never worried about the environment.' All women in this sample preferred to talk about family health issues rather than experiences of changes in physical environments.

Three OOM women referred to old sayings describing their links with the natural environment. Farming and gardening are not only essential to raising their families but are also a part of their traditions: 'A person needs to eat seven pounds of dirt before it will become mature. This is a part of life to be in contact with environment, soils, and water.' They trust that close contact with natural environments is beneficial to raising healthy families. We found that most OOM women did not consider themselves to be living in a highly contaminated environment nor did they express concern that pollutants might be dangerous to health. One OOM woman admitted: 'We do not know about these smog days and we do not listen to the radio. Our children always play or work outside.' Concepts of toxicity and pollution did not appear to be well understood; yet two women indicated awareness of the possibility of danger. One woman stated: 'Creek water is not good for cattle to drink.'

In the case of air quality, twelve women stated that they felt safe in the rural environment, living on farms. One woman explained:

I am still struggling to get my head around it exactly. I grew up with the idea, 'you get used to the smell and then you are OK.' I somehow really did. The other day during the summer I had my windows open most of the time because it is hot in my room. The smell came through the open window, and I was not sure it is gas or it is a smoke or this is from somebody's fireplace. But I figured I was feeling OK.

For OOM users of buggies, automobile emissions are a sensitive issue: 'We have better air here than people in the town. We are not exposed here to this car pollution.' One woman also noticed unsustainable driving practices, and spoke about inefficient use of motor transportation: 'There are so many cars at the roads and it is often only one person in one car with many empty seats. It would be less pollution if people did not drive so much or they drive together.'

Six of fifteen women commented about the quality of the air coming from the town, especially in the past: 'I did not like the smell.' Only two women stated that they were aware of the toxicity in the air: 'We know that the air can be toxic. They teach us not to spray pesticides on windy days in our orchard.' OOM women know that farming practices and open horse-drawn transportation can result in potential exposure to air-borne contaminants, yet they do not generally perceive their environment as dangerous to their health.

OOM women are aware of bacterial water contamination, as they are obliged to follow the provincial private wells water testing regulations. However, the water testing procedure is perceived as unnecessary and time consuming since it takes 'half a day to deliver a water sample by horse and buggy for testing.' The general comment is: 'If the water does not kill us – it must be O.K.'

Rural Pride

OOM women in our study reported strong feelings of safety within their communities. They did not appear to question their way of living or their roles. They presented their world views with the confidence that 'this way life should be.' They reported that they value their simple way of life and view their homes and farms as healthy places:

> We are healthy here. When I go to the city I am always thankful that I live on the farm. We are happy here at the farm. I hope that the environment will stay [healthy] for next generations and our grandchildren will be farming.

The women portrayed themselves as 'plain and simple' people whose community networks are also their religious community. Their spirituality contributes to a strong sense of unity, ethnic identity, and an 'affirmation of difference' that promotes a sense of deep comfort within their separate community. The women focus on preservation of their values and their way of living and are resourceful in doing so, sharing children's clothing and sewing their own dresses or purchasing second-hand clothes in town. Living a simple life is a virtue and is essential to their health and well-being in this community (Snyder & Bowman, 2004). 'Farmers are not as clean as city people. We do not use cosmetics, beauty products or colour our hair. We are forbidden to use photography. This is not important for us.' The book of rules was mentioned by one woman as integral to her well-being: 'I wear the same clothing as all other women. This gives me a sense of my identity. I follow the rules of *Ordnung*. This also reflects my spirituality.'

Guided by their religious beliefs, OOM women are strengthened by identifying themselves as different from other ethnic groups and general society. Their ethno-religious identity is embedded in their theology and spirituality. According to their beliefs, separation is biblically ordained (2 Corinthians 6:17, John 15:19); it is essential to live 'apart' from the general society and to protect the community against 'worldly influences.' Our participants were explicit that 'separateness' from the outside world was critical to their well-being and to 'living peacefully' at their farms. OOM women reported that their lives were enhanced by a community protective against unwanted influences: 'In our families, we pray and work together. We are safe at the farms here.'

Patriarchal relations determine that OOM women do not speak for themselves in public settings, but they do have collective power constructed through strong social networks with other women from their community. There is also evidence of changing attitudes and influences upon male community leaders to improve women's health in cooperation with social work professionals (Snyder & Bowman, 2004). One unmarried woman reported that she received 'permission to attend a workshop how to help women in abusive relationships.'

Implications

This exploratory research with OOM women in southwestern Ontario reports on their previously silent voices concerning their health experiences. Our study explores OOM women's perceptions of health and health hazards in one small community affected by environmental pollution.

The OOM women in our study are different from women of postmodern risk society, as described by Beck (1992) or other researchers who have reported on rural communities affected by environmental hazard (Mackenzie, Lockridge, & Keith, 2005). OOM women living with the well-known environmental hazards in the Elmira area do not worry about the quality of their local environment. They believe that scientific information is not important to their lives. Nor do they feel a responsibility to learn more or take action to mitigate possible health impacts. Since health understandings are mediated through cultural and religious beliefs, biomedical models of health are not relevant: 'We are not in control of our own health, God's will determines that.' The majority of women reported lack of awareness of toxicity concepts or of the possibility of long-term effects. Having a knowledge system largely based on religion contributes to their lack of awareness of or concern about local environmental hazards, which in turn may create less uncertainty and stress in their lives than would be the case with their non-OOM neighbours. The data demonstrate culturally unique understandings of health. To be healthy means to live in orthodox consistency according to the *Ordnung*. The principal orientation in OOM life is towards submission, which leads to humility, obedience, and adjusting one's personal will to God and to the community (Wengler, 2003). For the OOM women in our study, satisfactory fulfilment of their roles as mothers, wives, sisters, or workers in their community demonstrates personal well-being and mental and spiritual health.

OOM culture and social forces shape the health of that population differently than would be predicted by prevailing assumptions concerning some relevant socio-economic factors (limited education, low income, patriarchal relations, and lifestyle) (Canadian Institute for Health Information [CIHI], 2006). Rural pride has specific meaning for OOM women. In their humility and obedience, they have a deep spiritual sense of who they are and of the purpose of their lives. These women demonstrate a strong sense of their rural identity and strong cohesion. Our definition of affirmation of difference (from mainstream society), within the ethnographic context of this study, emphasizes women's efforts to maintain their traditional, plain way of living and their belief that this allows them to maintain good health.

The ethno-religious identity of OOM women means that they experience a unique landscape of health. OOM women report that they are empowered through their ethno-religious differences, which may mitigate some of the disadvantages of polluted environments. Research with conservative Anabaptists communities elsewhere confirms complex interactions between health, human biology, and culture, contributing to different health experiences from those of the general population. In one of the first systematic surveys of women in Amish culture, women reported less stress, fewer symptoms of depression, and better mental health compared with a general population sample in Central Pennsylvania (Miller et al., 2007). In that study, social support was a health determinant suggested to explain the better mental and reproductive health of the Amish women. According to the CIHI, OOM children living near Mount Forest, Ontario, are stronger and healthier than peers from the general society (Bassett et al., 2007).

Observed and reported differences in culture, gender relations, access to political power, and access to knowledge and resources, as well as economic disadvantages associated with OOM lack of participation in government-funded health insurance programs, are factors that, when combined, may be expected to negatively affect women's health and increase women's vulnerability to environmental hazards. In our study, however, women did not directly voice any concerns related to their gendered roles. Neither did the majority of participants voice income concerns directly, although one unmarried woman mentioned lack of financial stability and her ongoing need to reach out to the community for support.

We note, however, a decline in farming income in the Waterloo area and attendant rises in the cost of medical services (Woolwich Community Health Centre, 2005). As OOMs do not participate in the Ontario Health Insurance Program, they pay full cost for medical care. Four women reported having high medical bills, and two referred to visiting their grandchildren in Toronto's Hospital for Sick Children. These expenses were covered by all members of their community. In practical terms, these OOM women participate in programs and services only with the permission of church and community leaders – reflecting an understanding that their well-being and that of their families is best served by operating within rather than outside of the framework of patriarchal relations that is basic to their community and family relations.

In this rural community with its tradition of separation, changes are slow and carefully planned but are nonetheless welcomed. Access to health care in case of emergency has improved with adoption of telephones. Access to medical services is a known barrier to women's health in rural areas (Leipert & Reutter, 2005). In our study, six OOM women talked about their difficulties in getting help due to distance. The women noted that access to phones makes them more comfortable asking their neighbours for rides to medical care when needed. OOM women also valued the addition of electricity and running water in their homes

Women in our study did not query the affordability of medical services, noting that self-sufficiency, caring for their own, and being a 'brother keeper' are important community values (Gingrich & Lightman, 2006). Elsewhere, the growing cost of medical care has been identified as a threat to the financial stability of Old Order Mennonite and Amish communities in North America. Medical professionals in Pennsylvania are also aware of these issues and have advocated for changes in medical systems (Anonymous, 2008). In general, due to financial pressures associated with rural changes, our participants indicated a growing community tolerance for women working outside of the community. None of the married women participants were working off their farms; however, they contributed to family income by selling quilts and farm products, mainly eggs and vegetables. The unmarried women who participated in our study did housekeeping for parents, worked for non-Mennonite households, or worked in a local factory.

Our sample was not large enough for us to be able to speculate on whether OOM community members are experiencing the increased cancer rates associated with contaminant levels as high as those identified along the Canagagigue Creek, nor can we speculate on whether OOM members share the increased rates of respiratory ailments and birth defects claimed by advocacy groups for residents in the rest of the Elmira area. Despite these limitations, we argue that our research raises some compelling questions for researchers and practitioners about the relationships among culture, belief systems, knowledge, and conventional assumptions about environmental risk and population health.

The study also raises some important ethical questions and potential dilemmas about health promotion programs and health research. Other research suggests that raising awareness about possible health impacts may have negative consequences for the psychological well-being of vulnerable populations (Pidgeon, Simmons, Sarre, Henwood, & Smith, 2008) – a concern for us in planning our study and one that shaped our methodology and approach to interviews. At the same time, OOM community members have the same rights as all Canadians to information and services that allow them to make choices that may protect their families and enhance opportunities for health and well-being. For example, some OOM families in our study area have recently responded to broader community concerns about soil and water contamination by agreeing to fence along the Canagagigue Creek.

In closing, we argue that the growing costs of medical care, and some evidence regarding rising socio-economic barriers for the conservative OOM communities and Amish groups that currently opt out of government-supported subsidy programs, suggest that negotiating alternative means of providing primary health care and health promotion programs for and with these groups may become increasingly important. We recommend policy and program provisions that are respectful of the life choices of OOMs and other Anabaptist groups in various geographic areas of Canada. Their decision to live separately and their tradition of keeping women's voices out of public discourse do not justify a lack of attention or concern.

Conclusions

This exploratory study provides some evidence that health inequalities may be experienced differently by OOM communities, based on their ethno-religious beliefs and understandings about the nature of health. We do not suggest that such beliefs protect them from all environmental hazards. Although OOMs' constrained physical environments, patriarchal relations, and community isolation may be somewhat problematic, our research suggests that countervailing positive factors related to faith and a strong network of community support may provide compensatory strength, empowerment, and a strong sense of value and identity.

Our work suggests that principles of trans-cultural health care with conservative Anabaptists communities require clear recognition that their cultural definitions of health and understandings of community well-being are not based on biomedical and individualist perspectives. Our study explored women's understandings of determinants of health in one OOM community near Elmira, Ontario. Implications of our work suggest a need to further examine the concepts discussed here. More research is needed to determine to what degree the findings of this study are transferable across geographical communities and across women's experience as members of other ethno-religious minority groups.

References

Anonymous. (2008). Old Order Amish, Mennonites reject health insurance, face high costs for care at not-for-profit hospitals. Retrieved from www .medicalnewstoday.com/articles/113392.php.

Bassett, D., Jr., Tremblay, M.S., Esliger, D.W., Copeland, J., Barnes, J.D., & Huntington, G.E. (2007). Physical activity and body mass index of children in an Old Order Amish community. *Medicine & Science in Sports & Exercise, 39*(3), 410–15.

Beck, U. (1992). *Risk society: Towards a new modernity.* London: Sage.

Bennett, E. (2003). Emancipatory responses to oppression: The template of land-use planning and the Old Order Amish of Ontario. *American Journal of Community Psychology, 31*(1/2), 157–71.

Canadian Institute for Health Information. (2006). *How healthy are rural Canadians? An assessment of their health status and health determinants: Summary report.* Ottawa: Canadian Institute for Health Information.

Conestoga-Rovers & Associates. (2003). *Human health risk assessment for Canagagigue Creek.* Waterloo, ON: Conestoga-Rovers & Associates.

Epp, M. (2008). *Mennonite women in Canada: A history.* Winnipeg: University of Manitoba Press.

Gingrich, L.G, & Lightman, E. (2006). Striving toward self-sufficiency: A qualitative study of mutual aid in an Old Order Mennonite community. *Family Relations, 55*, 175–89.

Horst, I.R. (2000). *A separate people: An insider's view of Old Order Mennonite customs and traditions.* Waterloo, ON: Herald Press.

Kulig, J., Babcok, R., Wall, M., & Hill, S. (2006). *Growing up as a woman: The health perspectives of low-German-speaking Mennonite women.* Research Report. Lethbridge, AB: University of Lethbridge.

Leipert, B., & George, J. (2008). Determinants of rural women's health: A qualitative study in southwest Ontario. *Journal of Rural Health, 24*(2), 210–18.

Leipert, B., & Reutter, L. (2005). Women's health in northern British Columbia: The role of geography and gender. *Canadian Journal of Rural Medicine 10*(4), 241–53.

Little, J. (2002). *Gender and rural geography: Identity, sexuality, and power in the countryside.* Toronto: Prentice Hall.

Mackenzie, A.C., Lockridge, A., & Keith, M. (2005). Declining sex ratio in a First Nation community. *Environmental Health Perspectives, 113*(10), 1295–8.

Miller, K., Yost, B., Flahery, S., Hillemeier, M., Chase, G., Weisman, C., & Dyer, A.-M. (2007). Health status, health conditions, and health behaviors among Amish women: Results from the Central Pennsylvania Women's Health Study (CePAWHS). *Women's Health Issues, 17*, 162–71.

Peters, J.F. (2003). *The plain people: A glimpse at life among the Old Order Mennonites of Ontario.* Kitchener, ON: Pandora Press.

Philo, C. (1992). Neglected rural geographies: A review. *Journal of Rural Studies, 8*, 193–207.

Pidgeon, N., Simmons, P., Sarre, S., Henwood, K., & Smith, N. (2008). The ethics of socio-cultural risk research. *Health, Risk and Society, 10*(4), 321–9.

Snyder, L., & Bowman, S. (2004). Communities in cooperation: Human services work with Old Order Mennonites. *Journal of Ethnic and Cultural Diversity in Social Work, 13*(2), 91–101.

Wengler, L. (2003). *Unser Satt Leit:* Our sort of people. Health understandings in the Old Order Mennonite and Amish community. Master's thesis, University of Waterloo, Ontario.

Woolwich Community Health Centre (2005). *Community needs and capacity assessment: Final report.* St. Jacobs, ON: Author.

PART THREE

Gender-Based Violence

Wilfreda E. Thurston

Only one of the four chapters included in this section is focused on women's experiences of violence (Dyck, Stickle, and Hardy), but in keeping with the determinants-of–population-health framework, life course analysis, and gender-based analysis, together the four reveal the central role that experiences of gender-based violence (GBV) over the lifetime play in women's health and well-being. For rural women, personal experiences of violence and their responses are shaped by the rural geography and the availability of supportive social networks and social supports, including appropriate and gender-sensitive and safe services. Dyck, Stickle and Hardy, for instance, note that leaving home to avoid violence may mean leaving her place of work for the farm woman; Illauq notes that women in northern communities have few choices for leaving; and Montgomery, Forchuk, Gorlick, and Csiernik point out that women who leave for safety reasons often end up drifting among accommodations in towns and cities without adequate attention to their mental or physical health needs. Porter and Beausoleil place reproductive health in the context of GBV and other gendered discourses that promote sanctioning and control of women's bodies. Their interviews also reveal how women are silenced about the impacts on their bodies and minds, and how reproductive health is one window on women's sense of well-being. Together the chapters draw us to an understanding that the causes and effects of GBV are communal; that is, gendered norms and social practices, such as racialized sexism, sustain rates of GBV, and the effects can be community-wide post-traumatic stress disorder (Illauq), loss of women and children from the community (Montgomery, Forchuk, Gorlick, & Csiernik), and other losses to communal well-being. They illustrate why primary health care with an emphasis on holism and participation of community members in planning of services is so important for rural women. Services designed for towns and cities are not likely to respond to their needs. The chapters also show the relationship between colonization and Aboriginal women's experiences of GBV. Responses and services, therefore, both for individuals and for communities, need to be formed around an understanding of the context of each rural community, reflecting place as a determinant of population health.

9 Living with Their Bodies: Three Generations of Newfoundland and Labrador Women

Marilyn Porter and Natalie Beausoleil

In this chapter, we draw on a three-generational, comparative life story study that focused on Newfoundland and Labrador women's experience of their reproductive lives. We understood reproductive lives more broadly than as simply being about women's reproductive health, but rather as also encompassing family relations, learning about sex, attitudes to marriage and heterosexuality, body image, and much else. This broad focus also enabled us to approach how women themselves understood the events of their reproductive experience in the overall context of their lives. Women do not separate out either the events and processes in their biological reproductive lives or their physical and mental health from the rest of their lives. Our data, then, was not narrowly focused on health as such, and our conversations ranged much more broadly than most health-focused projects. We wanted to talk to women about how they saw their lives and how they saw health and reproductive issues fitting in with the rest of their lives. We wanted to identify how health problems arise, how unhealthy practices develop, and where the influences that encourage healthy living come from. In our approach to helping women live healthier lives, we must first understand how they view their bodies.

There are three reasons for our decision to start from women's experience of their bodies in order to better understand women's health. First, we wish to bridge macro and micro analyses of gender, health, and culture by paying attention to how women embody femininity in their everyday practices, in relation to their specific life contexts (Grosz, 1994; Young, 2005). Second, feminist scholars have long pointed to the control of women's bodies in general, and reproductive processes in particular, as a crucial mechanism of women's oppression; we ask if women still experience oppression or coercion through the body (Bordo, 1993; De Beauvoir, 1949). Third, recent scholarship emphasizes how the social production of ideal bodies in the name of health has become a key control mechanism for populations and individuals alike in contemporary western society (Turner, 1996; Wright & Harwood, 2009). As feminist scholars and activists, we need to understand how women experience and negotiate normative expectations of the body and health in the current social, political, and economic context. Thus we situate our discussion about rural women's health in Newfoundland and Labrador in the context of how they understand, discuss, and transmit views about their bodies.

Background: Rural Health in Newfoundland and Labrador

Newfoundland and Labrador is, essentially, a rural province. The federal Community Information Database (n.d.) identifies the only urban regions in the province as the metropolitan areas around St. John's and Mount Pearl, Gander, Grand Falls-Windsor, Corner Brook, Marystown, Stephenville, Happy Valley-Goose Bay, and Labrador City. Over 50% of the population live outside these centres, in rural areas. Most of the older women we talked to were brought up in very small and remote communities, and while some within the younger generations have moved to urban areas, many still live in rural areas. Though these areas are not as remote as they were – in terms of electronic communications, access to cars, etc. – such communities, especially in Labrador, are a long way from health centres and hospitals, and everyone in the province has to go to St. John's for major medical procedures. Rural-based occupations such as fishing, logging, and other resource-extractive industries are notoriously dangerous (Canadian Institute for Health Information [CIHI], 2006; *Globe and Mail*, 2006; Koehoorn, McLeod, Fan, Hurrell, & Demers 2009; Neis, 1998; Power, 2005; Wilkins & Mackenzie, 2007).[1] In addition, rural working people often have to commute long distances on poorly maintained roads in winter conditions (Harris, Alasia, & Bollman, 2008).[2] Most statistical data tend not to distinguish between rural and urban areas. Available data are broken down by province or by sub-provincial regions, both of which include rural and urban areas.[3] We know, for example, that farming, forestry, and mining have the highest occupational accident and fatality rates, and we know that rural people work mostly in primary, extractive industries, but we do not have the precise correlation of the two sets of data. While few women are engaged in such work, they are the main labour force in fish processing, which leads them to be exposed to less visible dangers, such as crab asthma (Neis et al., 2004).

We can get a better understanding of the involvement of rural men, in particular, in potentially dangerous occupations when there is a major tragedy, such as the Ocean Ranger sinking (1982) or the more recent Cougar Helicopter crash (2009), and can see how many rural communities have lost one or more people from their small populations. Equally, while the numbers are not statistically significant, small fishing boat accidents, with the loss of two or three men, can devastate small communities.

In addition to these adverse factors, rural populations tend to be less exposed to health education initiatives, be less well served by health professionals, and have less access to facilities such as swimming pools or gyms. They are also less likely to have access to healthy foods, such as salads, cheese, or nuts, some of which have to be imported and are expensive. In chapter 12 of this volume Montgomery, Forchuk, Gorlick, and Csiernik provide a detailed analysis of the difficulties women in rural and isolated communities face in accessing appropriate health and housing services, and Suthern et al. (2004), among others, have documented the disadvantages and difficulties faced by women in rural and remote communities. In fact, all the chapters in this section call into question the kinds of benefits that urban observers attribute to rural life, such as fresh air and close community relations.

Our study also noted the ways in which poverty and isolation combine to create significant health risks in Newfoundland and Labrador. The rates for diseases of the circulatory and digestive systems in this province tend to be higher than the national average (Community Accounts, n.d.). Some rural areas have twice the national rate of diabetes. Low income levels and low education levels also contribute to poor health status. In addition, there tend to be higher rates of other negative health behaviours such as smoking, poor diet, and lack of exercise in rural and especially remote areas (Grzetic, 2004; Kealey, Coombs, Turner, & Yeoman, 2006; Parrish, Turner, & Solberg, 2007). The ability of the provincial health system to cope with delivering health to a dispersed and rural population is constantly under threat. As the Coasts Under Stress team puts it: 'The health care system has been under considerable stress over the past several decades, and nowhere has this been more the case than at the level of remote coastal regions and communities' (Ommer, 2007, p. 184). To take one example, access to clean water is considered vital to community health, but the Canadian Medical Assocation reports that there are currently 228 communities in Newfoundland and Labrador under a boiled water advisory, third after British Columbia (530) and Ontario (679), both of which have much larger populations.

The study, entitled *Women's Experience of Their Reproductive Lives*, involved teams from Pakistan, Indonesia, and Canada. In the Newfoundland and Labrador section of the study we interviewed fifty-four women in twenty-seven families, and it is this material that we report on here. Our decision to work with three-generational families of women had two key objectives. One was to get as close as possible to a longitudinal approach in order to understand how women's lives had changed since the birth of our oldest participants. The other was to use the institution of the family to examine relationships between genera-tions of women, to hear how they interacted with each other, and to learn how knowledge and ideas were transmitted across generations. We recruited our participants using a variety of strategies, including snowball sampling. Given the small numbers of participants, we could not attain anything close to a representative sample, but we endeav-oured to talk to women and families that were broadly typical of the population, including all areas of the province, all social classes, immi-grant women, and members of an Aboriginal community. We were not looking for women with particular health issues, but rather women who had experienced 'normal' reproductive lives, although some of our participants did have health problems or difficult pregnancies and childbirth experiences. Our oldest participant was born in 1911, the youngest in 1985. We include the birthdates of the participants to give the reader some sense of when they grew up and thus what kinds of issues they may have faced during their reproductive lives. For exam-ple, our oldest participants used cut-up rags to stem their menstrual flow, while our youngest used the most modern of tampons; many of the older women were delivered by local midwives, while the youngest mothers had all had their babies in hospitals.

All the interviews were transcribed and, along with field and other notes, entered into NVivo, a qualitative analysis computer program (Richards, 1999)

Talking about the Body

We were particularly interested in the way in which ideas, values, and knowledge were transmitted within families. The family and the relationships between women constituted an important conduit, and ideas, values, and knowledge were transmitted both up and down the generations and at each point were contested and negotiated. We explore some of the ways this happened in terms of how the women of different generations talked about their bodies.

Our feminist approach to women's health recognizes that women are embodied beings, whose experiences cannot be fully understood by the sole use of epidemiological categories provided by a biomedical model (Gustafson, 2009). Moreover, women's ideas about and experiences of health are inextricably tied to their ideas about and experiences of the body. We view women's interpretations and experiences of health and bodies as socially, culturally, and politically shaped; health and the body are indeed social texts belonging to culture. Illnesses and diseases and problems in accessing quality health care affect women and other marginalized groups in particular ways. In contemporary Western society the dominant discourses of health focus on individuals' lifestyle and their achievement of a specific shape and appearance of the (gendered and racialized) body. Individual citizens are pressured to take personal responsibility for health through consumption of products and services as well as self-surveillance and control of the body. Discourses of health are fed by dominant discourses of beauty, individual responsibility, consumption, self, productivity, and meritocracy in contemporary Western society (Rail & Beausoleil, 2003). A key prescription for the 'ideal healthy body' is for women to be thin and men to be muscular; this must be achieved through diet and physical activity (Gard & Wright, 2005). Normative ideas of the healthy body are promoted not only through popular media but also by policy makers, health professionals and health organizations, large corporations, and schools (Evans, Rich, Davies, & Allwood, 2008; Wright & Harwood, 2009). A number of scholars have critiqued the dominant individualist approach to health, reminding us that the most important determinants of health (socio-economic status, education, employment, physical and social environment) have little to do with individual lifestyles and body shapes (Rail, 2009; Raphael, 2008). In this chapter, however, we are interested in how women take up, absorb, or negotiate the dominant discourses of the body and health in their everyday practices and sense of identity. We analysed women's stories of health, including how women know and care for their bodies, bearing in mind that these stories are linked to larger narratives of health and the body in contemporary Western society. Our study showed not only how women's attitudes to their bodies have changed over the generations but how women interact with each other and influence each others' views of their bodies.

Among the participants in our study, women of the middle and younger generations talked more explicitly and easily with us about their experiences with their bodies than women of the older generation. We found older women had a greater sense of the body as intimate and private, while body image (the perception and evaluation of one's body) has become common knowledge among young and middle-aged women.

One interesting example concerns an older participant Peggy (born 1914)[4] and her daughter Patricia (born 1956). In this case, we asked Patricia to interview her own mother, which allowed Patricia to challenge her mother in ways that were not likely to happen with an unknown interviewer. Even so, Peggy was clearly reluctant to talk about her experience with her body. Here is Patricia's account of her own body and her mother's response to it:

> Patricia (born 1956): Well you know I've always been a bigger person, you know, taller ... I've always been big. But I really didn't put on any weight until after my first pregnancy ... it never bothered me being a big woman, you know. And it's only in later years when I put on weight it seemed to really bother my mother. Because I think my mother must have had an obsession about her weight. She's short and she was always very round. I have one sister who is very slim. But the three of us [Patricia and two other sisters] are not, we're big. And my mother has continuously made remarks about that. So much so that I had fights with her about it. But she still doesn't get it, she still thinks she's saying it because she loves me, you know. And I said mother don't love me so much, it's killing me, your love ... But you know I sort of, I've gotten past it, I mean I suppose it has bothered me. But you know it's mom, it's just the way she is. It's more a reflection on how she feels.

As we will see, participants talk about the significant impact of other family members' comments on their body and appearance. The quotation above also raises the interesting question of silences among family members. Some issues stood out as we analysed our interviews: the importance of women's gazes in the family; weight control and health; growing up, body embarrassment, and body-based harassment; and self-esteem and the body.

Women's Gazes in the Family

Family members observe each other. Mothers, grandmothers, daughters, sisters, aunts, nieces, in-laws observe and comment on each other's body and appearance. In our study, women talked about their own bodies, but they also gave their opinions about their relatives' bodies. Indeed, some of the interviews that included two or three women in the same family contained discussions about each other's bodies and about the bodies of relatives who were absent. Sometimes, both mothers and daughters in our study devoted considerable energy and intelligence to interpreting what their relatives said, and what they did not say, about their bodies and sexualities. The discussions we had with women indicated how important this area was to them and to their relationships with their female kin. Their concern and interest in understanding each other's experience reflected the concerns they had for each other's health, especially as they often saw patterns of health and sickness in the family. Some participants heard comments received from other women in the family about their body and appearance as critical, especially those comments that revolved around body weight. For instance, Sarah talked about her daughter Susan in her absence, but while her granddaughter Samantha was present:

> *Sarah* (born 1935): I don't know about Susan, I don't think Susan's very comfortable because she's put on a lot of weight – wouldn't you say, Samantha?
> *Samantha* (born 1977): Yeah. She had a hysterectomy.
> *Sarah:* Yeah, she had a hysterectomy so she's put on a lot of weight, I don't think she's very happy with her body right now, I'm sure she'd like to be … But my other girls now they're slimmer.

This example shows us how the issue of body weight comes to symbolisz and encapsulate other concerns about health. It is as if the visible signs of the waistline come to represent all other symptoms of health and concerns about health.

Betty's perspective on intergenerational family dynamics is also mediated through concerns over weight and appearance:

> *Betty* (born 1983): I can remember my mom saying when … I was probably around seven and I can remember her saying, 'you know Betty you could

lose a lot of weight if you just drank water for a couple of days.' My family is obsessed with weight, it's very insane.

Natalie (interviewer): So your mother herself was constantly dieting – that's what you saw?

Betty: Yes.

Natalie: And your grandmother?

Betty: Everyone, all my aunts.

Natalie: So you saw that all the time?

Betty: Oh yeah and still all the time. Any time anyone in my family sees me, like it could be twice a day they'll see me and they'll say 'oh you've lost weight.' Or if it's my mom who sees me say, 'you gained weight Betty. What's the problem?' and when my aunts say, 'Oh you're losing weight' I say, 'I don't care, it's not an issue really.' It's always an issue. Or if Oprah's on the TV they'll say, 'Oprah gained a lot of weight' and I'll say, 'It's Oprah who cares' and then the next day Oprah will look exactly the same and she'll say, 'Oprah looks great, she's lost a lot of weight.'

Patricia and Betty are from different generations but they both want to foster a healthy body image for younger women and girls in their families. Patricia says she is worried about her younger daughter's body image, and Betty emphasizes her attempts to model body self-confidence for her young nieces. Another woman of the youngest generation, Lucy, is grateful that her mother has always tried to foster a positive relationship to the body, but she also talks about her mother's own struggles to attain a healthy body image.

Lucy (born 1985): When mom was 19 … she had a different body image. I know she did because we've talked about this. She was skinnier than I am but she always felt like she was fat. She was in nursing, she was in a health profession so she technically knew that she wasn't [fat] but she had a distorted body image, so then in the last few years now that she's older and started to gain weight she doesn't realize that she's gaining weight. She thinks that her body image that she had all twisted when she was young stayed distorted, so now that she actually could be considered fat or a little bit overweight, she doesn't see herself like that, like in her head she still sees herself as skinny. Whereas when she was skinny she thought she was fat, so it's all kind of twisted up like that. But I don't feel like that.

Families can therefore be sites of support or criticism, or both, but always centred on the appearance of the body, and in particular on whether it does or does not accord with the 'ideal weight.' Criticisms can be hurtful, and some women were very aware of the impact of what was said and done in front of other women and girls in their family.

When looking at each other and commenting upon each other's bodies and appearance women may be expressing love, support, negative judgment, and/or fear about bodily manifestations of health issues and aging. In contemporary Western society, the body can be 'read' for specific signs of health/illness and aging, and women watch for these signs in others in the family as well as in themselves (Beausoleil, 1998). Cultural and aesthetic judgments are inextricably involved in women's attitudes to bodily change accompanying aging. How women experience the relation between weight and health is also shaped by a specific culture and its bodily standards and aesthetics, which remain tied to an ideal of youthful beauty. This means that in Western culture, the natural processes of aging and changing bodies are often seen as failures that must be fought through individual discipline and self-control. The expectation for women (and men) is that as they age they have to work even harder at keeping the body 'young' and 'fit' (Beausoleil &Martin, 2002; Turner, 1995).

Weight Control and Health

Talking about weight and weight control spanned all three generations of the women we talked with. However, women did differ considerably in how far they themselves were actually worried about their weight. Some said they had always worried about weight. Others said they worried about it at specific times in their lives. A few said they had never really worried about their weight. Zelda, a participant of the older generation, is an example of one who says she has always worried about weight:

Zelda (born 1927): I've always felt I was too fat.
Marilyn (interviewer): You described yourself as hefty.
Zelda: Yes, and then when I was at university everyone was slim of course, and one of my friends had a purging diet and drank black coffee and ate prunes for breakfast, and someone else had something else, and I lost a lot of weight when I was at university. Of course I was younger and moving around much more and [when] I left university I was 113 pounds and still my waist wasn't small enough. All my life I've been very conscious of weight and I think that's something that kind of, the 50s and the 40s this

new look came in, and I think women's magazines besides having really good recipes they also had something about diet, and of course diet was the thing for years and years and years – not exercise – so you had this idea that you should be a certain way. I think I'm gradually growing out of it.

In contrast, Sarah, who was of the same generation as Zelda, said she never worried about her weight:

Sarah (born 1935): Oh no, I was just as confident as I ever was.
Marilyn (interviewer): So you're pretty comfortable within that particular body. Anything you'd like to change?
Sarah: Well, I'd like to be a little bit smaller [laughter] but other than that ...

Sarah's ambivalent position – not worrying about her body but not being completely satisfied with it either – is reflected by other women, such as Rebecca.

Rebecca (born 1948): Um, I was kind of small I guess when I was in high school I was petite. I still am ... I did gain some weight the last couple of years. I put on maybe about five pounds of dead weight since then [laughs] ... Well maybe I was 110 or 120 when I married and I think every ten years I put on an extra five that I don't take off.
Natalie (interviewer): But have you given much thought to it? Has it been an issue for you?
Rebecca: Well, I try to keep in shape somewhat but I guess just my heredity keeps me within a reasonable size. And I don't think too much about it. I do some exercises but I'm more interested in it for health ... And I guess if I gain a lot of weight, the summer comes now and I put on a bathing suit and I look at myself and I'll say, 'yeah you've got too much around there.' And sometimes when I go trying on clothing I think, 'oh I wish I was thinner here.' But it's not something that I dwell on that much, I guess. I haven't put on excessive weight and I don't like the fact that I'm too heavy here and here but it's not something that I spend a lot of time thinking about.

Other participants, especially of the second generation, talked about their desire to lose weight as a way to be healthy. For instance, Barbara sees her weight as a health problem and is trying to lose weight through exercising:

Barbara (born 1960): I have a [health] problem now with ... I put on a lot of weight with stopping smoking. Both my husband and I, we both put on at least thirty pounds ... We may have to try that [specific diet], we want to increase exercise and that's been a hard thing. He's just going through another job change. He left that job so that's been another level in our whole existence ... And that hasn't been helping with the weight.

There is no doubt that most of our participants considered physical activity essential to good health. Some participants enjoyed physical activity all their lives, while others were more active when they were younger but have now been overtaken by domestic responsibilities.

Julia (born 1969): No – well I've got kids! ... when I was younger I did exercise. I didn't know what it was to walk, I ran everywhere, even in my later teens, I was in basketball, and volleyball and cheerleading – cross country skiing, always involved.

Most of the women who talked about exercise simply saw it as a way to improve their health. Indeed, some saw that weight loss was not necessarily healthy.

Ilya (born 1974): In high school I remember a big thing about weight and stuff ... But then when I got in, I think it was grade nine when I started kind of a bad eating habit. I started, even though my mom made me lunches, I never used to eat them, I used to buy, this is bad though, I used to buy a bag of chips for lunch. And that's what I'd have for lunch every day. And I lost weight ... I used to, usually I'd skip breakfast or I'd have a piece of fruit, for lunch I'd have a bag of chips and water [laughter]. And then I'd have supper at home, like a regular meal ...

While participants in all three generations of our study talked about weight concerns and attempts to lose weight (or less commonly to gain weight), it was only the younger women who mentioned the dangers of dieting and losing weight and who were more aware of the reality of disordered eating and eating disorders than participants from the first or second generation.

Growing Up and Body Embarrassment

One of the most critical stages in women's knowledge about and awareness of their bodies comes with puberty and the onset of menstruation. While girls know that they are girls, and come to understand the social consequences of gender very early, puberty is often the first time that they have to come to terms with their approaching womanhood and what that might mean (Porter, 2006).

Accomplishing menarche successfully will lay the groundwork for the growing woman's healthy acceptance and understanding of her reproductive body. We expected that the younger women in our study would be better informed than their grandmothers because of sex education in schools and a more liberal attitude to sex. However, the situation is not this simple. Let us take, for example, the 'S' family:

Marilyn (interviewer): How did you learn about menstruating?
Sarah (born 1935): To tell the truth I didn't know. You know what I thought before I started to have my periods? I used to think that when you have your period it comes through your stomach ... Well, I guess I just heard from my girlfriends like that I had a couple of girlfriends that maybe was a year or so older than me. As a matter of fact that was the first one I told. I didn't even tell my mom, she found my pajamas. [Laughter] I didn't even tell her, you know? I just went right on down to my friend's house and told her something happened and she told me what it was. But I didn't ... You see when I was young there was no such thing as sanitary napkins ... She [mother] didn't explain it very much, just told me what was happening, that it was gonna happen every month, like you know when you want anything to come to her and she'd get it for you, that kind of thing, right ... Yeah, but I remember I used to use cloths, I know that. My mom used to have special flannel and that's what we used to use. [Laughter] Ah my. Some different now. You can advertise it on TV and everything now.

When we talked to Sarah's daughter Susan we found similarities in their experience.

Susan (born 1957): How did I find out? I don't know, I honestly don't know. I knew what it was when it came. But I honestly don't know how, it wasn't from my mother, that I do know. I guess it was just friends ... I went and told H–; I was more comfortable telling her than I was my own mother. I felt embarrassed and I don't know why. But that age, I was only twelve, that's who I told and she told mom.

Susan was better prepared for menarche, but the information did not come from her mother. Like many other women of all generations, Susan turned first to her friends. At that time there was no structure in place (in school, for example) to ensure that she was prepared. By the time Susan's daughter Samantha reached menarche, there was more information available and mothers felt more obliged to ensure that their daughters were prepared. So Samantha went into menarche with more information than her mother or her grandmother. But with the information Susan had also passed on her acute embarrassment about discussing matters of sex.

> *Samantha* (born 1977): Yeah because I was, as a child I was really embarrassed at the thought of puberty or sex ... anything that had to do with my body I always felt really ashamed. I remember the first time I found a hair under my arm, I was SO embarrassed and I don't know why I felt embarrassed, but I think it was the whole religion and sex and your body change. And I didn't like my body.

What is clear from this account of the transmission of information in the 'S' family is how embarrassment and negative feelings about sex broaden to become negative feelings about girls' bodies in general. This in turn generates silences around topics of sex and the body that prevent women from turning to other women in their families for guidance and support. We should also note that while the older two generations of the 'S' family grew up and lived in rural areas, Samantha has now moved to St. John's, where there is greater acceptance of sexual diversity and the issues facing people living with HIV. There are also activist groups working on sexual information and rights and providing support to women.

Self-esteem, the Body, and Shaping One's Life

For most of our participants, the most difficult period of their lives was menarche and the adolescent years. Our study confirms that adolescence is a crucial time for the shaping of girls' social identity through bodily attributes and that it is also a time where much of the oppression and marginalization of girls occur through their bodies (Larkin & Rice, 2005; Rice, 2007, 2009). Negotiating early sexual relations, friendships, school and family relations, and marriage or partnerships was clearly taxing. Some women also reported the difficulties of trying to obey religious edicts about sexual behaviour. The majority achieved a more easy relationship with their bodies as they moved into marriage or partnership and childbearing. For some women, however, the transition to acceptance has been much more difficult. This is especially so when they have to deal with severe poverty and social isolation in combination with addictions or violence.

Molly provides us with some insight into the scale of personal destruction that results from sustained sexual abuse.

Phyllis (interviewer): So, what did you learn about sex?
Molly (born 1965): Well, more or less I was [sexually abused] all my life. I knew a lot more than I should have done for my age like today ... I was sexually abused from the age of two. It went on as far back as I can remember, right back it went on until I was twelve years old. At first I didn't know and then about a couple of years after I was scared ... so like I knew and I was too scared to tell anyone and I was [mumbles] ... I knew a lot more than I should have known for my age. Ever since I could remember, one of my first childhood memories is somebody sexually abusing me.
Phyllis: From the age of two? Did it happen at home?
Molly: Yep. At home. So I lost my trust in a lot of people ... I closed up ... I'm still shy, have no self-esteem ... like my whole life was ruined ... from that moment on, I never ever wanted to charge anybody for anything in my whole life, and I never did. No matter how bad I was beaten, didn't matter what they did or if no matter what they done to me ... my nose was broke three times, never charged nobody for that, I didn't charge nobody for a lot of things because of the embarrassment at that time when I went to court and all them people looking at me and me there with that stupid, ugliest shit they were asking me is, and I was not yet ten years old. It scarred me ... I was always abused by every man I went with. I think it's more or less I looked for it. I'm sure I did. If somebody was treating me too nice I got mad ... I don't want to be with this person because they were too good for me or something like that.

Molly's story is an extreme example, but it helps us to see the integral connection between the way women see their bodies, their ability to develop a positive self-image, and their ability to take control of their lives (including their own health and that of their families). To have suffered sexual or physical violence as a young girl damages these abilities in ways that are very difficult to overcome (Croll, 2008).

Implications

We opened this chapter by describing our focus on women's experience of their reproductive lives as a means to understanding women's health. All of the women we talked to had medical histories, and some had severe ailments or problems with their pregnancies, even though we had made a point of trying to select women for the study who had relatively 'normal' reproductive experiences. Their doctors and other health professionals treated the symptoms they saw and advised women as best they could, and we have no quarrel with the care the women received. But we are aware of a disjuncture between the integrated nature of women's reproductive health lives and their own interpretation of them, on the one hand, and the partial, medicalized view that is seen by the health professional system and systematized in medical records, on the other.

If women are to be helped to take positive control over their own health, then the kind of qualitative research that we have presented here helps us to start from where women experience their own bodies. Talking about their relations to their bodies is one way in which women describe their lives. Talking about the body is also a way to talk about the changes in one's life, and the talk itself organizes one's life history in the process. In this chapter we have focused on one of the fundamentals of health – a healthy attitude to, and knowledge about, one's own body. We have seen that women are acutely aware of their bodies, but that they are often preoccupied with appearance and image. This is not surprising given the ubiquitous messages about health and the (gendered) body pressuring women to perform femininity through exhibiting (or trying to exhibit) specific body attributes. Such dominant discourses of health define some bodies as more healthy than others and generally conflate thinness and youth with health, fatness and old age with illness. Recently, a number of scholars have denounced these dominant definitions of health as sexist, ageist, racist, ableist, fat phobic, classist, heterosexist, and therefore based more on cultural and aesthetic criteria than on a sound understanding of the range of possibilities for women to experience 'healthy bodies' (Beausoleil & Ward, 2010; Rail & Beausoleil, 2003; Wright & Harwood, 2009). We see both the way in which the women we talked to tried to comply with idealized models of the female body and the way these models structured their discourse about their bodies as forms of covert control, which Foucault (1978) has so ably described. We have described how some women take up the view points and normalizing practices of health and the body spread through education, media, and health systems, or 'biopedagogies' (Harwood, 2009). We have also cited some examples of more obvious forms of coercion by means of child sexual or physical abuse, with their clear consequences of such women's difficulties in developing healthy attitudes to their own bodies or control over their own healthy living. That women so often express their hopes and concerns in terms of body image and weight control is not surprising given the dominant health discourses and their emphasis on lifestyle changes and individual will power as solutions to, or preventive measures for, health problems.

We interpret women's talk about their appearance, and especially their concern about weight, as a genuine concern for health as well as a code for discussions that they are too embarrassed to have. If sex is constructed as both negative and forbidden, and therefore as silenced, then girls enter puberty at a disadvantage. The information about their bodies is already tainted with their embarrassment about sex. Later, in adult life, they use this displaced focus on body weight to express their feelings and concern for each other.

The issues we raise in this chapter are not unique to rural women, although our data are drawn from women who live in rural areas. We think that rural women face issues about body in starker form than urban women because they face numerous challenges in their quest for healthy lives. They, and their menfolk, tend to be employed in physical occupations with a higher accident rate. The health and social network is spread thin and is often inaccessible. Resources, such as healthy food, adequate spaces for physical activity, and health education, are scarce. Rural poverty, certainly in Newfoundland and Labrador, is pronounced. All these factors affect rural women's ability to control their bodies and their health in profound ways.

Conclusion

From a socio-cultural and critical perspective it is crucial to separate weight and body image issues from health issues (Beausoleil, 2009; Beausoleil & Ward, 2010). Broad social, economic, and political determinants of health are more important than lifestyle for health promotion and the health of a population (Raphael, 2008). Our study shows how important the issue of health is to women and how much effort they are prepared to put into obtaining good health. Their narrative allows us to see some of the problems that women face in establishing the foundations for a healthy understanding of their bodies, itself a foundation for their own health and that of their families. Our responsibility is to argue for greater resources to be made available to rural women in order to facilitate healthier lives. Our responsibility is also to continue doing critical research in the fields of health and how women's bodies are 'produced' and experienced.

Notes

1 Injuries and poisonings had the highest of all mortality rates in rural areas, making them the most important cause of mortality in these areas (CIHI, 2006, p.129). Men are more vulnerable than women, and many of the injuries occur as a result of accidents at work.

2 In Newfoundland and Labrador the prevalence of moose is a particular danger, especially in the summer months. There are approximately 120,000 moose on the island, with 600 moose/vehicle accidents per annum, 18% of which result in injury, with about two fatalities per year (http://www.releases.gov .nl.ca/releases/2010/env/0322n01.html, www.releases.gov.nl.ca/releases/ 1997/forest/0711n02.htm).

3 This is despite recent efforts to develop a classification of MIZ (Metropolitan Influenced Zones), which was particularly useful to the researchers in the *How Healthy Are Rural Canadians* study (CIHI, 2006).

4 In these pages we have quoted from only a small fraction of the fifty-four women we interviewed in the study: *Family 6:* Barbara, Generation B, born 1960. *Family 1:* Sarah, Generation A, born 1935; Susan, Generation B, born 1957; Samantha, Generation C, born 1977. *Family 3:* Peggy, Generation A, born 1914; Patricia, Generation B, born 1956. *Family 8:* Lucy, Generation C, born 1985. *Family 9:* Ilya, Generation C, born 1974. *Family 13:* Julia, Generation C, born 1969. *Family 20:* Molly, Generation C, born 1965. *Family 15:* Betty F, Generation C, born 1983. *Family 4:* Rebecca, Generation B, born 1948.

References

Beausoleil, N. (1998). Corps, santé, apparence et vieillissement dans les énoncés de femmes francophones en Ontario. *Reflets, 4*(1), 53-74.

Beausoleil, N. (2009). An impossible task?: Preventing disordered eating in the context of the current obesity panic. In J. Wright & V. Harwood (Eds.), *Biopolitics and the 'obesity epidemic': Governing bodies* (pp. 93-107). London: Routledge.

Beausoleil, N., & Martin, G. (2002). Activité physique, santé et vieillissement chez des femmes francophones de l'Ontario. *La Revue Canadienne du Vieillissement/Canadian Journal on Aging, 21*(3), 443-54.

Beausoleil, N., & Ward, P. (2010). Fat panic in Canadian public health policy: Obesity as different and unhealthy. *Radical Psychology: A Journal of Psychology, Politics, and Radicalism, 8*(1). Retrieved from http://www .radicalpsychology.org/vol8-1/fatpanic.html.

Bordo, S. (1993). *Unbearable weight: Feminism, western culture and the body.* Berkeley: University of California Press.

Canadian Institute for Health Information (CIHI). (2006). *How healthy are rural Canadians? An assessment of their health status and health determinants.* Ottawa: Author.

Community Accounts. (n.d.). Newfoundland and Labrador Statistics Agency. Retrieved from www.communityaccounts.ca.

Community Information Database. (n.d.). Government of Canada Rural Secretariat. Retrieved from http://www.cid-bdc.ca/english/index.html.

Croll, M. (2008). *Following sexual abuse: A sociological interpretation of identity re/formation in reflexive therapy.* Toronto: University of Toronto Press.

De Beauvoir, S. (1949). *Le deuxieme sexe.* Paris: Gallimard.

Evans, J., Rich, E., Davies B., & Allwood, R. (2008). *Education, eating disorders and obesity discourse: Fat fabrication.* London: Routledge.

Foucault, M. (1978). *The history of sexuality: Volume 1: An introduction.* New York: Random House.

Gard, M., & Wright, J. (2005). *The obesity epidemic: Science, morality, and ideology.* London: Routledge.

Globe and Mail. (2006, September 25). Editorial.

Grzetic, B. (2004) Women fishes these days. Halifax, NS: Fernwood.

Grosz, E. (1994). *Volatile bodies: Towards a corporeal feminism.* Bloomington: Indiana University Press.

Gustafson, D. (2009). Underpinnings and understandings of girls' and women's health. In N. Mandell (Ed.), *Feminist issues: Race, class, and sexuality* (5th ed., pp. 272-97). Toronto: Pearson.

Harris, S., Alasia, A., & Bollman, R. (2008). Rural commuting. *Perspectives, November 9.* Statistics Canada, Catalogue no. 75-001-X. Retrieved from http://www.statcan.gc.ca/pub/75-001-x/2008111/pdf/10720-eng.pdf.

Harwood, V. (2009). Theorizing biopedagogies. In J. Wright. & V. Harwood (Eds.), *Biopolitics and the 'obesity epidemic': Governing bodies* (pp. 15-30). London: Routledge.

Kealey, L., Coombs, H., Turner, N., & Yeomans, S. (2006). Knowledge, power and health. In P. Sinclair & R. Ommer (Eds.), *Power and restructuring: Canada's coastal society and environment* (pp. 107-28). St. John's: ISER Books.

Koehoorn, M., McLeod, C. Fan, J., Hurrell, C., & Demers, P. (2009). *WorkSafeBC-CHSPR research partnership annual report: 2008-2009.* Vancouver: Centre for Health Services and Policy Research, University of British Columbia. Retrieved from http://www.chspr.ubc.ca/files/publications/2009/Partnership_AR_2008-09_FINAL.pdf.

Larkin, J., & Rice, C. (2005). Beyond 'healthy eating' and 'healthy weights': Harassment and the health curriculum in middle schools. *Body Image, 2,* 219-32.

Neis, B. (1998). Women's health and work restructuring in rural, resource-based hinterland areas. Unpublished presentation, Maritime Centre for Excellence in Women's Health, Halifax.

Neis, B. Cartier, A., Gautrin, D., Horth-Susin, L., Jong, M., Swanson, M., Lehrer, S., Bickis, U., & Howse, D. (2004). *Report on the SafetyNet snow crab occupational asthma study.* St. John's: Workplace Health, Safety and Compensation Commission.

Ommer, R. (with Coasts Under Stress Research Team). (2007). *Coasts under stress: Restructuring and social-ecological health.* Montreal: McGill-Queens University Press.

Parrish, C.C., Turner, N.J., & Solberg, S.M. (Eds.). (2007). *Resetting the kitchen table: Food security, culture, health and resilience in coastal communities.* Hauppague, NY: Nova Science Publishing.

Porter, M. (2006). First blood: How three generations of Newfoundland women learned about menstruation. *Atlantis, 31*(1), 45-54.

Power, Nicole. (2005). *What do they call a fisherman? Men, gender, and restructuring in the Newfoundland fishery.* St. John's: ISER.

Rail, G. (2009). Canadian youth's discursive constructions of health in the context of obesity discourse. In J. Wright & V. Harwood (Eds.), *Biopolitics and the 'obesity epidemic': Governing bodies* (pp. 141-56). London: Routledge.

Rail, G., & Beausoleil, N. (2003). Introduction: Health panic discourses and the commodification of women's health in Canada. In N. Beausoleil & G. Rail (Eds.), Health panic and women's health (Special issue). *Atlantis: A Women's Studies Journal, 27*(2), 1-5.

Raphael, D. (2008). Grasping at straws: A recent history of health promotion in Canada. *Critical Public Health, 18*(4), 483-95.

Rice, C. (2007). Becoming the fat girl: Acquisition of an unfit identity. *Women's Studies International, 30,* 158-74.

Rice, C. (2009). Exacting beauty: Exploring women's body projects and problems in the 21st century. In N. Mandell, *Feminist issues: Race, class and sexuality* (5th ed., pp. 131-60). Toronto: Pearson.

Richards, L. (1999). *Using NVivo in Qualitative Research.* London: Sage.

Sutherns, R, McPhedran, M., & Haworth-Brockman, M. (2004). Rural, remote, and northern women's health: Policy and research directions. Winnipeg: Prairie Centre of Excellence for Women's Health.

Turner, B.S. (1995). Aging and identity: Some reflections on the somatization of the self. In M. Featherstone & A. Wernick, (Eds.), *Images of aging: Cultural representations of later life* (pp. 245-62). London: Routledge.

Turner, B.S. (1996). *The body and society* (2nd ed.). London: Sage.

Wilkins, K., & Mackenzie, S. (2007). Work injuries. *Health Reports, 18*(3), 25-42. Statistics Canada, Catalogue 82-003.

Wright, J., & Harwood, V. (Eds.). (2009). *Biopolitics and the 'obesity epidemic': Governing bodies*. London: Routledge.
Young, I.M. (2005). *On female body experience: 'Throwing like a girl' and other essays*. New York: Oxford University Press.

10 Intimate Partner Violence: Understanding and Responding to the Unique Needs of Women in Rural and Northern Communities

Karen G. Dyck, Kelly L. Stickle, and Cindy L. Hardy

Intimate partner violence (IPV) poses significant health challenges for Canadian women residing in rural and northern (R&N) communities. Factors such as geographic isolation, longer emergency response times, limited or no public transportation, unique financial situations, limited health care resources, limited access to women's shelters, lack of privacy, and cultural factors have the potential to exacerbate the significant problems encountered by women in violent relationships.

This chapter provides readers with a summary of literature on IPV in R&N Canada, including prevalence, consequences, risk factors, barriers to accessing services, prevention, and intervention. Unique aspects of this chapter include incorporation of personal observations from the first author's clinical practice in R&N Canada within the review of literature, and utilization of the social ecological model as an organizing framework for understanding and responding to IPV in R&N Canada.

Defining 'IPV' and 'R&N'

IPV is the occurrence within an intimate relationship of threats or acts of physical aggression, psychological abuse, sexual coercion/abuse, and other controlling acts (Heise & Garcia-Moreno, 2002). In this chapter, the focus is on violence directed towards women within the context of heterosexual marital or common-law unions.

Recognizing the lack of consensus in the literature regarding the most appropriate definitions of 'rural,' 'northern,' and 'remote,' this chapter summarizes Canadian studies in which participants were identified as dwelling in rural, northern, or remote communities. The authors recognize the considerable heterogeneity that exists among

R&N communities and urge caution in generalizing findings across diverse communities.

The Scope of the Problem

The prevalence and consequences of IPV in Canada have been documented in telephone surveys of large nationally representative samples. Despite biases due to exclusion of women who do not speak either English or French and women who do not have telephones, telephone surveys are preferable to police records, which underestimate the true incidence of violence against women because only a small portion of such violence is ever reported to police (Statistics Canada, 2006).

A recent telephone survey estimated the five-year prevalence of IPV as 7% in 2004 (Statistics Canada, 2005). Urban and rural areas in Canadian provinces had similar rates of IPV (Statistics Canada, 2005). Higher five-year prevalence rates of IPV were reported by Aboriginal women (24%) and women residing in the territories (12%), whereas lower rates were reported by immigrant women (5%; Statistics Canada, 2006). Rural Aboriginal women reported more than twice the rate of violence reported by urban Aboriginal women, whereas urban non-Aboriginal women reported somewhat more violence than rural non-Aboriginal women (Brownridge, 2003). Aboriginal women were significantly more likely than non-Aboriginal women to report more severe forms of violence and to be murdered by their intimate partners (Statistics Canada, 2006).

IPV has significant consequences for women, children, families, and society: psychological (e.g., post-traumatic stress disorder, depression, anxiety, erosion of child's connection to family and culture), physical (e.g., injuries, health conditions, poor health), and economic (e.g., reduced economic and financial security, lost productivity, financial costs associated with health/mental health service use) (Campbell, 2002; Dahlberg & Krug, 2002; Rodgers, 1994; Statistics Canada, 2005; Thurston, Patten, & Lagendyk, 2006; Walmsley, 2005). The few studies exploring the impact of IPV in rural Canadian communities (Hornosty & Doherty, 2002; Martz & Saraurer, 2000; Thurston et al., 2006) have generally reported consequences similar to those reported in national studies. Chapter 11 in this volume offers an in-depth account of the trauma experiences of Aboriginal women in remote communities. Together these findings reveal the high cost of IPV and highlight the importance of addressing this significant health issue.

An Organizing Framework for Understanding IPV

The social ecological model (e.g., Bronfenbrenner, 1979) has been used as a framework to understand the complex interplay of individual, relationship, community, and societal factors influencing violence (e.g., Dahlberg & Krug, 2002). This model provides a framework for organizing and understanding multilevel factors within the R&N context relative to risk factors, barriers to services, and potential prevention and intervention strategies.

Risk Factors Associated with IPV

When considering risk factors, it is important to use caution in generalizing from one group to another, as studies with specific subgroups of women (e.g., rural, Aboriginal) in Canada are lacking. One author who explored risks for Aboriginal women concluded that risk factors generally operate in the same direction for Aboriginal and non-Aboriginal women but that many Aboriginal women experience more of the risk factors and the impact is generally greater. The author concluded that differences between Aboriginal and non-Aboriginal women on measured risk factors do not fully account for the significantly higher IPV prevalence rates for Aboriginal women, suggesting existing research has not identified and measured all relevant risk factors (Brownridge, 2003).

Individual

Current literature has identified young age (eighteen to twenty-four years), heavy drinking, and witnessing or experiencing violence as a child as factors associated with an increased risk of men abusing their female partner (MacMillan & Wathen, 2001; Rodgers, 1994; Statistics Canada, 2006). Factors associated with a woman's increased risk of experiencing IPV include young age (under twenty-five years), low socioeconomic status, less than high school education (except for Aboriginal women, among whom greater education is associated with increased risk [Brownridge, 2003]), unemployment, and witnessing abuse during childhood (MacMillan & Wathen, 2001; Rodgers, 1994; Romans, Forte, Cohen, Du Mont, & Hyman, 2007; Statistics Canada, 2006). Poor self-rated health and activity limitations are also associated with increased risk of IPV (Forte, Cohen, Du Mont, Hyman, & Romans, 2005; Romans et al., 2007).

A number of risk factors are over-represented in R&N communities, including low income, low educational attainment, and high unemployment (Canadian Institute for Health Information [CIHI], 2006; Nagarajan, 2004). Rural Canadians are more likely to report their health status as fair or poor (CIHI, 2006). Alcohol and substance abuse are more prevalent in some communities (Dell & Garabedian, 2003; Stockwell et al., 2007).

Relationship

Marital conflict, unequal status within the couple, partner's use of psychological or emotional abuse, being separated or in a common-law relationship, and having children in the home have been identified as relationship-level risk factors (MacMillan & Wathen, 2001; Romans et al., 2007; Statistics Canada, 2006; Wathen et al., 2007). Unwanted pregnancy, increased number of pregnancies, and increased number of stressful life events were associated with increased risk of abuse during pregnancy (MacMillan & Wathen, 2001). Canadian farm women have identified poor economic conditions, long hours of labour, high debt loads, and few solutions as additional triggers for family violence (Scott & VanDine, 1995).

It has also been suggested that traditional norms concerning marriage and the family and patriarchal attitudes that devalue and objectify women may be more prevalent in rural communities (e.g., Hornosty & Doherty, 2002; Leipert & Reutter, 1998). Although interviews with rural women who experienced IPV highlight the presence of patriarchal attitudes in rural Canada (e.g., Riddell, Ford-Gilboe, & Leipert, 2009), empirical data exploring rural and urban differences in such attitudes are lacking. Further, it is important to acknowledge that males can occupy traditional roles without engaging in inappropriate behaviour (Scott & VanDine, 1995).

Community

Poverty and weak community sanctions against IPV, such as fewer formal legal sanctions, fewer supports for women, and less moral pressure for neighbours to intervene, are commonly identified community-level risk factors for IPV (Heise & Garcia-Moreno, 2002). The exact relationship between poverty and IPV remains unclear. Poverty may contribute directly to increased risk of IPV, and it may have indirect influence through other factors such as hopelessness, overcrowding, stress, frustration, and sense of inadequacy, or by causing additional barriers for women who wish to change or leave violent relationships.

Within the R&N context, Canadian women generally have limited access to appropriate services, including physical and mental health care, justice, law enforcement, and shelters (Hornosty & Doherty, 2002; Leipert & Reutter, 1998; Taylor-Butts, 2007). Further, rural women have expressed concerns that service providers may be friends with the perpetrator or his family, which may contribute to providers' not taking complaints of violence seriously or may deter professionals and others in the community from offering help to the woman (Hornosty & Doherty, 2002). These factors may, in turn, be interpreted as representing weak community sanctions against IPV.

In her professional practice in small R&N communities, the first author has found the high prevalence of IPV in some communities has significant implications for the community's definition of abuse and norms regarding relationships. For example, in one small community where violence was quite prevalent, women often minimized their experiences of violence or did not perceive violence as abuse when compared with more extreme forms of IPV (e.g., those involving weapons) occurring in the community. Other women talked about how friends and family members discouraged them from leaving their violent partners by contrasting their experiences to more severe IPV and using this as a means of stressing 'how lucky' they were. Riddell and colleagues (2009) obtained similar feedback from rural women who had left abusive partners. Women spoke about exposure to statements supporting male power and control, including ones from their fathers supporting the abuser. Such comments amount to weak community sanctions against IPV and can lead women to believe they should stay with their violent partners.

Additional community-level factors have been suggested as determinants of IPV within Aboriginal communities (Bopp, Bopp, & Lane, 2003). These include such factors as the wellness of the community, including extent of healing from historical trauma; community leadership; public policy; the quality of relationships between community members and police; community awareness and vigilance; geographical and social isolation; and the spiritual and moral climate of the community.

Societal

The World Health Organization (WHO) identified traditional gender norms (e.g., the idea that men have economic and decision-making power in the household) and social norms supportive of violence (e.g., the idea that violence is an acceptable way of resolving conflict) as societal risk factors for IPV (Heise & Garcia-Moreno, 2002). According to the WHO, IPV is most prevalent in societies when women begin to assume non-traditional roles or enter the workforce. Within the Canadian context, the experience of colonization and the resulting historical trauma and social dislocation for Aboriginal people have been recognized as significant factors accounting for the higher prevalence rates of violence against Aboriginal women (Bopp et al., 2003; Brownridge, 2003; Ipsos-Reid, 2006). Present-day government policies and programs, the continued marginalization of Aboriginal people in society as a whole, and national and global trends that undermine Aboriginal community values and dynamics are identified as societal-level factors influencing violence against Aboriginal women (Bopp et al., 2003).

It has been argued that government policies and programs are not responsive to the unique economic, social service, and law enforcement challenges facing R&N communities (Hornosty & Doherty, 2002; Scott & VanDine, 1995). Canadian farm women expressed concern that limited understanding (e.g., mistaken beliefs about lack of violence in rural areas), negative stereotypes (e.g., viewing rural peoples as uneducated and resistant to change), and assumptions about farming made by the general public, professionals, policy developers, and service providers contribute to women's stress and act as barriers to effective solutions to IPV in rural areas (Scott & VanDine, 1995).

Barriers to Accessing Services in R&N Communities

In keeping with the social ecological model, it is important to consider factors within the R&N context that have potential to exacerbate the significant problems encountered by women in violent relationships and create additional barriers to accessing appropriate services or leaving the relationship. For example, geographic isolation can make it more difficult to access natural supports and make it easier to hide violence from others, which in turn can delay or prevent the intervention of others (Hornosty & Doherty, 2002). Women in R&N communities may be more fearful of experiencing serious harm or death due to the greater availability of guns (Doherty & Hornosty, 2007; Royal Canadian Mounted Police, 2002). This heightened fear together with the longer response time for emergency services (Hornosty & Doherty, 2002; Scott & VanDine, 1995) can have significant implications for a woman's willingness to access appropriate services. The small-town atmosphere and the greater availability of guns can also heighten fear about repercussions for leaving violent relationships, as women who choose to leave their relationship but remain in the community can be easily found by their partner (Martz & Sarauer, 2000). This fear is well justified, as research indicates that women who leave their partners remain at risk for violence, and in fact may experience an increase in the severity of violence (Rodgers, 1994).

Financial dependence on the perpetrator is often heightened in R&N communities due to limited employment opportunities. Poverty was identified as one of the most problematic factors for women from rural Saskatchewan leaving abusive relationships (Martz & Sarauer, 2000). Hornosty and Doherty (2002) reported that almost all of the women they interviewed from rural New Brunswick were financially dependent on their spouse, and many had never participated in the paid labour force. Financial dependence presented an additional challenge for those women because they did not have access to employment insurance, pensions, jobs, or job training.

Farm women are often in business with their partner, and leaving the relationship would essentially mean leaving their business (Hornosty & Doherty, 2002; Scott & VanDine, 1995). The emotional attachments farm women have to the farm and the animals are additional factors that may prevent women from leaving an abusive relationship (Scott & VanDine, 1995). Farm women from rural New Brunswick spoke about feeling re-victimized by service providers and urban women who made them feel guilty for not acting on their rights because of their attachment to the farm or farm animals (Hornosty & Doherty, 2002).

In many R&N communities affordable housing is often limited or lacking (Martz & Sarauer, 2000; see also chapter 12). The lack of women's shelters in R&N communities (Taylor-Butts, 2007) also has significant implications. As discussed in chapter 11, even when shelters are located in R&N communities, insufficient safeguards exist to promote a truly healing environment. As a result, many women are faced with having to leave their existing social support systems in order to access a women's shelter. This has significant implications for children, who may be forced to leave their friends and attend a new school. As discussed in chapter 12, frequent relocation may also erode sense of identity and family and peer supports. These concerns can influence a woman's decision to access shelter services. Women who do access urban shelters may perceive staff as being unaware of and insensitive to their unique experiences and find the services do not adequately meet their needs (Hornosty & Doherty, 2002).

Public transportation is often limited or unavailable in R&N communities, and this can affect a woman's ability to access formal services and social support or for her to physically leave a violent situation (Martz & Saraurer, 2000). Even if public transportation is available, limited services and shelters and a lack of awareness of services pose additional barriers to accessing appropriate services (Martz & Saraurer, 2000; Scott & VanDine, 1995).

Responding to IPV can be particularly problematic when the perpetrator is a prominent member of the community or has a personal relationship with service providers (Martz & Saraurer, 2000). The first author has observed this problem in her experience as a 'fly-in' therapist in a remote northern community. Women in the community often reported that having access to a counsellor who did not know their partner or reside in the community positively influenced their decision to access services.

Concerns about anonymity and confidentiality are frequently identified as barriers to accessing services in rural communities (Hornosty & Doherty, 2002). It has been the first author's experience that women in R&N communities may be fearful about professionals maintaining their confidence, particularly when the professional knows the perpetrator. Women might be fearful that their husband will find out that they are accessing services, either by seeing them enter the office or by having another community member see them and inform their husband. As discussed in chapter 11, cultural practices may also prevent Aboriginal women from discussing their partner with others, including professionals. The first author's experience further suggests that women who do access services may discontinue services prematurely if they become concerned about the service provider's safety.

Although this section has focused on community-level factors and their impact on relationship and individual factors, it is important to recognize the impact that societal factors (e.g., government policies and funding) have on many of these issues (e.g., availability of alternate housing, access to employment insurance).

Prevention and Intervention

Canadian anti-IPV policies and government spending focus mainly on criminal justice and public health approaches (Paterson, 2009). The criminal justice approach focuses on arrests and charges against perpetrators and provision of support and transition services for women experiencing violence. The public health approach is characterized by funding for research and awareness education, along with provision of prevention programs and services for women experiencing violence. These approaches have been criticized for focusing primarily on protection of women and for assuming that leaving the violent relationship is the only option available (Paterson, 2009). Rural women have reported using placating strategies with their violent partners, as part of an intentional, long-term approach in which they may take several years to accrue sufficient supports, resources, and sense of control before leaving abusive situations (Riddell et al., 2009). The 1999 General Social Survey revealed that many women experiencing violence relied solely on the support of friends (17%) and family (16%) to cope with and prevent further IPV, while 11% used public services such as shelters and only 7% called the police (Paterson, 2009). The low usage rates reported by women (Paterson, 2009; Riddell et al., 2009) are evidence that existing approaches are not meeting the needs of R&N women, and emphasize the need for policy reform to address barriers unique to R&N settings.

Well-designed, culturally targeted public awareness campaigns have been effective at informing and changing the public's attitude towards the problem of IPV, while also informing women experiencing IPV of available services (Campbell & Manganello, 2006). In the 1990s in Canada, a wide variety of programs, including public awareness campaigns, addressed the issue of violence against women (Du Mont, Forte, Cohen, Hyman, & Romans, 2005). These programs appear to have had a positive effect. In 1999, as compared to 1993, women were significantly more likely to have disclosed IPV, were more likely to know about available services, and were more likely to have accessed resources (Du Mont et al., 2005).

To date, most IPV prevention programs have targeted individuals and couples (Wathen & MacMillan, 2003). Because IPV often co-occurs with child abuse and because children who witness IPV are at increased risk of experiencing or perpetrating IPV as adults, these two types of abuse share common risk factors and developmental pathways (Capaldi, Kim, & Pears, 2009). Thus, teaching parents to use positive non-violent parenting practices (e.g., Triple P Program [Sanders, Markie-Dadds, & Turner, 2003]) would be expected to reduce the child's risk for IPV in adulthood. Similarly, school-based programs that promote empathy and social skills and reduce bullying and aggression (e.g., Roots of Empathy Program [Gordon, 2005]) would be expected to reduce risk of IPV. In fact, a recent BC coroner's jury recommended that all students from kindergarten to grade 12 receive programming focused on relationship skills to reduce IPV (British Columbia Ministry of Public Safety and Solicitor General, 2009).

Most IPV prevention efforts focus on dating and relationship skill development in adolescence (e.g., Fourth R Program [Wolfe et al., 2009]). Rigorous evaluation demonstrated that when delivered during Grade 9 health classes, the Fourth R Program reduced dating violence 2.5 years after participation in the program (Wolfe et al., 2009). The availability of programs such as Triple P, Roots of Empathy, and Fourth R varies widely across R&N communities in Canada, but these public health and school-based programs have the potential to be delivered in most communities.

Interventions for IPV have focused on both partners in the intimate relationship. The necessity of identifying appropriate resources for perpetrators is recognized in social ecological models (Bopp et al., 2003; Pauktuutit Inuit Women of Canada, 2006); however, because our focus is on women, interventions for perpetrators will not be addressed here. There has been very little peer-reviewed, empirical research regarding the effectiveness of IPV interventions, and much of what has been reported is either of poor quality or from non-rural or non-Canadian populations (e.g., Annan, 2008). The brief review that follows focuses on interventions that are available in or have been recommended for R&N Canada.

Routine IPV screening of all women during medical and mental health visits, regardless of the reason for the visit, has been recommended by some (Hornosty & Doherty, 2002; Wathen, Jamieson, & MacMillan, 2008). Screening has not been associated with any short-term harm (MacMillan et al., 2009), and may have some longer-term benefits with respect to influencing socio-cultural norms and reducing IPV in R&N Canada. However, there is insufficient evidence to recommend for or against routine screening (MacMillan et al., 2009). Instead, clinicians should ask questions about exposure to IPV as part of their diagnostic assessment of women displaying any indication of abuse (MacMillan & Wathen, 2001).

Women who receive counselling in shelters are likely to experience less violence post-shelter than women who go without counselling (Sullivan & Bybee, 1999; Sullivan, Campbell, Angelique, Eby, & Davidson, 1994; Wathen & MacMillan, 2003). The Canadian Network of

Women's Shelters & Transition Houses (http://endvaw.ca) offers an Internet-based support network providing regional, searchable links to shelters and other useful information and resources, including how to make an escape plan and tips to keep abusers from tracking Internet activity. There are other websites that provide similar resources.[1] Such resources will reach more women as Internet access becomes more widely available in isolated R&N communities.

Access to appropriate counselling services in R&N communities is often limited (Havelock, 2006). The University of Manitoba's R&N Psychology Program is an initiative aimed at increasing services for R&N residents, including those affected by IPV (Dyck, Cornock, Gibson, & Carlson, 2008). This program places clinical psychologists and pre- and post-doctoral residents in R&N Manitoba. As a member of this program, the first author has provided counselling and assessment services to women and children affected by IPV, facilitated Triple P groups, consulted with local clinicians working with those affected by IPV, and provided workshops to shelter staff.

Women in R&N communities who seek public services to deal with IPV report varying degrees of satisfaction. For example, some rural women have reported finding it helpful to speak with a physician or nurse whereas others reported feeling as though their problems were being medicated by doctors or that they were inappropriately referred to marriage counselling (Hornosty & Doherty, 2002; Riddell et al., 2009). Current research suggests rural women tend to find counselling services through domestic violence and mental health programs to be helpful (Martz & Sar, 2000; Riddell et al., 2009). However, women also reported instances where they felt re-victimized and blamed for the violence by counsellors and other professionals (Riddell et al., 2009). As discussed in chapter 11, fly-in counsellors, high staff turnover, and inexperienced or culturally incompetent counsellors pose additional challenges to women seeking support in remote communities. Going to a shelter, filing a petition for a protection order, and accessing legal aid are other strategies that have been rated as helpful by rural women. Interestingly, the perceived helpfulness of strategies such as placating and resisting appears to decrease as the intensity of the violence increases (Riddell et al., 2009).

Recommendations for Programming and Research

Consistent with the multilevel approach imbedded within the social ecological model, the WHO has recommended that IPV-specific programs integrate with youth violence and family support programs, and that access to informal sources of support such as community networks of safe havens (e.g., in private homes or churches) be enhanced (Heise & Garcia-Moreno, 2002). This is consistent with the collaborative inter-sectoral approach recommended for small communities in Canada (Thurston et al., 2006). Moreover, there are suggestions that access to private resources such as income, employment, and childcare be enhanced by community involvement programs that strengthen social networks. As highlighted in chapters 11 and 12, some women in some communities will benefit from such approaches, but others may not. At the same time, increased funding for shelters and transitional housing, reformed criminal justice policies, and policy changes to fund resistance programs should be made available, with acceptance that some women may choose to remain in their relationships and resist violence (Paterson, 2009).

Ultimately, R&N communities are unique, and each will require a unique approach (Health Canada, 1996; Stith, 2006).The most effective resources may be early intervention and prevention programs, and increased public awareness of the prevalence and consequences of IPV (Hornosty & Doherty, 2002; Mason & Pellizzari, 2006) such that sociocultural norms change (Heise & Garcia-Moreno, 2002). Programs such as Triple P, Roots of Empathy, and the Fourth R have shown promise and have the potential to be delivered in most R&N communities. Government policy changes are needed to address additional risk factors (e.g., unemployment, poverty) that may be commonplace in many R&N communities and to ensure that R&N women experiencing IPV have access to resources that are effective at preventing further abuse (Wuest, Ford-Gilboe, Merritt-Gray, & Lemire, 2006).

Considering the challenges related to unique features of R&N communities, such as weapon availability and limits on confidentiality and anonymity, all service providers working in those communities should be trained to respond carefully and sensitively to IPV in R&N contexts. Service providers, including doctors, nurses, social workers, teachers, and clergy, should be trained to ask about IPV in formal and informal settings (Hyman, Forte, Du Mont, Romans, & Cohen, 2009) and to provide discrete opportunities for disclosure (Riddell et al., 2009). They can help women manage risk (e.g., by promoting safe gun storage) and assist in accessing available resources (Hornosty & Doherty, 2002; Mason & Pellizzari, 2006; Nason-Clark, Holtmann, Fisher-Townsend, McMullen, & Ruff, 2009). Evaluation of short- and long-term benefits of screening and risk assessment should be supported in R&N communities adopting such strategies. Service providers should be held accountable for not responding or inappropriately responding when they are aware of IPV (Riddell et al., 2009).

Harper (2006) and Hornosty and Doherty (2002) have presented guidelines for Aboriginal communities and rural and farming communities, respectively; in both cases improving response times for emergency services and locating shelters or safe houses within easy access of potential users are considered critical. Riddell and colleagues' (2009) findings further stress the need to address systemic barriers that prevent R&N women from accessing services.

Conclusion

Clearly, the prevalence and consequences of IPV emphasize the need for evidence-based interventions to support women experiencing IPV. Risk factors for and mental health implications of IPV among subgroups of R&N Canadian women have yet to be evaluated (Wathen, Jamieson, & MacMillan, 2008). We need a better understanding of the internal and motivational stages of change that women traverse on their journeys to safety and healing (Burke, Mahoney, Gielen, McDonnell, & O'Campo, 2009). Well-designed studies are needed to evaluate the effectiveness of current prevention and intervention programs, to test supporting theories, to understand how to best educate and inform the public and encourage community support, and to identify strategies that will help women and service providers in R&N communities identify and respond to IPV (Mackay, 2008). Despite these needs, progress is being made and will continue with the efforts of researchers, practitioners, policy makers, and women themselves.

Notes

1 Further examples of available Internet resources are found at the following websites: Pauktuutit Inuit Women of Canada (http://www.pauktuutit.ca), International Directory of Domestic Violence Agencies (http://www.hotpeachpages.net/canada/canada1.html), and Public Health Agency of Canada (http://www.phac-aspc.gc.ca/hp-ps/index-eng.php).

References

Annan, S.L. (2008). Intimate partner violence in rural environments. *Annual Review of Nursing Research, 26*, 85–113.

Bopp, M., Bopp, J., & Lane, P. (2003). *Aboriginal domestic violence in Canada.* Ottawa: Aboriginal Healing Foundation.

British Columbia Ministry of Public Safety and Solicitor General (2009). *Verdict at Coroner's Inquest: File No: 2007:168:139/40/41/42/43* Retrieved from http://www.pssg.gov.bc.ca/coroners/schedule/docs/verdict-chun-park-lee-2009-dec-18.pdf.

Bronfenbrenner, U. (1979). *The ecology of human development.* Cambridge, MA: Harvard University Press.

Brownridge, D. (2003). Male partner violence against Aboriginal women in Canada. *Journal of Interpersonal Violence, 18*, 65–83.

Burke, J.G., Mahoney, P., Gielen, A., McDonnell, K.A., & O'Campo, P. (2009). Defining appropriate stages of change for intimate partner violence survivors. *Violence and Victims, 24*, 36–51.

Campbell, J. (2002). Health consequences of intimate partner violence. *The Lancet, 359*, 1331–6.

Campbell, J.C., & Manganello, J. (2006). Changing public attitudes as a prevention strategy to reduce intimate partner violence. *Journal of Aggression, Maltreatment & Trauma, 13*(3), 13–39.

Canadian Institute for Health Information (CIHI). (2006). *How healthy are rural Canadians? An assessment of their health status and health determinants.* Ottawa: Author. Retrieved from http://www.phac-aspc.gc.ca/publicat/rural06/pdf/rural_canadians_2006_report_e.pdf.

Capaldi, D.M., Kim, H.K., & Pears, K.C. (2009). The association between partner violence and child maltreatment: A common conceptual framework. In D.J. Whitaker & J.R. Lutzker (Eds.), *Preventing partner violence: Research and evidence-based intervention strategies* (pp. 93–111). Washington, DC: American Psychological Association.

Dahlberg, L.L., & Krug, E.G. (2002). Violence – A global public health problem. In E.G. Krug, L.L. Dahlberg, J.A. Mercy, A.B. Zwi, & R. Lozano (Eds.), *World report on violence and health* (pp. 2–21). Geneva: World Health Organization. Retrieved from http://whqlibdoc.who.int/publications/2002/9241545615_eng.pdf.

Dell, C.A., & Garabedian, L. (2003). *Canadian Community Epidemiology Network on Drug Use 2002 national report: Drug trends and the CCENDU Network.* Ottawa: Canadian Centre on Substance Abuse. Retrieved from http://www.ccsa.ca/2003%20and%20earlier%20CCSA%20Documents/CCENDU-National-2002-e.pdf.

Doherty, D., & Hornosty, J. (2007). *Exploring the links: Firearms, family violence, and animal abuse in rural communities. Executive summary.* Retrieved from http://www.crvawc.ca/documents/Exploring%20the%20Links%20 Firearms,%20Family%20Violence%20and%20Animal%20Abu.pdf.

Du Mont, J., Forte, T., Cohen, M.M., Hyman, I., & Romans, S. (2005). Changing help-seeking rates for intimate partner violence in Canada. *Women & Health, 4,* 1–19.

Dyck, K.G., Cornock, B.L., Gibson, G., & Carlson, A. (2008). Training clinical psychologists for rural and northern practice: Transforming challenge into opportunity. *Australian Psychologist, 43,* 239–48.

Forte, T., Cohen, M., Du Mont, J., Hyman, I., & Romans, S. (2005). Psychological and physical sequelae of intimate partner violence among women with limitations in their activities of daily living. *Archives of Women's Mental Health, 8,* 248–56.

Gordon, M. (2005). *Roots of empathy: Changing the world child by child.* Toronto: Thomas Allen.

Harper, A.H. (2006). *Ending violence in Aboriginal communities: Best practices in Aboriginal shelters and communities.* Ottawa: National Aboriginal Circle Against Family Violence.

Havelock, J. (2006, 8 May). Rural, remote, and northern women's mental health. In Ad Hoc Working Group on Women, Mental Health, Mental Illness and Addictions,*Women, mental health and mental illness and addiction in Canada: An overview* (pp. 42–5). Retrieved from http://www.cwhn.ca/ PDF/womenMentalHealth.pdf.

Health Canada. (1996). *Family violence in Aboriginal communities: An Aboriginal perspective.* Retrieved from http://www.phac-aspc.gc.ca/ncfv-cnivf/pdfs/ aborigin.pdf.

Heise, L., & Garcia-Moreno, C. (2002). Violence by intimate partners. In E.G. Krug, L.L. Dahlberg, J.A. Mercy, A.B. Zwi, & R. Lozano (Eds.), *World report on violence and health* (pp. 87–121). Geneva: World Health Organization. Retrieved from http://whqlibdoc.who.int/publications/2002/9241545615_ eng.pdf.

Hornosty, J., & Doherty, D. (2002). *Responding to wife abuse in farm and rural communities: Searching for solutions that work.* Retrieved from http://www.uregina.ca/sipp/documents/pdf/Regina%20revised% 202002.pdf.

Hyman, I., Forte, T., Du Mont, J., Romans, S., & Cohen, M.M. (2009). Help-seeking behaviour for intimate partner violence among racial minority women in Canada. *Women's Health Issues, 19,* 101–8.

Ipsos-Reid. (2006). *Aboriginal women and family violence final report.* Retrieved from http://publications.gc.ca/pub?id=324717&sl=0.

Leipert, B., & Reutter, L. (1998). Women's health and community health nursing practice in geographically isolated settings: A Canadian perspective. *Health Care for Women International, 19,* 575–88.

Mackay, K. (2008). To screen or not to screen: Identification of domestic violence in Canadian emergency departments. *Canadian Journal of Emergency Medicine, 10,* 329–30.

MacMillan, H.L., & Wathen, C.N. (2001). *Prevention and treatment of violence against women: Systematic review and recommendations* (CTFPHC technical report no. 01-4). London, ON: Canadian Task Force on Preventive Care.

MacMillan, H.L., Wathen, C.N., Jamieson, E., Boyle, M.H., Shannon, H.S., Ford-Gilboe, M., Worster, A., Lent, B., Coben, J.H., Campbell, J.C., & McNutt, L.-A. (2009). Screening for intimate partner violence in health care settings: A randomized trial. *Journal of the American Medical Association, 302,* 493–501.

Martz, D.J.F., & Saraurer, D.B. (2000). *Domestic violence and the experiences of rural women in East Central Saskatchewan.* Retrieved from http://www.pwhce.ca/pdf/domestic-viol.pdf.

Mason, R., & Pellizzari, R. (2006). Guidelines, policies, education and coordination: Better practices for addressing violence against women. *Canadian Woman Studies, 25*(1/2), 20–5.

Nagarajan, K. (2004). Rural and remote community health care in Canada: Beyond the Kirby Panel Report, the Romanow Report and the federal budget of 2003. *Canadian Journal of Rural Medicine, 9,* 245–51.

Nason-Clark, N., Holtmann, C., Fisher-Townsend, B., McMullen, S., & Ruff, L. (2009). The RAVE Project: Developing web-based religious resources for social action on domestic abuse. *Critical Social Work, 10*(1). Retrieved from http://cronus.uwindsor.ca/units/socialwork/critical.nsf/main/E193B211B874DBFD852575E70022A92B?OpenDocument.

Paterson, S. (2009). (Re)Constructing women's resistance to woman abuse: Resources, strategy choice and implications of and for public policy in Canada. *Critical Social Policy, 29,* 121–45.

Pauktuutit Inuit Women of Canada. (2006). *National strategy to prevent abuse in Inuit communities and sharing knowledge, sharing wisdom: A guide to the national strategy.* Ottawa: Author.

Riddell, T., Ford-Gilboe, M., & Leipert. B. (2009). Strategies used by rural women to stop, avoid, or escape from intimate partner violence. *Health Care for Women International, 30*(1/2), 134–59.

Rodgers, K. (1994). Wife assault: The findings of a national survey. *Juristat, 14*(9), 1–21.

Romans, S., Forte, T., Cohen, M., Du Mont, J., & Hyman, I. (2007). Who is most at risk for intimate partner violence? A Canadian population-based study. *Journal of Interpersonal Violence, 22,* 1495–1514.

Royal Canadian Mounted Police. (2002). *Urban and rural firearm deaths in Canada*. Retrieved from http://www.rcmp-grc.gc.ca/cfp-pcaf/res-rec/urb-eng.htm.

Sanders, M.R., Markie-Dadds, C., & Turner, K.M.T. (2003). *Theoretical, scientific and clinical foundations of the Triple P – Positive Parenting Program: A population approach to the promotion of parenting competence* (Parenting Research and Practice Monograph no. 1). St. Lucia, Australia: University of Queensland, Parenting and Family Support Centre. Retrieved from http://www.gov .mb.ca/triplep/for_practitioners/articles.html.

Scott, W., & VanDine, C. (1995). *Family violence in rural, farm, and remote Canada*. Fredericton: Canadian Farm Women's Network.

Statistics Canada. (2005). *Family violence in Canada: A statistical profile 2005* (Catalogue no. 85-224-XIE). Ottawa: Minister of Industry.

Statistics Canada. (2006). *Measuring violence against women: Statistical trends 2006* (Catalogue no. 85-570-XIE). Ottawa: Minister of Industry.

Stith, S.M. (2006). Introduction. *Journal of Aggression, Maltreatment & Trauma, 13*(3), 1–12.

Stockwell, T., Pakula, B., Macdonald, S., Buxton, J., Zhao, J., Tu, A., Reist, D., Thomas, G., Puri, A., & Duff, C. (2007). *Alcohol consumption in British Columbia and Canada: A case for liquor taxes that reduce harm* (CARBC Statistical Bulletin no. 3). Victoria: University of Victoria. Retrieved from http://carbc.ca/portals/0/resources/AlcoholBulletin0712.pdf.

Sullivan, C.M., & Bybee, D.I. (1999). Reducing violence using community-based advocacy for women with abusive partners. *Journal of Consulting and Clinical Psychology, 67*, 43–53.

Sullivan, C.M., Campbell, R., Angelique, H., Eby, K.K., & Davidson, W.S., II. (1994). An advocacy intervention program for women with abusive partners: Six-month follow-up. *American Journal of Community Psychology, 22*, 101–22.

Taylor-Butts, A. (2007). Canada's shelters for abused women, 2005/2006. *Juristat, 27*(4), 1–20. Retrieved from http://www.statcan.gc.ca/pub/85-002-x/85-002-x2007004-eng.pdf.

Thurston, W., Patten, S., & Lagendyk, L. (2006). Prevalence of violence against women reported in a rural health region. *Canadian Journal of Rural Medicine, 11*, 259–67.

Walmsley, C. (2005). *Protecting Aboriginal children*. Vancouver: UBC Press.

Wathen, C.N., Jamieson, E., & MacMillan, H.L. (2008). Who is identified by screening for intimate partner violence? *Women's Health Issues, 18*, 423–32.

Wathen, C.N., Jamieson, E., Wilson, M., Daly, M., Worster, A., & MacMillan, H.L. (2007). Risk indicators to identify intimate partner violence in the emergency department. *Open Medicine, 1*, 113–22. Retrieved from http:// www.openmedicine.ca/article/view/63/62.

Wathen, C.N., & MacMillan, H.L. (2003). Interventions for violence against women: Scientific review. *Journal of the American Medical Association, 289,* 589–600.

Wolfe, D.A., Crooks, C., Jaffe, P., Chiodo, D., Hughes, R., Ellis, W., Stitt, L., & Donner, A. (2009). A school-based program to prevent adolescent dating violence: A cluster randomized trial. *Archives of Pediatrics and Adolescent Medicine, 163,* 692–9.

Wuest, J., Ford-Gilboe, M., Merritt-Gray, M., & Lemire, S. (2006). Using grounded theory to generate a theoretical understanding of the effects of child custody policy on women's health promotion in the context of intimate partner violence. *Health Care for Women International, 27,* 490–512.

11 There's a Nightmare in the Closet!: Post-traumatic Stress Disorder as a Major Health Issue for Women Living in Remote Aboriginal Communities

Beverly Illauq

Post-traumatic stress disorder (PTSD) is being referred to more frequently than ever before by this generation of health practitioners in rural and northern Canada and by their research counterparts. The author believes that this is a reflection of a more informed health system as much as it is a result of more circumspect inquiry into the serious and tenacious social and medical ills that are endemic to remote Aboriginal communities, particularly in Canada's North.

In an effort to increase awareness of both the prevalence and the intensity of PTSD amongst women in remote Aboriginal communities, I have chosen to write an auto-ethnography from a qualitative research perspective in order to better expose the reader to a personal experience of the multiple layers of PTSD resident in one family of one small Arctic settlement. Gleaned from over thirty-five years' experience living as a wife and mother of an Inuit family and working in remote Aboriginal communities in northern Quebec and what is now Nunavut, the content of this article reflects real events in real time. It is for the reader to allow this interior view of complex PTSD to inform future perceptions about the role of traumatic response in the delivery and efficacy of health services delivery to women living in remote Aboriginal communities.

Background

It was a comment that I had heard often in the school staffroom: 'She could do so well, if only ...,' followed by one of the stock rejoinders: if only she would leave that jerk; if only she stopped drinking; if only she would do something for herself; if only she'd get her act together; if only she weren't so slow. As an educator and a mother in an Inuit family in our remote Arctic community, I have often been stung by comments such as these.

We professionals from southern Canada so quickly judge the young women, the mothers, and the elderly living in our country's remote Aboriginal communities. *Mea culpa!* I too used to walk into a classroom and critically broad-brush my students and their families.

Then I married into the community and began, myself, to live the daily dramas that inevitably unfold that are the trauma fallout of accelerated colonization. And I fell silent. I could not pass verdict on my relatives as I drank tea and listened to a litany of deaths from an elder, or washed dishes in the house of a neighbour whose son had just been murdered, or listened intently to the high-frequency radio detailing the overturned boat and the figure, that I hoped was my husband, crouched on the beach.

At times I lashed out in defence of myself and our community, from the agony of my soul. But more often I too began numbly buying into the myth that I should 'just get over it.' Finally, like so many other women in the 1990s, after fifteen years of freezing them out, I began to seek answers to the questions that would not go away: Why do I feel this way? Why can't I (professional woman that I am) do life properly? What hope is there for my children? What's wrong with our family? Why are my children trying to commit suicide?

These questions were the leading edge of a healing journey that has led me to understand my own 'nightmare in the closet,' my own post-traumatic stress disorder. In healing, I have been able to tame that set of monsters and shadows that plague individuals exposed to extreme, interconnected, and complex levels of trauma; a set of monsters and shadows that fragment our personalities, our lives, our families, and our communities. I wish to share my findings in this chapter as we look at the unique relationship women in remote Aboriginal communities have with trauma, and particularly with post-trauma response.

A Turning Point

The news was electrifying. An Inuit mother in our community had been found by a family member hanged in her closet. I remember exactly where I was sitting in our kitchen with my infant son on my lap when the news was delivered. It was shocking. Just the day before she and I had been talking at the store about our babies. An acute trauma response set in and I woodenly tried to continue

with life, I and approximately half of the community of six hundred in our re-
mote Inuit settlement. For three days, until the funeral was over, the seasonal
Christmas celebrations were suspended. Visiting, subdued talk, sessions of pri-
vate and public weeping, and all kinds of speculation replaced the usual rau-
cous community games, and a round-the-clock watch was set up at the family
home where the suicide had occurred. In time, we all went back home, but we
did not forget. Each birthday that came and went, each celebration in her
daughter's life as it unfolded, each person named for her, reminded us poi-
gnantly of this woman's tragedy.

This vignette accurately describes my first direct encounter, as a
teacher in a remote Aboriginal community, with acute PTSD resulting
from suicide. I remember finding the weight of the incident particularly
difficult to bear. Suicide in any culture is an unfathomable tragedy. It is
a signal that life has become extremely cumbersome or lonely, dark or
fragmented, and leaves in its wake family and friends reeling from feelings of guilt, grief, and anger. As a southern Canadian, I had experienced the suicide of a classmate in high school, and as an adult had
shared the grief of friends whose son had shot himself. But they had
both been young men, and their suicides were relatively isolated incidents in relatively stable southern communities. This woman, however,
was an integral member of our family, a mother (by definition in Inuit
tradition a community nurturer and care giver), a sister, and a cousin of
over two hundred people who were grieving her death. This was the
death of a person who, with all of us, was a survivor of many past traumas, both present and intergenerational, who had chosen to exit the
survival bond that had so carefully been fostered in order to survive
previous scenarios of violence and accident. For me as a southern professional, the incident was unconscionable and the response to this suicide in our remote Aboriginal community was beyond comprehension.
It left me with two key questions I have heard echoed many times by
other Aboriginal and non-Aboriginal teachers, medical personnel, civil
servants, and service providers: What is happening here? and Why?

What Is Happening Here?

PTSD-Level Trauma

At the time when the above vignette occurred, in the mid-1980s, trauma
was largely a medical term, associated with the lacerations, broken
bones, and concussions of hospital emergency rooms. Recently, how-

ever, trauma has come to be more commonly associated with its second definition, that of 'an emotional shock that has lasting effects on the victim' (Gage Canadian Dictionary, 1983), and is becoming a word generally equated with intense stress.

I discovered the term 'PTSD' quite by accident, and that discovery became for me and my family the way out of a downward spiral towards death. In 1995, my hunter and outfitter husband was in a tragic boating accident in which tourists lost their lives. I found it extremely difficult to deal with my husband's violent dreams, sleeplessness, crying spells, driven morbidity, binge drinking, and angry outbursts. I reached out to the settlement's health centre for help. I was told that it was his problem, and that I had nothing to do with it. However, it *was* my problem; my husband's behaviour was jeopardizing the safety of our family. I was desperate. A referral from the Regional Department of Health resulted in a conversation with a navy medic in Halifax. It was he who informed me that I was not going crazy, and that there was a name for the chaos that we were dealing with: post-traumatic stress disorder. This conversation marked the beginning of a quest to heal our family from multiple and complex layers of PTSD.

Parameters of PTSD

Today many descriptions of PTSD exist and each, whether formal or informal, can help a PTSD survivor further describe and clarify what is happening to her or to a loved one suffering from this mental disorder. The *DSM-IV* (American Psychiatric Association, 1994), however, provides a definitive clinical explanation of PTSD and defines criteria for diagnosis. In section 309.81 it lists fifteen possible stress experiences that have been found to precipitate PTSD, starting with military combat and ending with 'learning that one's child or spouse has a life-threatening disease.' Interestingly, two of the other stress experiences cited,, 'learning about the sudden, unexpected death of a family member or a close friend' and 'childhood sexual molestation or abuse,' were factors in the above suicide vignette. The *DSM-IV* also makes a statement of symptoms, specifically that:

> characteristic symptoms [follow] exposure to an extreme traumatic stressor involving direct personal experience of an event that involves actual or threatened death or serious injury, or other threat to one's physical integrity; or witnessing an [extreme traumatic] event ... of another person; or learning about ... [an extreme traumatic event] ... experienced by a

family member or other close associate (Criterion A1). The person's response to the event must involve intense fear, helplessness, or horror (or in children, the response must involve disorganized or agitated behaviour) (Criterion A2). The characteristic symptoms … include persistent re-experiencing of the traumatic event (Criterion B), persistent avoidance of stimuli associated with the trauma and numbing of general responsiveness (Criterion C), and persistent symptoms of increased arousal (Criterion D). The full symptom picture must be present for more than 1 month (Criterion E), and the disturbance must cause clinically significant distress or impairment in social, occupational, or other important areas of functioning (Criterion F). (DSM-IV, sec. 309.81)

It is clear that the suicide vignette described above fits the *DSM-IV* PTSD definition. The first criterion of exposure, the second of a response of horror, helplessness, and fear, and the third of persistent re-experiencing of the traumatic event were all immediately evident in the following players in the drama: the person who found the victim; other family members and friends; anyone who had spoken with the victim over the past week (approximately two hundred people); and the child of the victim. Furthermore, the victim herself, who was the victim of recurrent child and adult sexual abuse, likely experienced these symptoms.

The fourth criterion, the avoidance and numbing of stimuli associated with the trauma, the fifth of increased arousal, or hyper-vigilance, and the sixth of symptom persistence for more than one month were more evident in some involved with the suicide than others. Interestingly, my own symptoms related to this trauma persisted for years. I was unable to process this death fully until twenty years later, after I had been safely away from the location of the death for four years and had psychological support in place to process the trauma completely.

The seventh criterion, of disturbance 'in social, occupational, or other important areas of functioning,' is much harder to assess, because of the multiple layers of trauma that previously and subsequently aggravated the effect of this suicide in the community. These trauma layers included other suicides, several other assaults, including ongoing sexual abuse and domestic violence, and unexpected deaths. Clearly, then, even though it was not identified as such at the time, this suicide triggered a widespread PTSD response in the whole community, that manifested itself in many forms of dysfunction, primarily at the individual level but also at the levels of family and community.

Unpredictability of Trauma Response

In order to fully understand PTSD as a health issue for women in remote communities, we must also understand the unpredictability of trauma response. To the same traumatic incident, some individuals respond hardly at all and seemingly forget the incident, while others react 'acutely' with symptoms surfacing in their lives immediately. Still others, and particularly children, experience what the *DSM-IV* terms 'PTSD with Delayed Onset,' where symptoms resulting from the incident become a problem for trauma survivors at least six months and sometimes years later. For some witnesses, PTSD-type behaviours and reactions will dissipate quite quickly, whereas for others the problem does not 'just go away' and becomes chronic and sometimes progressively debilitating. Although many studies have been conducted, the factors controlling this kind of unpredictability are still unclear. The *DSM-IV* simply states, 'The likelihood of developing this disorder may increase as the intensity of and physical proximity to the stressor increase' (sec. 309.81). Given the close-knit nature of Aboriginal communities where family and kinship ties are so important and so strong, and where abusers and victims live within the same small community, it is possible that whole communities are almost continually struggling with multiple layers and various intensities of PTSD, making it very challenging to establish effective and lasting treatment programs.

The *DSM-IV* further states, 'The disorder may be especially severe or long lasting when the stressor is of human design (e.g., torture, rape)' (sec. 309.81). Our Elders Committee members once told me they perceived that at least 85% of our community's members had been sexually assaulted. A study published in 2008 indicates that 'almost half of sexually abused girls experience Post-traumatic Stress Disorder' (Bernard-Bonnin, Hébert, Daignault, & Allard-Dansereau, 2008, p. 479). Thus, it would seem clear that there is a correlation between the pandemic nature of both sexual assault and PTSD in at least some remote Aboriginal communities.

Primary, Secondary, and Tertiary Traumatization

In my lived experience, and corroborated by Matsakis (1996), there are at least two levels of traumatization, primary and secondary, and I believe that there is a tertiary level of traumatization as well. Because of the interconnectedness of Aboriginal communities, these three levels must be considered in order to understand the prevalence of PTSD in remote communities.

It is clear that anyone who has been a victim of domestic violence, sexual assault, or a vehicular accident will suffer primary traumatization, by being the direct object of the traumatic stressor. Primary traumatization can clearly lead to chronic PTSD, with all of its symptoms – dreams, social disconnections, and increased arousal and vigilance – as well as its accompanying personality disorders. Secondary traumatization is more elusive, but nevertheless produces traumatic response in people. Sometimes called 'Compassion Fatigue' (Figley, 1995), secondary trauma refers to the sympathetic trauma response one experiences due to involvement with the victim, particularly as a primary care giver. Given the nurturing role traditionally assigned to women, this level of trauma can be even more overwhelming than primary trauma for mothers in Aboriginal families, particularly in families with intergenerational issues of abuse, addictions, and unresolved grief. In the suicide vignette, both primary and secondary traumatization were clearly present.

There is also another level of traumatization that I believe bears attention. Although I have not seen it mentioned in traumatic stress literature, I have observed a third level of trauma, or tertiary trauma, in Aboriginal communities in particular. It is my opinion that given the interrelatedness of Aboriginal communities, individuals are also traumatized when they simply hear of the sudden death or injury of someone in their own or in another community, no matter how close the relationship. This occurs, for example, when a rescue is underway, and people with the rescue channel installed on their high-frequency radios are able to listen to detailed proceedings of the rescue, with the effect that one is vicariously present at the accident scene and participates at some level in the recovery procedures. Tertiary trauma is also experienced by those who were not part of the incident but who become vicariously present at the trauma scene simply through a retelling of the event. In some cases it appears that rampant self-destructive or numbing behaviours, such as substance abuse, clinical depression, or attempted suicide, follow incidents of such tertiary traumatization.

Victimization

One final aspect of PTSD-level trauma that seriously affects women must be acknowledged here, that of victimization. Matsakis (1996)

identifies three levels of victimization that operate in traumatized individuals: the shattering of assumptions, secondary wounding, and
victim thinking. Matsakis indicates that victims of a traumatic event
suffering from PTSD are not only struggling to regain equilibrium on a
personal level, but are also often struggling with equilibrium at a societal level and are often re-victimized by people around them. Sadly,
often members of the helping professions, who in frustration tell them,
'Just get over it already!', impose further disconnection and its subsequent isolation on the trauma victim.

With the suicide of our relative, I experienced all three levels of victimization. My previously held assumptions that this small Inuit ham-
let was idyllic and safe were shattered within minutes of being informed
of the death; this was first-level victimization. I experienced secondary
wounding as well. Secondary wounding can emerge as denial, minimi-
zation, justification, or blame from a friend, relative, health care worker,
or other helping professional. My southern family members commiser-
ated with me for a day or two, then questioned why I was so sad about
the incident and mocked the slow-down in the community resulting
from the suicide. Finally, I also struggled with 'victim thinking' when I
began excusing my own dysfunction with details of the demise of this
one suicide victim and other members of my family.

The Extent of PTSD-level Trauma
in Remote Aboriginal Communities

I feel that very few people understand the extent of PTSD-level trauma
in remote Aboriginal communities. In 2006, when I began to seek ag-
gressive medical help for my twenty-one-year-old son who was suffering from complex PTSD, a cross-country search revealed two Canadian
centres that were equipped to treat PTSD in military personnel and
only one centre that would treat trauma disorder in civilians, that is,
University of British Columbia Hospital. Unfortunately, when the intake worker heard the trauma history of my son, she commented that
the centre was equipped to deal with clients with one to a maximum of
three concurrent traumas but not clients with PTSD as complex as that
of my son. She referred to other young Aboriginal males who presented
similar compounded PTSD and whom the clinic found nearly impossible to treat.

For many years I too simply survived, assuming that the chaotic patterns that were entrenched in our family's life through trauma were

normal. After all, other Inuit families experienced much the same things on a regular basis. Finally, by moving away to safety, I had opportunity to reflect on the various layers of trauma in my own life.

To describe for the reader how much trauma a woman in a remote Aboriginal community generally accommodates, I refer to my own lived experience. As a teacher, a counsellor, and a mother in an Inuit hunting family over the past twenty-five years, my experience is, if anything, less trauma filled than the lives of Aboriginal women who have lived their whole lives in a remote community. Elders, for example, seem to have no end of stories that deal with traumatic incidents, through which they have survived, although not always thrived.

Ours is an Inuit family of eight people consisting of an Inuk father (hunter, outfitter, guide, Canadian Ranger), age fifty-six; a Caucasian mother (teacher, counsellor, Wellness Centre coordinator), age fifty-five; a son, age twenty-four; an oldest daughter, age twenty-one; a middle daughter, age seventeen; a youngest daughter, age twelve; the son's spouse, Inuk, age twenty-three; a grandson (son's child), age five; and a granddaughter, (oldest daughter's child), age fifteen months. In many ways, our family's profile is typical of Aboriginal families: grandchildren living within their grandparents' household; family members transferring between their remote home community and a southern urban setting; and a family in which the mother worked full time to fund the father's hunting equipment and supplies, until such time as she became too ill to do so. I had moved to the North to work as a teacher, met my husband, and had gladly become an Inuit family member.

While studies show lifetime prevalence rates for PTSD ranging from 1–14%, studies of at-risk individuals have yielded higher prevalence rates ranging from 3–58% (*DSM-IV*, sec. 309.81). I submit that most women living in remote Aboriginal communities have much higher rates of PTSD than most individuals living in southern Canadian urban centres. For example, by age fifty-five I had experienced twenty-eight primary PTSD-level traumas. Various childhood experiences and teenage rape had initiated my PTSD symptoms and made the chaos of a trauma-infested lifestyle seem normal. However, most of the PTSD-level traumas that I have experienced, including personal assault, multiple suicides, searches for missing family members, and serious vehicular incidents, have occurred within the context of my role as a woman in an Aboriginal family. By comparison, family members, friends, and associates in southern Canada can sometimes identify two or three traumatic events over the course of their own lives, and very few can understand the PTSD-level traumas that my family members contend with on a daily basis.

In addition, I have experienced innumerable secondary and tertiary traumas as a result of dealing with events (even more extreme than my own) experienced by my husband and my older children. For example, when I discovered that our three oldest children had been sexually molested by multiple abusers at babysitters' homes, it was deeply disturbing and interfered with my parenting at many levels. I responded, not by binge drinking or gambling, but by immersing myself in busy-ness, working full time as a teacher, operating three businesses concurrently, and sitting on several committees, all while mothering four young children.

In regard to levels of trauma in younger women, it is helpful to review the trauma profile of our eldest daughter. By the age of thirteen, when she left the community, our daughter had experienced innumerable traumas including repeated sexual abuse, involving twelve adults, and the suicides of seventeen friends/cousins. She had been the driver in two serious snowmobile accidents and had been in several life-threatening situations while camping with our family. She had also dealt with such secondary traumas as witnessing domestic violence on a regular basis and having her father rescued six times, and her brother once, from the Arctic Ocean by the Coast Guard.

Although I did not understand it at the time, I recognize now that our daughter was experiencing a great deal of disorder resulting from the layers of trauma that had built up in her life by the time she was a young teenager. At the time, I was so numb to the dysfunction within our family, so out of order myself, and so busy surviving hour by hour in a household that was in daily chaos, that I did not 'catch on' until it was almost too late; it was only when my daughter was trying to commit suicide that I awoke to the fact that our community was toxic for her. Along with my son's first two suicide attempts, this helped me realize that our family was dysfunctional and needed immediate and effective help. Finally, my pain was so great that it overcame the fear and numbness that manifest as PTSD symptoms. It was at that point that I left my husband to heal with his own people and took our children to a southern urban centre to embark on a seven-year healing journey back into a reasonably functional family life.

Emotional and Mental Manifestations of PTSD

Given these levels of trauma, is it any wonder that so many women in remote Aboriginal communities manifest emotional, mental, and social disorders? Since I was diagnosed with PTSD seven years ago, I have accessed the care of over thirty health professionals to heal my own 'fragmented drivers.' I have been diagnosed with, and have had to work through, a variety of psychological, emotional, and psycho-somatic symptoms and conditions, including excessive irritability and rage and the resulting impairment of relationships with others. Depression, anxiety disorder, insomnia, flashbacks, hyper-vigilance – the list of my own challenges reads much the same as the Associated Features and Disorders list for PTSD (*DSM-IV*, sec. 309.81). However, through many healing modalities, I have learned to recognize the triggering of the PTSD nightmare. I now know how to gently ground my emotions and thinking to continue life with restored relationships and without the rage, hyper-vigilance, and depression that have sat on my shoulder for years.

I recall that before I began my healing journey, when I was still in denial that anything was wrong, I generally put up a good front, although I would clean wildly, teach like crazy, work through the nights, kick the dog, and mother at arms' length. Taking the PTSD nightmare out of the closet was 'not pretty' and was very expensive, and most of all it took huge amounts of energy just to survive through this time when I was learning again how to live. The good news is that with persistence, prayer, and a wide variety of resources I was able to heal to the point that I am now, again, a reasonably functional human being, with a will to live and to work.

Physical Manifestations of PTSD

Although a growing body of research links PTSD to poor physical health, the National Centre for PTSD at the US Department of Veterans Affairs reports that 'existing research has not been able to determine conclusively that PTSD causes poor health' (Jankowsi, 2009). However, in my lived experience in the Canadian Arctic, I have observed that there are a variety of ways that PTSD, and perhaps more specifically the traumas underlying PTSD, affect the health of women living in remote communities.

The most common trauma-related ailment requiring medical intervention may be 'nonspecific pain,' manifesting in headache, stomach and abdominal pain, and a variety of musculoskeletal pains that cannot be attributed to injury or a specific disease process. Breathing difficulties, traditionally associated with fear and with unexpressed emotion, are very common amongst women in northern communities, along with auto-immune diseases such as arthritis, eczema, psoriasis, and Type I diabetes mellitus. In addition, substance abuse is a prevalent health problem in remote communities as men, women, and children endeavour to self-medicate against their many physical and emotional symptoms. For example, 58% of Inuit are heavy smokers, as compared with 17% of all Canadians, and have the highest rate of lung cancer in the world (Tait, 2006, p. 14, sec. 4.1.4). Given that smoking is the most common drug being used to 'calm the nerves,' there is a clear correlation between trauma and illnesses resulting from substance abuse.

It is interesting to note that for the three young women in my own family, personal healing work has had a big impact on their rates of illness; all three have been able to stop drinking, have had their symptoms of daily headache syndrome resolved, and have experienced improved intestinal health as their lives have calmed down and their PTSD symptoms have dissipated. It is my observation that when PTSD is addressed as an underlying cause of illness, the stress on medical services decreases significantly.

Why Is PTSD Such a Major Health Issue?

Questions echo around northern communities, from staff rooms to legislatures: what has happened to the women of remote Aboriginal communities? Why can't women who live in Aboriginal communities just 'kick out the jerk' or 'get their lives together'? Why are suicides and addictions such a problem for so many women in remote communities? More specifically, the question is: why is PTSD such a major health issue for women, for women in Aboriginal communities, and especially for women in *remote* Aboriginal communities? Although it is beyond the scope of this chapter to address this problem thoroughly, I submit the following observations as a starting point for future discussions.

We Are Women

Just by virtue of being women, we are more prone to a PTSD response to trauma. The American Psychological Association states, 'Research indicates that women are twice as likely to develop Posttraumatic Stress Disorder (PTSD), experience a longer duration of posttraumatic symptoms, and display more sensitivity to stimuli that remind them of the trauma' (American Psychological Association, n.d.). Clearly, women anywhere, remote Aboriginal areas included, need to be attended by health professionals who have a good knowledge of PTSD, not only for purposes of diagnosis of this disorder but also for guidance through treatment.

Although men are also victims of domestic violence, it is well known that the majority of physical domestic violence victims are women. Furthermore, a social worker who teaches a Domestic Violence Victim Resource Group in Regina estimates that at least 95% of all victims of domestic violence were previously victims of sexual abuse (I. Klassen, Family Services Regina, personal communication, 6 Feb. 2007). This indicates that domestic violence survivors are most often multiply traumatized women. Given the high rates of both domestic violence and sexual assault crime in remote northern communities, it is clear that women in these areas are bound to exhibit higher rates of PTSD than their male counterparts.

The fact that women are known as the nurturers and care givers also makes them more vulnerable to trauma, particularly through secondary traumatization. In hunting cultures in particular, men are often subject to dangerous activities, resulting in shooting accidents, wilderness travel accidents, and extreme weather conditions. Even if a young spouse is present, it is most often up to the mother or grandmother to take on the role of primary care giver if an accident does occur, sometimes to the detriment of her own health and the well-being of her children.

As the partners of men whose identity has been so badly eroded by the effect of colonization, women also bear the burden of at once being both the counsellor and champion and at times the 'beating post' or sex object of men who suffer from chronic PTSD as a result of residential school abuse or other forms of trauma they have encountered. Typically, a woman in a relationship with such a man defers to her spouse's dysfunction, is often co-dependent to his addictive behaviours, and stays with the father of her children because leaving is too frightening to consider. Indeed, co-dependence has become an addiction diagnosis itself, and in some jurisdictions is treated as seriously as alcoholism and drug addiction. It is clear, then, that women, especially those living in Aboriginal communities where cultural erosion is rampant, are at risk of developing PTSD just by virtue of fulfilling their role as women in the community.

We Have Aboriginal Traditions and Histories

Aboriginal cultural traditions also have a direct bearing on the levels of PTSD experienced by women in remote communities. It is clear that family and kinship ties are extremely strong in both the First Nations and Inuit cultures, not only through blood relationships but also through naming relationships. While this fact is the backbone of Aboriginal societal values, it is clear that being intimately involved with so many people in a community can lead to much higher rates of traumatization. A suicide, for example, deeply affects not only the close family members of the victim, but also all extended family members in the home community, and members in all communities where the victim is known or has distant relatives, or has kinship ties because of naming traditions.

Levels of intergenerational trauma can also be more deeply ingrained in Aboriginal communities than in non-Aboriginal ones. It could be said that the collective memory that gives birth to rich oral histories also intensifies traumatization, writing traumas indelibly into the intergenerational stories and making the effects of the trauma much harder to forget as a society. This is perhaps one reason why residential school abuse is so hard to heal within second-, third-, and fourth-generation survivors.

Another significant factor in Aboriginal communities that contributes to high trauma levels, and so to high PTSD levels, is the number of pandemics that swept through Aboriginal camps and settlements early last century. The survivors of these epidemics, many of whom are now elders, often suffered serious levels of PTSD, without diagnosis and with very little treatment available. Parents who had thus suffered often passed on trauma-induced behaviour patterns to their children, such as insomnia, depression, addictions, or disorder and abuse in family and kinship patterns. Unfortunately, this scenario is more common than not, and affects women just as much as if not more than men because of the nurturing and care-giving role that women play.

An Aboriginal tradition that feeds the PTSD 'nightmare in the closet' is the taboo against talking about others, and one's spouse in particular; my mother-in-law, for example, instructed me that if I talked about my husband to anyone, I would be giving his life away. As a result of this deeply ingrained moral code, many women in Aboriginal communities, myself included, have been unable to talk to anyone about their traumas and have chosen self-destructive behaviours instead, such as suicide, substance abuse, and other addictions. Such customs are not easily changed. Healing programs must address these underlying issues, such as breaking the silence to end the violence, in a culturally sensitive way, and not seek simply to stop domestic violence or alcohol

and drug abuse. Unless long-term, culturally appropriate, and supportive healing programs are in place, cease-and-desist addictions programming will be ineffective and will sometimes escalate self-destructive
behaviours within a remote Aboriginal community.

While I have suggested that there are some Aboriginal traditions
that maximize PTSD-level traumas, it must be recognized that there
are also Aboriginal mental health practices that have traditionally
helped individuals deal with trauma. I believe that storytelling is the
most important of these. Unfortunately, given the high population
densities of present-day settlements and reserves, the crowded, life-
draining dwellings, and the prevalence of electronic entertainment
and informational devices, storytelling along with many other cathar-
tic traditions have stopped. As a result, community populations become more intent on simply surviving the high levels of mental anxiety
and depression that build up in such crowded living conditions than
on storytelling sessions that traditionally helped mitigate trauma and
post-trauma disorder.

Our Communities Are Remote

Finally, I address remoteness as a serious contributing factor to high
levels of PTSD. Many women in remote communities, myself included,
often feel trapped. For example, although we had the whole of the tun-
dra and the Arctic Ocean at hand, very few women from our community would venture more than an hour or two away from the settlement
by snow machine or by all-terrain vehicles, simply because of the environmental risk factors. It often happens that women in remote, fly-in
communities in particular are unable to leave the settlement or the reserve unless they are flown out for medical reasons. Even in communities with road connections to larger centres, distances can be prohibitive
for travel outside the community. This stasis can be very difficult to ac-
commodate mentally. Even in nomadic times and before mechanized
land and air travel, women often travelled more than they do now, and
had a better chance of keeping fit mentally as a result.

In addition to the fact that travel outside the community is often re-
strained by either cost or environmental concerns, very few women
have any place to go to heal. As a woman with family members living
in southern Canada, I had options when I realized that I and my children needed to seek refuge and respite. In spite of having connections
with several family and friends, however, my options were very limited

because of the chaotic state the children and I were in. Yet I recognize how fortunate I was; most of my extended family members in the North have little safe refuge, particularly for the long term, and have minimal access to good, long-term trauma treatment. Safe shelters typically cannot be provided within a region where community and family members are usually present. It is a great challenge in remote areas to build enough safeguards and healthy new connections into a shelter program to ensure that sustained healing treatment for PTSD can occur.

Unfortunately, this remoteness also makes it difficult for any kind of mental health services to be offered in the communities themselves. I recall that eight years ago when my own life began to crumble, the Baffin Region of Nunavut had only one qualified mental health professional on staff, a psychiatrist who admitted that he alone could do very little to help patients in settlements outside of the capital of Iqaluit. At that time, the only regular mental health services in the communities consisted of young psychologists from an institution in Toronto. They would make a two-day visit to the community once every six months, spend an hour with each of the twenty or so patients on their list, usually with translators, prescribe medications or recommend further treatments, and then leave the community. Compared to the five years of psychotherapy sessions and two years of intensive core issues work I needed to heal well, such transient mental health services clearly do very little towards effectively treating PTSD.

The relative isolation of many settlements and reserves also lends itself to high rates of secondary wounding of trauma survivors by well-meaning health professionals. Although many health professionals hired to work in remote Aboriginal communities are well qualified for general mental health work, they very rarely have the knowledge or experience needed to provide the many complexities of PTSD healing work. Unfortunately, this situation is often compounded by lack of knowledge of the cultural complexities of an Aboriginal community. As a result, many patients exhibiting PTSD symptoms such as insomnia, depression, anxiety disorder, or flashbacks are mistakenly given anti-depressant drugs, which in my experience aggravate rather than diminish PTSD symptoms, at times leading in the long term to more frequent and more serious self-destructive behaviours.

In addition, because PTSD often manifests itself in disordered relationships, a trauma survivor greatly needs an ordered relationship with someone outside of the trauma bond. Because all community members are by association fellow trauma survivors, the only non-traumatized people available are often the culturally incompetent professionals who come and go from the community. Relationships with such people often flourish for a time, but when transient professionals' work terms are completed, they leave the community and very often break the fragile trust relationship proffered by trauma victims. It is debatable, therefore, whether such relationships are in the long term more productive than counter-productive, in terms of healing from PTSD.

Clearly, a community's remoteness, the traditional Aboriginal elements, and the fact that women are PTSD victims more often than men all play a major role in the severity of PTSD as a major health issue for women living in remote Aboriginal communities.

Conclusion

In conclusion, it seems that there is a much higher rate of PTSD-level trauma occurring for women living in remote Aboriginal communities than for most non-Aboriginal women living in southern Canadian urban areas. Because of the extreme levels of traumatization, PTSD is a very real health issue for most women living in these communities, whether as a result of primary, secondary or tertiary traumatization. Furthermore, PTSD has been found to be a major factor affecting the emotional, mental, and physical health of women living in remote Aboriginal communities. Finally, secondary wounding and victimization contribute to the intensity of the problem. I have shown that PTSD is a greater problem for *women*, for women in *Aboriginal* communities especially, and most particularly for women living in *remote* Aboriginal communities.

PTSD, as a major health issue for women living in remote Aboriginal communities in Canada, must be treated seriously and its healing actively encouraged, so that it does not remain the 'nightmare in the closet' that continues to undermine the functionality and well-being of its victims. Many questions still urgently require answers: Who will take on the formidable task of becoming responsible for the healing of trauma survivors? What kinds of healing modalities are most effective? Where should long-term treatment of PTSD survivors be delivered? When a community-level trauma occurs, how can it best be handled to minimize PTSD symptomatology? These and a myriad of other questions must be pursued by the academic, medical, and human services sectors in order to prevent the loss of individual lives and to restore health and wellness to family units and whole communities, especially in remote Aboriginal communities.

References

American Psychiatric Association. (1994). *Diagnostic and statistical manual of mental disorder* (4th ed.). Washington, DC: American Psychiatric Association.

American Psychological Association. (n.d.). *Facts about women and trauma.* Retrieved from http://www.apa.org/about/gr/issues/women/trauma.aspx.

Bernard-Bonnin, A.C., Hébert, M., Daignault, I.V., & Allard-Dansereau, C. (2008). Disclosure of sexual abuse, and personal and familial factors as predictors of post-traumatic stress disorder symptoms in school-aged girls. *Paediatrics & Child Health, 13*(6), 479-86.

Figley, C.R. (Ed.). (1995). *Compassion fatigue: Coping with secondary traumatic stress in those who treat the traumatized.* Psychological Stress Series. New York: Routledge.

Jankowski, K. (2009). *PTSD and physical health.* Washington, DC: National Centre for PTSD, U.S. Department of Veterans Affairs. Retrieved from http://www.ptsd.va.gov/professional/pages/ptsd-physical-health.asp.

Matsakis, A. (1996). *I can't get over it: A handbook for trauma survivors* (2nd ed.). Oakland, CA: New Harbinger.

Tait, H. (2006). *Aboriginal peoples survey, 2006: Inuit health and social conditions* (Catalogue no. 89-637-X – No. 001). Ottawa: Statistics Canada, Social and Aboriginal Statistics Division.

12 Rural Women's Strategies for Seeking Mental Health and Housing Services

Phyllis Montgomery, Cheryl Forchuk,
Carolyne Gorlick, and Rick Csiernik

Although the majority of Canadian young and adult women are housed, 2.1 million females, or 16%, live in accommodations that are below national adequacy, suitability, or affordability standards (Canada Mortgage and Housing Corporation [CMHC], 2002a). Women with health challenges, and particularly those in rural locations, were more likely to experience housing needs (CMHC, 2002a, 2002b). The relationship between women's health and housing in rural areas is complicated by a number of related social and health issues. In addition to rural women's experience of intimate partner violence (IPV) as presented in chapters 10 and 11 of this volume, evidence also exists that such women have higher prevalence rates of poverty and unemployment and lack a continuum of health and social services in comparison to urban areas (Canadian Institute for Health Information [CIHI], 2006; Ontario Women's Health Council, 2002; Sutherns, McPhedan, & Haworth-Brockman, 2004). Within this context, women living with mental health issues may experience increased risk for homelessness (CIHI, 2007). According to the Ontario Women's Health Council (2002), little is known about women's homelessness or those at risk for homelessness in rural communities. This remains an area warranting further exploration.

The purpose of this chapter is to describe how Canadian women with mental illness who are homeless, or who are at risk of being homeless, and their service providers manage within a rural context. In response to a primary inquiry about how rurality influences women's abilities to 'make do to have a life,' this chapter includes a brief overview of the literature, a description of the approach used to reveal women's rural landscape, and an account of the strategies they use to manage within and as a result of this context.

Background

A comprehensive review of the academic literature yielded eight peer-reviewed studies involving samples of Canadian rural adult women experiencing mental illness and homelessness, including being at risk for homelessness. None of the identified studies contained specific empirical data related to the three topics of interest: rural women, mental health, and homelessness. In Brannen, Johnson Emberly, and McGrath's (2009) systematic review of evidence examining rural Canadians' sources of stress, they reported that there were no specific studies regarding housing as a stressor despite the research addressing poverty associated with the economic, social, and demographic restructuring of rural communities. Two additional studies involved samples of rural women living with IPV and their reliance on social services such as shelters (Jategaonkar, Greaves, Poole, McCullough, & Chabot, 2005; Thurston, Patten, & Lagendyk, 2006). Another three studies described the health status of rural women (Bédard, Gibbons, & Dubois, 2007; Leipert & Reutter, 2005; MacMillan et al., 2008), two of which specifically dealt with mental health. The final two studies addressed structural-geographical implications for women's sense of autonomy and women's efforts to remain invisible, blaming themselves for their lack of housing (Chouinard, 2006; Whitzman, 2006).

Collectively, the reviewed literature did not specifically define 'rural,' with the exception of Whitzman (2006). Across the studies, specific information about mental illness among the different subgroups of vulnerable rural women was difficult to glean. A shared finding, however, was a complex relationship between rural location and women's efforts to cope with enduring health challenges.

Methods

Retrospective interpretation (Thorne, 1998), a type of qualitative secondary analysis, was used to understand how the rural context influenced consumers' and service providers' experiences of 'doing things that needed doing.' This work expands on an aspect of the original five-year, mixed-method study (Forchuk et al., 2006). The sample for this secondary analysis included a total of sixty-two participants: forty-eight women consumers and fourteen service providers. They participated in one of twenty-five group interviews about experiences in seeking and securing housing, barriers and solutions to housing challenges, and housing preferences. From the transcripts of the group interviews, the extracted data sets were indexed by the location of the group and subject to inductive context analysis (Elo & Kyngas, 2007; Sandelowski, 1995; Sandelowski & Barroso, 2003). Category labels often were expressed in the women's own words to respect their linguistic meanings (Bushy, 2005). To address credibility, the authors regularly articulated the constructions of their data perceptions in an effort to support their evolving analysis and decision-making processes (Thorne, 2008).

The following sections include actual excerpts from the data illustrating the actions of staying and drifting and the phenomenon of improvising. The slash '/' within excerpts represents incomplete sentences or fragmented ideas, content included within square brackets '[ ]' provides clarifying information, and ellipses '...' indicate excluded material.

The Rural Landscape

The rural landscape was romanticized neither by women nor by service providers. Instead, it was generally characterized as deprived of essential material and human resources, impeding women's efforts to protect and sustain their health and housing. Deprivation was represented in a number of socio-structural forms, including IPV, use of substances, housing stock, poverty, food security, employment opportunities, social inequality, accessibility/availability of mental and social health services, and often non-existent or unaffordable public transportation. The latter is illustrated by this woman's historical account:

> Originally when the CNR [Canadian National Railroad] closed the rail line / there was an agreement with the community / it was for moving products from place to place and passenger service. And closing up the small trunk lines / the rail lines to stop running through Ontario, through [name of a small community] were supposed to provide bus service. Greyhound took that over and they downloaded it onto other carriers ... they just gradually cut everything out. So in other words the federal government downloaded it to provincial, the provincial downloaded it down to private and then it just disappeared. So I don't know what is going to happen ... you can't get at the services because you can't afford a taxi so you don't have people going there ... This is a tough one in a small community.

In such dynamics of hardship, women experiencing mental health challenges, stigmatization, and isolation as well as substandard housing or homelessness were confronted with a dilemma. They struggled with an ongoing internal dialogue over their limited options in an effort to make a better life. To best 'make do,' should they stay in their rural community or drift elsewhere? Should they seek supports within their present rural community to address the immediacy of their needs, or should they relocate to seek the promise of secure individual, family, and community resources?

Strategies of Managing

The active practices of staying and drifting were undertaken as a means to obtain the best possible living conditions, material and non-material, within their rural context. Common to both staying and drifting were the creation of informal social structures to secure needed resources in the absence of satisfactory formal health and social services. Common to both groups of women, those who stayed and those who drifted, was exposure to multiple push-and-pull counter-forces. Women who stayed experienced a predominance of pull forces holding them within their communities. Although women who drifted also experienced pull forces, in their case the counteractive push forces were more powerful, resulting in out-migration. Both groups of women struggled to achieve optimal life circumstances, requiring them to engage in improvising activities, which they described as maximizing their creative use of existing resources while concurrently seeking new resources in an effort to 'have a better life.'

Staying

One group of women living with illness and precarious housing stayed in their rural community, establishing and sustaining social ties with family, other women with health challenges, and service providers. Such relationships supported their intra- and inter-dependent abilities to improvise in a social and economic context described in terms of 'cut-backs,' 'cut-off[s],' or 'cut-down[s].' Long-standing and compassionate relationships with others, including specific service providers, were binding for some women. Others talked about being bound by their care work with other vulnerable women. They were motivated by concern for these women's well-being, and social and individual caring had become significant in their daily lives. Their caring work involved making themselves, their home, and/or their material possessions (such as the telephone) available for women in need, organizing social and leisure activities, volunteering, providing information about services, driving others to appointments, or visiting others in hospital. These carers engaged in practices that affected other women's lives. The following is an example of a discussion among women describing their commitment to care work:

> *Woman 1:* What has happened is I think I'm the 911 after the hospital closes and on weekends and it falls to me for my town.
>
> *Woman 2:* With some of our group members / you become the frontline because they know that in an emergency on a Sunday afternoon then who are they going to call? And they trust you.
>
> *Woman 3:* With our group we go bowling, we have a potluck at Christmas time and we usually invite other groups at that time ... And we usually have a good turnout. We have our turkey and the ham, taters / I call them taters but its potatoes.
>
> *Woman 4:* ... now over the summer, we've had two meetings in each month ... they have a concert in the park and we've been going down there. We have pot lucks, we go mini-golfing, we bowl, we have a movie once a month ... we try for a walk / we try to / we try to do a lot of different [activities].

The dependability and trustworthiness of these peer care providers created places of affiliation for other women, either face to face or via regular telephone contact. The relationship was reciprocal: 'they support us as well as we [carers] are support[ing] for them.' Mutuality among the group members lessened women's risk of becoming exhausted or overburdened by others' needs.

Caring work by peers offered women expanded choices for promoting their health. For example, one woman said that peer support offered her an opportunity to 'come out of [her] shell.' Women with social connections sought opportunities among available alternatives that may have been unknown to them as isolated women. The following example illustrates another woman's deliberate choices about her involvement in the community:

> I'm an Anglican, a practicing Anglican. I haven't been going [to the church] too often right now because my priest is on holidays. I preferred him to be there / I'm more comfortable when he's there ... and I am waiting for the fall to come so that I can go on Tuesdays and Sundays because they have

the service on Tuesdays. I am waiting till the potluck suppers start up again in the fall ... So that maybe I can get a ride up to the potluck suppers ... [At a consumer agency] it's a lot of sports activities and I cannot do them ... and there is not enough crafts or others activities to interest me to go. There is that fellow that does wood working and he may be coming back / and if he comes back, then I will go up while he is there and attend every time.

This example highlights that staying engaged in meaningful and fulfilling rural community activities plus access to resources such as social networks and transportation were important for mental well-being. In turn, these resources, activities, and social connections were sufficient to persuade some women to remain in their community. In addition to improvising for themselves, women continued improvising for their peers. This was a means to collectively improve their life circumstances through a sharing of limited tangible resources. There was another group of women, however, who did not have this sense of community affiliation. Instead, they perceived themselves, and were referred to by some service providers, as 'drifters.'

Drifting

A second group of rural women characterized themselves as 'always on the edge' – emotionally, economically, socially, and geographically. Marginalized, these women were increasingly vulnerable to pressures often perceived as being outside their control. According to service providers, these pressures were compounded by women's lack of 'permanency' in home, social, and employment situations. Rural women's access to dependable material and social resources was tenuous, often more so than that of their partners. For some, improvising became increasingly challenging and at times unfeasible. Lack of material resources and limited social networks were two conditions that initiated drifting between locations and services in the hope of securing a better life.

In general, most of the women who drifted away lived in poverty with a mental illness and were on their own or exclusively responsible for their children. Some of these women had been threatened with separation from their children or had already become separated. As one woman succinctly stated, 'ODSP [Ontario Disability Support Program] keeps us pretty poor / right, right down in the poor class. You don't have nothing.' Motivation for a 'new and better life' became derailed by unmet needs for mental and physical health services, housing, and social support. Moving from one geo-social space to another often thwarted women's hopes for securing tangible and intangible resources as well as receiving timely service responses. Drifting lessened their hope to 'stay in one steady place.' For some, the drifting patterns occurred during much of their lives as they attempted to remain 'creative,' improvising as necessary in their relocated circumstance, and drifting when essential.

For many women, drifting and improvising occurred simultaneously, with one process at times being more pervasive and persuasive than the other. For example, a homeless woman of colour described her state of improvising to minimize her risk of 'automatically being turned away' from a potential accommodation:

> [My first child has] blonde hair and blue eyes and [my second child] has the same complexion as me and I had a hard time getting housing if I brought my [second child] but not my [first child]. So, it was a fight all around because if I brought my [second child] then it would automatically be 'No. You are turned down.' If I brought my [first child] they would be looking at me as if like ok, 'She's with a white man.' She is accepted type of thing.

In common usage, the term 'drifting' suggests passivity. Yet, as the above data describe, drifting involves action (such as seeking accommodation) in addition to re-action ('a fight all around') when resources are scarce or withheld. From this perspective, drifting is like moving within a strong current that pulls and pushes a woman forward and keeps things from being fully under her own control.

Drifting was not necessarily a new strategy for rural women coping with difficult circumstances. For some women drifting was an aspect of their histories. As stated by one service provider: 'We see a great deal of mental health issues that have come from the women being abused from the word go. They just drift from/you know/from family abuse origins to um, abusive partners.' As adults, women continued to rely upon drifting following a crisis situation. 'Just to get a roof over their heads' post-crisis was challenging for service providers in view of women's material deprivation, long-standing IPV, or mothers' fear of child removal by services. As a service provider observed:

They [rural women] don't have an option and not until they are at the point where they know they are going to die / when they know / when he's at the point that he's going to kill her / then they leave finally. But until that they are so angry and they need to stay.

For other women, transitions from drifting to improvising were dependent upon a series of fortunate events, including their readiness to move, the road conditions, the season, the availability of transportation, and most importantly, timely access to services and material resources. As described by one women moving into her new accommodation:

In July I'll have nine years sober and uh with / the um mental illness / they just uh / like that was the cliché that you know alcoholics or people with mental illness don't pay their rent. They trash the apartments ... I was really lucky because I didn't have to pay last month rent. I just paid first month and I didn't have to sign a lease.

Many women drifted across geographical boundaries in their search for resources. Their drifting and improvisation routes included within and into as well as out of rural communities. Some women preferred to remain within the bounds of their rural community, drifting or 'couch surfing' among family and friends. Others moved into rural places from urban places seeking less costly housing, escaping the urban drug culture, and wanting to provide their children with a more nurturing environment. Such expectations, however, were not fully actualized. For example, although rent for a rural dwelling may have been less in dollar terms, the women were unable to secure employment, afford food, or access transportation to mental health programs. This is illustrated in the following woman's account:

I like the situation I'm going to be moving into / it's a small town / it's a lovely little one-bedroom apartment / it's nicely decorated. I just like it. My only concern is that in a year I'm going to have to find a job somewhere and I will probably have to move because I don't see that there will be very many jobs in that small town.

The negative implications of the migration of younger rural residents; a shortage of community capital; unsatisfactory location, quantity, or quality of housing; and restructured mental health service delivery generally resulted in increased numbers of women breaking ties to their rural place. Women's motivation to drift from their rural to an urban location was based on the assumption that increased health and social services would be more readily available to them in an urban area. They believed they had a greater chance of securing resources in a timely manner in an urban rather than their rural place. As explained by a rural service provider:

[W]e don't have geared-to-income housing and different things. Our waiting lists are months, years longer than [name of urban centre]. So for women to get housing that they can afford when they are on OW [Ontario Works] / they have to move to [urban centre] and leave their family and support system and start a new life / a new life.

Unfortunately, the anticipated positive outcomes of relocating to an urban area to secure services were often not realized. This was a disappointment for many women, as they 'ended up' in shelters. One woman stated:

When I was in [a rural community] I was eighteen on the [housing] list. I came here [an urban centre] I went down to twenty-five, which is understandable cause I went from one town to another and all towns are different so yeah you go there and expect to drop down right / and now I'm thirty-two on the list. Now how did I get bumped down? I shouldn be going up the list / the longer you are there the more you should go up? ... I'm still going down [the list] instead of going up.

Some women began to question if they should return to their rural community or move to another urban centre, especially to provide for material needs. Vulnerable and poor women's frequent drifting between two places became a undesired yet necessary lifestyle, as illustrated in individual phrases such as 'This time I'm from [name of a location]' or 'I heard that in [name of city] there is [a particular type of service].' With increasing dependence on shelter care, women's drifting patterns were more influenced by service regulations, such as length-of-stay policies, than a desire to reside in one particular part of a community or another. Service policy in this context functions to impose drifting while making individual improvising difficult. For example, relocation within a community from one shelter to another in some circumstances disrupted women's access to their peer supports and disabled improvising strategies.

In seeking a new home, women weighed the physical distance to their destination in terms of its financial and transportation implications. Even if an accommodation became available, women could not necessarily afford the costs associated with an initial viewing to determine its suitability. This often results in blind acceptance of housing situations. For women separated from their children, maintaining parenting responsibilities at a distance could become not only challenging but prohibitively costly. Visits to family or friends, regardless of distance, became unlikely after women moved from a rural to an urban setting. As one woman said:

> There was not enough [social services] like there are in [name of urban centre]. That's why they [her family] sent me here because I needed to get out of that town ... but I'm up here / pretty strange experience / not have a Christmas with your family or anything. Couldn't go down there [to rural home community] / couldn't see my daughter ... I haven't been down home once you know.

This women's drifting, like others, was associated with a force – 'they sent me here.' The types of push and pull forces are described in detail below. In both women's and service providers' accounts, the transition from drifting to improvising was a back-and-forth movement often occurring simultaneously and fuelled by a unique combination of push and pull forces.

Pull forces. Pull and push factors in relation to drifting and improvising were often described as two counter-poles on a magnet. A pulling factor could be a promise of available quality housing and accessible medical, social, and employment opportunities. Correspondingly, a pushing factor could be a crisis associated with poor housing and inaccessible medical, social, economic, or work opportunities requiring relocation. For example, for some women, receiving Ontario Works functioned as a pull factor by assisting and encouraging them to secure employment. For others, however, Ontario Works served as a pushing force when they were unable to gain employment in their rural community due to lack of childcare services.

The research data reveal that the strongest pull force was women's intention to escape their rural place of residence for reasons of security, self-efficacy, and, in many cases, safety. Their expectations were 'choice,' 'sense of peace,' 'a chance,' 'available services,' acceptance, and wellness.

As clearly stated by one woman, her aspiration was to secure 'a life [and] a home,' thereby making drifting an intended action of improvising rather than a passive occurrence. For example:

> I am here [name of a shelter in an urban centre] / because I was living in [name of rural community] / to start a new life and to find a job and a place … I ran out of [motel] rooms uh money … And plus I have my [children] here and that is why I came back here [to urban centre] to start over. So that is why I'm here … to start a bigger and better life I hope. I find it very nice in [this shelter]. You get all three full-course meals … it's awesome like you know but I'd really rather not be here. I want my own home.

As the above illustrates, women with limited material and social resources initially rely upon services to meet basic needs such as food and shelter. Women recognized that available shelter services offered only temporary physical, emotional, psychological, and informational support, a place for respite before beginning a 'better life.' Arrival at their final destination, a place 'where they were meant to be,' represented more than just access to material possessions. As one woman living with her son explained:

> I live in a house or I live where there is ten people but it's all separate entities /it's a small town … you have to be careful about complaints … I've considered moving / he [son] doesn't want to move / I don't want to be in the small town that I am in / it's a vicious circle, I'm driving my own self nuts / I have a lot of ah, qualities that were good. They're stagnant. I used to be able to do um, crafts, I was able to be able to do just minor things. Now, I get started with stuff, and I think what am I doing here, like, I used to like my freedom / all I want to do is feel better. You know as far as meds / my doctor doesn't want to change them, you know, so the scenario goes around and I get my case worker, and we don't get anything resolved.

This suggests that a dwelling was not necessarily the same as a home. In addition to the physical structure, a home was characterized as a place where women could exercise choice.

For women with and separated from their young children, drifting and improvising was fuelled by the opportunity to provide safer and more consistent accommodation for their children's well-being. Parenting in a suitable place offered the possibilities of women building social ties with other women. Otherwise, women separated from their children expressed concern that their children may also experience drifting, especially if they had been placed in environments that women did not sanction or viewed as culturally insensitive. One woman said:

> The CAS [Children's Aid Society] right now / they have a problem with stabilization. Well, they are the ones that are making me unstable OK and they are the ones that have transferred my children eight times. Eight times now, just recently for the eighth time / I requested for my children to be placed [in a familiar rural community] because I know everybody and they [CAS] ended up placing them with [other] people / excuse me but I would like my children's heritage involved with them.

Push forces. Drift push forces consisting of family, rural socio-cultural, and service organizational factors (Table 12.1) played a role in constricting women's improvising alternatives as they sought 'options' for growth. Most forces were external, intermixing to challenge women's efforts to achieve upward mobility. Drifting without actual opportunities for improved well-being fuelled a 'never-ending' circular pattern. This was illustrated by women's use of phrases such as 'in and out of services,' 'coming and going,' 'on and off,' 'back and forth,' or 'running in circles.' Repetitive in comparison to positive movement, this circular pattern made it difficult for women to actually position themselves beyond their stressful situations and made improvising difficult and elusive. The momentum of the push forces was strengthened by dynamics such as persistent illness, addiction, IPV, lack of support from small social networks, and poverty. Despite frequent moves, women were essentially 'going nowhere.'

'Ingrained' gendered ideologies influenced drifting patterns. For example, rural women were typically expected to undertake traditional roles of wife and mother. Situated within traditional gendered roles, these women found their forward mobility constrained when their voiced concerns for health or safety were not fully acknowledged by social supports and service providers. Vulnerable women realized employed partners provided a place for them to reside in comparison to non-accessible or non-available accommodations. Oftentimes, disappointing service responses, avoidance of shame, and protection of their privacy combined to lead women back to unsuitable dwellings and dependent relational situations.

Table 12.1. The Push Forces of Drifting Identified by Women and Providers

Categories	Illustrations
Family • Seeking services and safety • Lessening sense of shame • Protecting self and children from violence	'And the church has an expectation that we stay married and my congregation believes that and how do I break away from that without you know shaming myself / my family / my peers / that's a huge battle.' (woman)
Socio-cultural • Poverty • Ideology • Stigmatization • Lack of school or employment opportunities • Lack of privacy • Lack of housing and range of housing	'Or even [women in IVP situation] calling the police or calling other service providers / their partner may have grown up knowing police officers. The police may or may not believe him. "No I know him. I played hockey with him. He's not like that. He wouldn't do that." … The woman is pre-judged. She's hysterical. Then sometimes they end up back with an abusive partner / whether he's the same person or a new person.' (service provider)
Service organizational • Shortage of providers • Need for ongoing provider development • Lack of accessibility • Under-serviced • Long waits and wait lists • Policy expansion beyond crisis orientation • Policy to address social exclusion • Policy to optimize equitable funding	'The system is setting them up for failure / so it sets them up to fail. There is no other way. They come here for food. They go to the food bank for food. They go to the churches for food … women are resorting to community churches to support and pay a lot of their bills / or hydro bills or rent because they don't have government subsidy like [name of urban centre] … they start doing the rotations of the churches.' (service provider)

Community service providers identified one of their primary roles as 'navigator or transition advocate.' To assist women to 'move beyond a survival mode of existence,' providers guided women through multiple service structures for health, material, economic, and employment resources. Service providers advocated for women to purposefully drift away from their rural community as a means to secure resources. In some cases, in collaboration with women, service providers orchestrated drifting to ensure women's safety. Service providers 'forced them' or 'told them' to move away from their rural community and encouraged them 'never to come back.' Displaced women were now confronted with a new challenge, to contend with urban lifestyles in the absence of their 'heirlooms' and familiar social ties. Women's aspirations for a 'chance in life' characterized by a sense of well-being decreased, especially when they became caught in what they described as the 'shelter shuffle.'

The organization of rural health and social services contributed to some individual providers demonstrating a heightened sense of responsibility to assist vulnerable women, going beyond the minimal expectations of their work role. As an exemplar, in response to the perception of fewer community mental health services, police officers have become more involved in rural emergency services. Police also provide transportation to and from emergency services for the group of women involved in this study. Augmenting service providers' responsibilities had associated costs, such as time consumption, being 'run ragged,' inter-agency conflict, overemphasis on crisis services, or increased personal risk secondary to 'lack of specialized training.' Emphasizing crisis-oriented rather than public-education or community-care approaches fuelled long waits for services and lessened women's efforts at continuous enablement. A positive outcome of extending service providers' responsibilities was a commitment to strengthen a 'joint team' response, especially service providers who perceived the service structure as being problematic rather than 'just' the individual.

Ironically, the structure of services was described as 'failing' women most in need by minimizing their control and choices. Despite service providers' 'best efforts' to assist women in meeting their needs, including a recommendation to relocate, they were cognizant of the increased probability of women's drifting and improvising, that is, moving 'from shelter to shelter ... anywhere there is room.'

Implications

In this study, women with mental illness and precarious housing situations described two prominent responses used to improve their health and housing circumstances in relation to their rural environments characterized by structural deprivation. Embedded in the rural social and political structures were chronic stressors such as poverty, stigma, and health and social inequities. These particular types of contextual stressors are insidious and unavoidable, as they are an aspect of everyday life (CIHI, 2007; CMHC, 2002b). Their presence posed barriers for meeting

health and social needs for the individual woman, with broader implications for the community. A growing body of research shows that
women are particularly susceptible to the consequences of rural disadvantage (Sutherns et al., 2004). This is in part related to vulnerable
women's reliance upon health and social services, and is further compounded by their compromised socio-economic status, as evidenced by
the women in this study. The effects of rural structural disadvantage on
women's health and access to quality housing identified in this study
emphasize the need to explore effectual and sustainable mechanisms
for gendered-based health and housing initiatives. This study supports
the need for comprehensive system-level processes to honour vulnerable rural women as they seek accessible, acceptable, and coordinated
services in their effort to stay secure.

For the women in this study who stayed, available peer support mediated the negative influences in their rural environments. They an-
chored themselves to familiar lifestyles by maintaining involvement in
their social network. The strength of their long-standing social relations
led not only to their assisting others through improvising but also to
their assisting themselves. Staying and engaging in care work for others is a theme reported in other rural Canadian literature (Brannen et
al., 2009). Creating and sustaining an arena for tangible and intangible
support acknowledges their resourcefulness. Although the results of
this study serve to highlight women's efforts to persevere in challenging rural settings, those results must be translated into action. Despite
the evidence that peer support is a means for women with mental illness to build an ally base (Chernomas & Clarke, 2003), for rural professions, expanding collaborative partnerships with peer support carers
may be a preliminary strategy to understand how vulnerable women
navigate health and social services.

For other women in this study, drifting between places was undertaken as a strategy to improve their lives. For some, drifting may be a
familiar pattern, a means of securing an acceptable existence that acknowledges their histories of trauma (Ontario Women's Health Council,
2002). The notion of drifting is not a new concept in the mental health
literature. The interaction between mental illness and socio-economic
factors often results in downward social mobility as opposed to stases or
a rise in social status (Fox, 1990). Findings from this study further suggest an existential dimension to the construct of social drifting towards
homelessness. Drifting for these women was a means to escape concrete,
chronic individual and rural stressors with the hope of arriving at a

place of purposeful well-being for themselves and, in some cases, their children. Frequent relocation, however, seemed to erode their sense of identity and the familial and peer supports that existed within their past rural home. The servicing of rural women in urban centres challenges providers to address the existential dimension that women are seeking once the basic material needs are met. This study raises the issue of meaningful place and purposeful improvising on the part of rural women as they seek a 'new life' in the absence of optimal services.

More effort is needed to understand and address the push and pull forces that initiate drifting. Drifting is an active strategy on the part of women, an activity sanctioned or 'pushed' by rural professionals as a means to address immediate needs of women. Drifting, however, does not address the burden imposed on the next community's resources, nor does it guarantee an improved life situation for the women who drift. Overall, the consequences of drifting for women, providers, and the health and social systems are counterproductive to achieving the goals of each. Immediate responses are needed to minimize the continued personal and social costs of out-migration. As the burden increases, the emerging service provider pattern of shortened tenures within rural communities may escalate. A rural lens could facilitate the structuring of services to 'pull' women experiencing overwhelming health, housing, and financial problems close to their families, support networks, and professional services and to maintain them in their rural community.

Conclusion

This study's findings present an opportunity to explore additional research specific to rural women: What differences are there between rural women who are able to stay in their community and those who engage in drifting? Is there a difference in the severity of their health and housing issues? The dearth of current national evidence undermines the significance of the struggles experienced by women with mental health challenges as they actively attempt to achieve and sustain optimal life circumstances.

References

Bédard, M., Gibbons, C., & Dubois, S. (2007). The needs of rural and urban young, middle-aged and older adults with a serious mental illness. *Canadian Journal of Rural Medicine, 12*(3), 167–75.

Brannen, C., Johnson Emberly, D., & McGrath, P. (2009). Stress in rural Canada: A structured review of content, stress levels, and sources of stress. *Health & Place, 15*(1), 219–27.

Bushy, A. (2005). Needed: A more inclusive research paradigm to learn about the health needs of rural women. *Women's Health Issues, 15*(5), 204–8.

Canada Mortgage and Housing Corporation. (2002a). *Special studies on 1996 census data: Housing conditions of women and girls, and female-led households.* Research Highlights Socio-economic Series 55-9. Retrieved from http://www.cmhc-schl.gc.ca/odpub/pdf/63007.pdf.

Canada Mortgage and Housing Corporation. (2002b). *Housing options for women living alone in rural areas.* Research Highlights Socio-economic Series 12. Retrieved from http://www.cmhc-schl.gc.ca/odpub/pdf/63055.pdf.

Canadian Institute for Health Information (CIHI). (2006). *How healthy are rural Canadians: An assessment of their health status and health determinants.* Ottawa: Author. Retrieved from http://www.phac-aspc.gc.ca/publicat/rural06/pdf/rural_canadians_2006_report_e.pdf.

Canadian Institute for Health Information (CIHI). (2007). *Mental health and homelessness.* Ottawa: Author. Retrieved from http://secure.cihi.ca/cihiweb/products/mental_health_report_aug22_2007_e.pdf.

Chernomas, W.M., & Clarke, D.E. (2003). *Social support and women living with serious mental illness.* Winnipeg: Prairie Women's Health Centre of Excellence. Retrieved from http://www.uwinnipeg.ca/admin/vh_external/pwhce/pdf/socialSupport.pdf.

Chouinard, V. (2006). On the dialectics of differencing: Disabled women, the state and housing issues. *Gender, Place and Culture, 13*(4), 401–17.

Elo, S., & Kyngas, H. (2007). The qualitative content analysis process. *Journal of Advanced Nursing, 62*(1), 107–15.

Forchuk, C. ,Turner, K., Hall, B., Wiktorowicz, M., Hoch, J.S., Schofield, R., Nelson, G., Evoy, L., Levitan, E., Ward-Griffin, C., Perry, S., Csiernik, R., & Speechley, M. (2006). *Research Report. Partnerships in Capacity Building: Housing, Community Economic Development, and Psychiatric Survivors.* London, ON: University of Western Ontario.

Fox, J.W. (1990). Social class, mental illness, and social mobility: The social selection-drift hypothesis for serious mental illness. *Journal of Health and Social Behavior, 31*(December), 344–53.

Jategaonkar, N., Greaves, L., Poole, N., McCullough, L., & Chabot, C. (2005). 'Still out there': Experiencing substance use and violence in rural British Columbia. *Canadian Woman Studies, 24*(4), 136–41.

Leipert, B.D., & Reutter, L. (2005). Women's health in northern British Columbia: The role of geography and gender. *Canadian Journal of Rural Medicine, 10*(4), 241–53.

MacMillan, H.L., Jamieson, E., Walsh, C.A., Wong, M.Y.Y., Faries, E.J., McCue, H., MacMillan, A.B., & Offord, D.R., with the Technical Advisory Committee of the Chiefs of Ontario. (2008). First Nations women's mental health: Results from an Ontario Survey. *Archives of Women's Mental Health, 11*, 105–15.

Ontario Women's Health Council. (2002). *Health status of homeless women: An inventory of issues*. Toronto: Author.

Sandelowski, M. (1995). Qualitative analysis: What it is and how to begin. *Research in Nursing & Health, 18*, 371–75.

Sandelowski, M., & Barroso, J. (2003). Classifying the findings in qualitative studies. *Qualitative Health Research, 7*, 905–23.

Sutherns, R., McPhedan, M., & Haworth-Brockman, M. (2004). *Rural, remote and northern women's health: Policy and research directions - Summary report*. Winnipeg: Prairie Women's Health Centre of Excellence.

Thorne, S. (1998). Ethical and representational issues in qualitative secondary analysis. *Qualitative Health Research, 8*(4), 547–55.

Thorne, S. (2008). *Interpretive description*. Walnut Creek, CA: Left Coast Press.

Thurston, W.E., Patten, S., & Lagendyk, L.E. (2006). Prevalence of violence against women reported in a rural health region. *Canadian Journal of Rural Medicine, 11*(4), 259–67.

Whitzman, C. (2006). At the intersection of invisibilities: Canadian women, homelessness and health outside the 'big city.' *Gender, Place and Culture, 13*(4), 383–99.

PART FOUR

Population Health, Health Promotion, and Public Health

Wilfreda E. Thurston

In each of the chapters in this section, women defined their health broadly as a combination of social, physical, spiritual, and psychological well-being. Not surprisingly, then, the intersection of gender with other determinants of a populations' health becomes clear. These chapters highlight the need to consider these when developing health promotion and public health interventions. We see that macro-level policies have an impact on our everyday life. Restructuring of the rural economy is gendered and therefore has differential impacts on women and men that are hidden in apparently gender-neutral policies. Heather, Skillen, Cross, and Vladicka note that the paid and unpaid work of women is central to rural economies and that cutbacks in services, particularly health care, disproportionately affect women. The gendered norms of rural life establish expectations that challenge the health and well-being of rural populations. For farm women, unusual stress is one outcome as well as reduced capacity to participate in organizations that might represent their interests. Gerrard and Woodland discuss how gender affects rural women's resiliency, both individual and collective, in the face of chronic stress, through gender politics, or in the negotiation of power. They found that resiliency is shaped by relations and the context surrounding women and that gender is a barrier, but one that is being challenged and resisted by women. Using the framework of the Ottawa Charter for Health Promotion, they recommend community-level interventions to benefit rural women. Etowa, Thomas Bernard, Clow, and Wiens provide insight into the largest populations of multi-generation African Canadians in Canada. The history of settlement and enduring racism is central to the experience of rurality and health for these women. These authors also introduce the notion of age and a life-course perspective in understanding groups of women. Novik also addresses the history of settlement and life course in her study of the experiences of Ukranian immigrants to Saskatchewan. Gendered history, culture, colonization, and geography are discussed again by Moffit as key elements in the health of northern women as they experience pregnancy and childbirth and by Stiles, Dukeshire, Paulsen, Goodridge, Hobson, MacLaughlin, MacNeil, and Rangel in studying leisure activities in rural areas. The chapters also note that women in rural communities have identities as rural or farm women and loyalties to communities that may be important assets in designing population health promotion, illustrating why the principle of community participation in health sector planning is key to primary health care.

13 Being a Good Woman: The Gendered Impacts of Restructuring in Rural Alberta

Barbara Heather, D. Lynn Skillen, Jennifer Cross, and Theresa Vladicka

From 2001 to 2003, Skillen, Heather, and Cross researched rural Alberta women's lives after restructuring in health care services and agriculture. Their findings form the basis for this chapter, which investigates how rural expectations and practices of gender, in a social context of change and uncertainty, affect the health of farm women who are also working off-farm as nurses.

Background

During the 1990s rural women's work and home environments were radically changed by the reorganization of federal and provincial agriculture and health care policies. Farmers had already responded to new technology, and the rise of more accessible global markets, with new practices and products (Lobao & Meyer, 2001; National Farmers' Union, 2003), but also had to cope with the impacts of federal restructuring under the North American Free Trade Agreement. This restructuring included the end of subsidies such as lower grain freight rates, and smaller grain elevators closing in favour of larger elevators in fewer places. At the same time as the costs of farming (such as seeds, fertilizer, and equipment repair or replacement) were increasing, income (including product sales and government subsidies) declined (Meyer & Lobao, 1997; Swisher, Elder, Lorenz, & Conger, 1998). Smaller farms are struggling to survive, while large farms, including agribusinesses, are seeing increased profits. Alberta lost 7.9% of its farms between 2001 and 2006, but the acreage farmed increased by 1% (Statistics Canada, 2006a) because small farms closed and the land was taken over by large farms such as agribusinesses.

Rural economies are significantly affected by the paid and unpaid work of women (Alasia, 2010; Lobao & Meyer, 2001). Rural culture is one of reciprocal relationships and conservative gender roles. Women are expected to carry out their family work but also to assist on the farm and volunteer in the community. Lowered farm income often means that women not only carry out these responsibilities but also take up off-farm employment or increase existing paid hours. While their paid labour is of value to communities, which may have a smaller labour pool (especially professionals) on which to call (Alasia & Magnusson, 2005; Statistics Canada, 2006b), taking on paid work creates a triple day for women, as they work in the home, on the farm, and as a paid employee (Mackenzie, 1994).

One common avenue for employment of women in rural Alberta has been the health care system. When the Alberta government changed the structures of health care delivery in 1994, the paid work of rural nurses, many of whom are also farm women, was significantly altered. The government collapsed twenty-seven small health units into seventeen health authorities, moving professionals with specific expertise to regional centres. Others, either reassigned or remaining behind in their own community, were often separated from supports and sources of expertise. Many were given new job descriptions with additional responsibilities, and were required to be accountable through the keeping of more written records. As well, the changes left many communities with no medical professionals or with one nurse. With no doctor and no public transportation, all community members, but especially the non-drivers such as elderly residents, turned more often to the nurse for information and assistance.

Restructuring in the agricultural and health sectors therefore affected the lives and the health of women as wives, mothers, farm women, health system employees, and members of rural communities.

Gender in rural areas is a deeply entrenched proscriptive and prescriptive norm. The good male farmer is tough, hard working, and in control of his environment (Alston & Kent, 2008; Ni Laoire, 2005). The good woman is caring, nurturing, and domestically proficient. She is expected to be there for her children and also to extend her caring role beyond her home (Constantine, 2001; Little, 2002). Being a good woman in a farm setting is being one who cares for and contributes to her family, her farm, and her community. She is always multitasking and 'always on' (Heather, Skillen, Young, & Vladicka, 2005, p. 9). Being a good woman in a community that has lost its health services is being one who both gives medical advice and sometimes physically takes a patient to the regional health centre. Combined with the additional workloads, being a good woman in order to fit into a beloved community can have significant impacts on health and well-being.

Methods

The research was an exploratory, descriptive project involving interviews with rural women the majority of whom were farm women and nurses. This allowed us to gain a unique insight into the lives of farm women-nurses after both of their industries experienced restructuring. We also conducted seven focus groups at which preliminary findings were tested. Individual interviewees were asked to tell us how they defined work and how they would describe being healthy, after which we asked them how they perceived their paid and unpaid work and its impacts on their sense of well-being (Skillen, Heather, & Young, 2003).

Work

Participants' definitions of work varied from 'what I am paid for' to 'what I don't like doing,' but participants were clear that their work activities had taken over time that was once available for relaxation and that they were experiencing higher rates of stress in consequence. Due to that lack of leisure time, they also said their work was to some extent injurious to their health. They spoke of being a good woman, or following expected gender roles in order to fit into their community, while at the same time they struggled for control over and balance in their lives.

When additional income was needed, nurses went back to work or increased their off-farm work hours. Paid work gave them additional resources in the form of income and collegiality. One participant said: 'My nursing work is work but it's my salvation, it's play. [It's my salvation from] the stresses of farming and [it is] other people to talk to. On the farm you're more isolated.' When health care services were regionalized, however, nurses who remained in the smaller centres found themselves working alone again.

As farm income decreased, off-farm income went increasingly towards farm bills rather than to leisure activities. Further, farm women found themselves needed as farm labour more than before, since the male farmer could not afford to hire help. Their working hours and responsibilities both increased at a time when the changes at their paid workplace meant they no longer had colleagues who could cover for them when they needed to be at the farm, such as at harvest time or when grain was being trucked to a more distant elevator by their husband. Farm women were finding that off-farm work – their 'salvation' time away from the farm – was being eroded as they tried to juggle farm needs and work responsibilities. The farm was intruding on their nursing work. There are multiple layers here. As farm income declined, the farm woman's paid labour, initially intended to ease the strain on household finances or to pay for a vacation, increasingly went to pay farm bills. When the farm absorbs the off-farm income, off-farm work becomes 'for the farm,' not 'for the self.' Together with changes at their workplace (discussed below), which left them feeling isolated once again, they had lost their sense of independence, of providing money for extras, including relaxation time for themselves. They had lost the income that gave them a little freedom, and the farm work was becoming more burdensome. A participant said: 'In every single aspect it seems like, with all that I have to do, I feel like in many ways I am gypped from having leisure time and having social time, 'cause there's not much left over of the day.' Some of the participants who still had children at home said they rose at about 6 am, packed lunches, made breakfasts, and sent the children off to school before leaving for their paid work. They came home at 6 pm to make dinner and assist with homework or other of their children's activities, after which they would go out to work on the farm. They rarely seemed to get to bed before midnight.

Multiple gendered identities were evident among participants (Brandth, 2002, 2007). They had many roles, each of which brought out a different identity. In the home a farm woman was the mother, wife, domestic organizer, and also bookkeeper for the farm. Outside she was the farm labourer, doing what hired labour had once done, on top of growing and preserving vegetables and fruit. In the community she was a nurse, called upon for her knowledge about health matters, and a volunteer. At work she was a professional, with responsibilities towards her colleagues as well as her patients. The ethic of caring involved in being a good woman is completely compatible with being a nurse, one said. However, relationships with colleagues are also based on that ethic of caring, doubling the focus of their responsibilities. For example, participants were conscious that if they took time off from their nursing job, there were no replacements called in, and that meant a colleague had to do the work of two people. Alternatively, some participants said their work would be waiting on the desk when they returned, making time off difficult to take. They interpreted this as the administration taking advantage of them because they were women and because they cared, that is, they would get the work done rather than risk any loss of services for their patients.

Farm women's work was more varied than that of farm men. Participants juggled household management, farm work, and care for family and community members with the demands of their paid work. They drew on resources, including the change of pace and affirmation that comes from working for pay, but also resented the losses, including time for themselves, time to be with family and friends, money to spend on family and self, loss of collegial relationships, and a loss of identity if the farm finally had to be sold. This last may be more important than it seems, since women's work tends to be undervalued and invisible[1] (Chafetz, 1984, 1990). When their farm was sold, one woman said she really felt the loss of identity – when she went into the local village, for example, she was no longer included in discussions about farming because she was no longer 'a farmer.' Losing recognition as a farm woman is losing another layer of recognition and becoming more invisible in the community.

Health

The women we interviewed defined health holistically. They talked about health as physical, mental, emotional, social, and spiritual in its dimensions. They described health as having the support of family and friends or as being in control of what they did, helping, contributing to the community, and having the ability to live day to day. In general, what they said about health as an ideal did not match their reports on their own health status. They were skipping meals just to get something done and going short on sleep, such that it was sometimes described in terms of a luxury. One participant, describing the lack of sleep and time for herself, said: 'I was out in the field crying, and I was picking up the little bits of swath and trying to throw it into the next swath,' and another, referring to her ideal of self-care, said: 'Sometimes the stressors every day change that wellness model that I have in my head.' The health needs of others came before their own. One participant said: 'I think nurses tend to lose themselves.'

For public health and home care nurses, work involved what they called 'add-ons,' that is, additional work, especially paperwork, that had come with regionalization. Farming also required more careful re-cord keeping, and this was generally women's work. One said: 'I'm not handling things at home very well. I'm so far behind it's actually quite pathetic ... I've even thought "now am I bordering on depression?"' Many women talked of 'spillover' between work and home. They were unable to leave paid work at work and farm work at home. A nurse recounted how things were before regionalization: 'It was like one big happy family, and we compared notes, and we worked together ... [now] we very seldom see some of those people.' They drew on their resources – education, family, and community members – to keep go-ing, but many said they were tired.

Participants were keenly aware that expectations of them were too demanding and that they were hurting physically and mentally as a result. Farming has always had an element of unpredictability, but that had increased with the variability of both costs and income. That was adding to their stress and fear that their farm would fail. They would see other farms closing down, attend the auctions that resulted, and wonder if their farm could be next (see, for example, Statistics Canada, The Daily, 16 May 2007). Nurse-farm women often acknowl-edged benefits such as from their educational background, for exam-ple, noting how training to be a nurse had also taught them to be organized, but pointed as well to the overload of expectations and demands with which they were struggling. Even before returning to paid work, one said: 'I certainly was out there picking rocks and haul-ing bales and ... having the female things in the house ... so I think there is more expected of women than there is of men.' Adding off-farm work to this made balancing farm, family, and paid work in-creasingly hard, but the women saw themselves as having no choice. The farm had to be prevented from failing. They included a sense of control in their definition of being healthy, but now they recognized they no longer had that control.

Internationally, family-run farms are struggling for survival (Boyce 1999; Christison, 2000), and if they fail, they affect the surrounding communities in terms of spin-off jobs such as retail sales or professional occupations (Alasia & Bollman, 2009; Alasia & Magnusson, 2005; Statistics Canada, The Daily, 17 July 2006). The struggle to save the farm, and through that to save the community they loved, was more impor-tant to the women we interviewed than their own well-being. It was this factor that drew our attention to the gendered implications of re-structuring and the resulting stress.

. Men and women experience stressors in gendered ways and also may respond to them differently (Constantine, 2001; Singh & Siahpush, 2002; Thurston, Blundell-Gosselin, & Rose, 2003). How individuals respond to stress affects outcomes. The participants in our study were becoming overwhelmed by their paid and unpaid workload. With no time to volunteer for women's organizations, such as Women of Unifarm or the local Women's Institutes,[2] our participants were losing touch not just with colleagues after restructuring of their workplace but with friends and neighbours, who in the past they had spent time visiting around the kitchen table or at community events. Financial stress and overwork, as well as loss of their professional and community networks, left farm women and nurses feeling not only a loss of control over their lives but also disempowered without the voice that their women's organizations had given them. In addition, where once their paid work had been a break from the stresses of the farm, and a place where their skills were recognized and valued, it was now also a source of stress.

Being a Good Woman

When women choose to live in a rural area, they may accept the more traditional view of gender and take that up as a part of how they see themselves. For the participants in this research, it had become part of their identity as a rural woman and as a farm woman or nurse. They took great pride in their ability to perform all of the expected roles. Because they loved a rural lifestyle and being part of their local community, they consciously emphasized gendered aspects of their sense of themselves, but remained aware that often their sense of self was becoming submerged in being a good woman. It is when they were tired and stressed that they realized how many and how demanding were their multiple roles.

One of the breaking points for farm women-nurses seemed to be farm safety issues. Many farm women were the safety coordinators for their district, but they had trouble getting their own menfolk to follow safe practices. They were frightened and frustrated with husbands who drove brakeless trucks and combines held together with wire, or who used dangerous chemical sprays without the proper protective gear, such as protective eye glasses. They said their husbands did not think there was anything to worry about – they knew what they were doing. It was almost a measure of masculinity not to pay attention to the dangers of their practices, and of femininity to worry and try to change those practices. An ethic of caring shaped much of how the women described and managed their relationships at home, at work, and in the community. However, that ethic of caring, which is part of being a good woman, also affected their health.

All of the participants were experiencing the effects of restructuring at home and at work as increased workload, although not all responded to those changes negatively. There were, however, stressors and responses to stress that were common to most participants and that were permeated by assumptions about, and responses to, gender and health. One surprise in the findings from this research was the strength of ideas about gender in the women's responses to restructuring, and the extent to which the women themselves were aware of how gender was shaping their responses. Yet they continued to overwork in order to be good women. As one said: 'Like I probably haven't thought about it because my environment is a fixed thing ... so I don't think of it as something that I would have a choice about, that it is affecting my health.' Another participant explained:

> There's times when I resented the farm because I'd do my eight hours a day and then still have to go home and cook. The kids had needs, plus there was the hired men to feed and they were there at 6 pm no matter when you got home. Farm women had three meals a day and two coffees to do but men expect the same when you work off-farm.

Being a good woman was recognized as a risk factor for ill health, but continued to be valued even while that value was based on a social context recognized as a man's world. Many times we heard 'the farm is his really' from farm women, the majority of whom held legal co-ownership. One said:

> Farming in and of itself is very much a man's world ... [the farm is ours] but he ultimately makes the, you know, the major farm decisions. We talk about them but he ultimately makes them I guess ... I guess I am thinking that I am always worrying and thinking about [multiple things for the family and the farm] and he's just thinking about what has to be done in the fields and he doesn't worry about what has to be done in the house ... he organizes what he has to do and I organize everything else.

While the male farmer focused on his farm work, being a good woman (both to a farmer husband and in a rural community) meant being able to multitask. In turn this multitasking might mean deferring or denying one's own needs and meeting expectations in the community, at work, and at home, while also being unpaid help on the farm:

> [I have been raised to do unpaid work]. I mean that I just was. I believe I was never really given the opportunity to question whether or not that was appropriate or whether I should embrace this effort because that's just who I was ... [there is agreement that] that's women's work if you like and this is my lot in life and this is what I do.

In such a context, women's needs are denied:

> It's all those feminist things if you like, about maintaining a sense of balance. I think nurses tend to lose themselves and so, you're a mummy, you're a nurse, but sometimes you forget who you are in the middle of all that, you know.

Struggling for Control and Balance

Women's paid work has been indispensable on farms for a long time (Ghorayshi, 1989) but is now contributing on more than one front. The farm woman is the care giver in the home, the organizer of family work, and usually the bookkeeper for the farm. In addition, the paid work she does enables her husband to continue working on the farm by paying the bills (Shortall, 2002). Consequently she may keep taking on more work (paid and unpaid), increasing her stress and vulnerability to health breakdown. There is unlikely to be any time for self when a woman works not just a second shift (Hochschild & Machung, 1989) but a triple day (Mackenzie, 1994). While most women doing paid work and family work are working a double day – coming home from paid work to organize family activities and do domestic labour – on the farm the wife also steps in to do some of the work previously done by hired labour, but which the couple can no longer afford. She will come home from her paid work, cook dinner, help the children with homework, and then go outside to herd cattle, feed pigs, or work in her garden.

The participants in this study appeared to be continually trying to work faster and harder in the belief that it would let them catch up with, and be in control of, the endless cycle of work. Although never explicitly stated, an element of conscious self-sacrifice emerged in the way that the women kept on working beyond their physical or mental limits. Most of the women talked about work overload. They acknowledged pile-up of their often conflicting responsibilities as mothers, farm labour, and nurses, as well as community members. They faced an increased workload not only at home but also at work. They had become the local 'go to' person in the absence of a local doctor, without any professional support for that role. They talked about additional expectations and responsibilities and said: 'So you make time, it's over and above everything else.' But they also admitted: 'Life is very tiring … that's a high stress [when farm is busy] that's a high stress then … I still do my work, nursing, well, but I have to really concentrate.'

Participants were not only working long hours, juggling many roles, but also living with too many unknowns. They talked about a sense of losing control of their lives, and the implications of that for their health status. They had not only lost a sense of control but also a sense of themselves, of who they were beyond being 'a good woman.' One said: 'Yeah, there's an emptiness inside but you're doing, you're being a wonderful woman, a wonderful mother, a wonderful employee, and wonderful.' Uncertainty is part of farm life, but it had now increased with the loss of subsidies, variations in demand for products, increasing costs, and so on. A farm woman with a sense of control knows when she will rest, knows the work will be finished at some foreseeable point. Participants could not be sure of that any more. They kept on working, trying to do more in less time, in an attempt to get back that sense of control. In this context, getting rest and living healthily was something to be deferred until later, but they did not know when that 'later' would be. Restructuring has added deeper levels of uncertainty. One participant said: 'The unpredictability makes it hard to plan.' Another stated: 'Stress around finances is the biggest thing.' A further comment was that 'self-confidence and worth get chipped away when seeing friends having to sell farms and wondering "when is it my turn?"'

Data from this research showed that rural women were proud of their ability to manage a heavy workload and of their contributions to farm and community. Similarly in health care, nurses talked about doing more with less. One nurse said: 'There wasn't more time added to my schedule. It was just more work.' Both as farm women and as nurses, participants portrayed themselves as working endlessly: 'Everyone has jobs outside the farm now … you're just working and running.' They were working endlessly, and dealing with loss. They were mourning the loss of others' farms, their colleagues, their organizations, and time to get together with others. They were losing friends and community services as others' farms were sold and businesses closed. They had lost their women's organizations because no one had time to run them anymore. They no longer had time for coffee with a neighbour. They no longer had time to read. All of this was affecting their overall health and wellness.

It was noticeable, also, that when women did not feel taken for granted they perceived the endless work as less hard on them. A feeling that they were consulted at work or were treated as an equal partner in the farm, for example, could make the work worthwhile, whereas being taken for granted added to the stress of a heavy workload: A participant commented on her farm work:

> Yeah, so all the bookkeeping and in fact, to make even a lot of, you know, decisions, he would send me to a sale to buy a combine, I mean that kind of stuff. So I feel very valued and I think that gives you satisfaction even though it's a big responsibility and it could be burdensome but if you feel valued then it doesn't seem to be as hard work or it doesn't bother you as much. So that's probably an important part of the whole picture, is to be valued ... And so sometimes I resent all the book work but ... because you feel valued then it's not so bad. And in a way, if you're doing the books then you know what's going on.

Increased workload, loss of a sense of control, a feeling of losing a sense of oneself while trying to get the work done all contribute to stress and to health issues.

Health impacts ranged from the physical to the mental. 'I'm probably about twenty pounds overweight,' said one. A second said: 'I feel frustrated at this time because you know, where I wanted to gear down and work less hours I'm finding ... I'm working full time [and that] is harming because it isn't what it should be.' Another participant said: 'I don't always have what it takes at the end of the day,' Participants dreamed of having more time to themselves. They were well aware of the impact that their workload had on their health, but regarded this as a temporary situation. Participants acknowledged that not all their workload-coping strategies were good ones. The exigencies of survival were in continual conflict with emotional and physical health needs. Some smoked; others were overweight. Several disclosed specific health issues such as depression, arthritis, cancer, and migraines. Days taken off paid work, ostensibly for rest, often included catching up with work at home. Men, they said, had less trouble keeping boundaries in place, whereas they felt they had made a commitment to their lifestyle and therefore had to do what needed to be done – all of it. That could mean going without sleep, missing meals, not taking care of their health, and not having time alone. They considered that to be part of their chosen lifestyle, but resented the lack of recognition for their efforts, the silencing of their voices, and their lack of visibility:

> Maybe I'm sounding negative but women just aren't, in rural Alberta, aren't really a voice, you know? ... farming is in and of itself very much a man's world. It's more the woman is the caregiver and support person. Not really a person we would be concerned about. Well if they aren't functioning we couldn't do this.

They knew that they deserved recognition and respect for what they did, but said that those rights came last – they would address them 'later,' because 'you, you come last.'

Implications

Lobao and Meyer (2001) write that while much research has been carried out on the effects of macro-level economic conditions, less has been carried out on the impacts of economic conditions at the micro level. Individual health impacts of economic change have been largely ignored. As noted by Gerrard and Woodland (chapter 14), determinants of health include economic and environmental factors such as income, social support networks, education, employment, and working conditions. The farm women-nurses we interviewed clearly reflect these factors. Loss of farm income, due to government policy and economic change, led to a decision to enter the workforce or increase additional working hours without laying down other expected roles. Their education gave them access to what are known as 'good jobs,' that is, jobs that had a good rate of pay and benefits, but restructuring of health care services in Alberta had undermined the atmosphere and organization of the work. In none of this were they consulted, which Gerrard and Woodland identify as another stressor. Their social status as not only women but farm women was threatened at the same time as gender roles dictated they not give up any of their activities. In other words, the women we interviewed were revealing significant health issues related to stress and overwork, undertaken because the work had to be done *and they were the ones to do it*. Men had to keep on farming. Women had to do everything else. In rural areas, where change has come from political responses to a globalizing economy, women appear to be caught in a combat zone between their desire to save both farm and community and the need to regain a sense of control and balance, at the same time as they have lost their political voice.

For the present, the participants in this study were focused on being a good woman in the way that their rural culture expected. They were doing the best they could to keep their farm and save the community because their buy-in to the rural and farm lifestyle was of greater importance than their own well-being. They cited a loss of leisure time, of access to their support networks, and in many cases a loss of control not only over their activities but also attributed to loss of power over decisions made by employers and governments. These are determinants of health and well-being identified more than once in this book. The resulting stress sometimes had serious health implications for them. 'Outcomes of such stress can include compromised physical and emotional health, increasing the risk of morbidity and mortality. These factors, combined with less access to health care, may compound the vulnerability of rural residents' (Ames, Brosi, & Domiano-Teixeira, 2006, p. 119).

Conclusion

Stress has received insufficient attention in relation to the effects of gender. Seen here in a rural setting, gender is encapsulated as 'being a good woman,' and is shown as having major implications for well-being. For rural women, expected gender roles are literally dangerous to their health. Gender is a major source of stress when multiple identities and the roles attached to them need all the women's time and energy at the expense of leisure, social networks, and access to political power. Well-being takes second place to being a good woman and to maintaining a well-connected life.

This was a small research project. More research needs to be done in Canadian rural areas generally. Specifically, the ways in which government policy and economic changes have health implications for those affected by them, and the gendered nature of that impact, especially among farm women and nurses working in rural health services, require further investigation. While aimed at greater efficiency, competitiveness, and cost reduction, government policies may have unintended consequences that could become a cost factor themselves.

Acknowledgments

This project was funded by the National Network on Environments and Women's Health (NNEWH). NNEWH is financially supported by the Centres of Excellence for Women's Health Program, Women's Health Bureau, Health Canada. The views expressed herein do not necessarily represent the views of NNEWH or the official policy of Health Canada. Research assistance was provided by Julie A. Gilbert, MN, and Yvonne Hauck, PhD.

Notes

1 Many early feminist academics (e.g., Chafetz, 1984, 1990) drew attention to the invisibility of women's work. This refers to the way in which writing about occupations such as farming assumes it is men's work. Until very recently, banks would not give loans to farm women for the farm unless their husbands co-signed, but would give loans to the men without their wives' signature even when the farm was in both their names (see Mackenzie, 1994).
2 See Langford (1997) for an account of farm women's organizations.

References

Alasia , A. (2010). Population change across Canadian communities, 1981–2006: The role of sector restructuring, agglomeration, diversification and human capital. Retrieved from Statistics Canada, *Rural and Small Town Canada Analysis Bulletin, 8*(4), March 2010.

Alasia, A., & Bollman, R.D. (2009). Off-farm work by farmers: The importance of rural labour markets. Retrieved from Statistics Canada, *Rural and Small Town Canada Analysis Bulletin, 8*(1), March 2009.

Alasia, A., & Magnusson, E. (2005) Occupational skill level: The divide between rural and urban Canada. Retrieved from Statistics Canada, *Rural and Small Town Canada Analysis Bulletin, 6*(2), February 2005.

Alston, M., & Kent, J. (2008). The big dry: The link between rural masculinities and poor health outcomes for farming men. *Journal of Sociology, 44*, 133–47.

Ames, B.D., Brosi, W.A., & Damiano-Teixeira, K.M. (2006). 'I'm just glad my three jobs could be during the day': Women in a rural community. *Family Relations, 55*, 119–31.

Boyce, J.K. (1999. The globalization of market failure? International trade and sustainable agriculture. Retrieved from www.peri.umass.edu/fileadmin/pdf/published-study/PS3.pdf

Brandth, B. (2002). On the relationship between feminism and farm women. *Agriculture and Human Values, 19*, 107–17.

Brandth, B. (2007). Gendered work in family farm tourism. *Journal of Comparative Family Studies, 38*(3), 379–93.

Chafetz, J.S. (1984). *Sex and advantage*. Totowa, NJ: Rowman and Allanheld.

Chafetz, J.S. (1990). *Gender equity: An integrated theory of stability and change*. Newbury Park, CA: Sage.

Christison, B. (2000, 5 July). The impact of globalization on family farm agriculture. Speech presented at the RIAD International Forum, Porto Alegre, Brazil. Retrieved from www.inmotionmagazine.com/bcbrasil.html.

Constantine, M.G. (2001). Stress in rural farm women: Implications for the use of diverse mental health interventions. *Journal of Psychotherapy in Independent Practice, 2*(2), 15–22.

Ghorayshi, P. (1989). The indispensable nature of wives' work for the farm family enterprise. *Canadian Review of Sociology and Anthropology, 26*(4), 571–95.

Heather, B., Skillen, D.L., Young, J., & Vladicka, T. (2005). Women's gendered identities and the restructuring of rural Alberta, Canada. *Sociologia Ruralis, 45*(1/2), 86–97.

Hochschild, A.R., & Machung, A. (1989). *The second shift*. New York: Avon.

Langford, N. (1997). *Politics, pitchforks and pickle jars: 75 Years of organized farm women in Alberta*. Calgary: Detselig.

Little, J. (2002). Rural geography: Rural gender identity, and the performance of masculinity and femininity in the countryside. *Progress in Human Geography, 25*(5), 665–70.

Lobao, L., & Meyer, K. (2001). The great agricultural transition: Crisis, change and social consequences of twentieth century farming. *Annual Review of Sociology, 27*, 103–24.

Mackenzie, F. (1994). 'Is where I sit, where I stand?' The Ontario Farm Women's Network. *Journal of Rural Studies, 10*(2), 101–15.

Meyer, K., & Lobao, L. (1997). Farm couples and crisis politics: The importance of household, spouse and gender in responding to economic decline. *Journal of Marriage and the Family, 59*, 204–18.

National Farmers' Union. (2003, 20 November). *The farm crisis, bigger farms, and the myths of 'competition' and 'efficiency.'* Saskatoon: Author.

Ni Laoire, C. (2005). 'You're not a man at all!' Masculinity, responsibility and staying on the land in contemporary Ireland. *Irish Journal of Sociology, 14*(2), 94–114.

Shortall, S. (2002). Gendered agricultural and rural restructuring: A case study of Northern Ireland. *Sociologia Ruralis, 42*(2), 160–75.

Singh, G.K., & Siahpush, M. (2002). Increasing rural-urban gradients in U.S. suicide mortality, 1970–1997. *American Journal of Public Health, 92*(7), 1161–7.

Skillen, D.L., Heather, B., & Young, J. (2003). Reflections of rural Alberta women: Health, work and restructuring. In P. Van Esterik (Ed.), *Head, heart and hand: Partnerships for women's health in Canadian environments* (pp. 107–26). Toronto: National Network on Environments for Women's Health, Women's Health Bureau, Health Canada.

Statistics Canada. (2006a). *Snapshot of Canadian agriculture.* Retrieved from www.statcan.gc.ca/ca-ra2006/articles/snapshot-portrait-eng.htm.

Statistics Canada. (2006b). *The financial picture of farms in Canada.* Retrieved from www50.statcan.ca/English/agcensus2006/articles/finpic.htm.

Statistics Canada. (2007). *Census of agriculture: Farm operations and operators.* Retrieved from www.statcan.gc.ca/daily-quotidien/70516/dq070516a-eng.htm.

Statistics Canada. *The Daily.* http://www.statcan.gc.ca/dai-quo/.

Swisher, R.R., Elder, G.H., Lorenz, F.O., & Conger, R.D. (1998). The long arm of the farm: How an occupation structures exposure and vulnerability to stressors across role domains. *Journal of Health and Social Behavior, 39,* 72–89.

Thurston, W.E., Blundell-Gosselin, H.J., & Rose, S. (2003). Stress in male and female farmers: An ecological rather than an individual problem. *Canadian Journal of Rural Medicine, 8*(4), 247–54.

14 Gender Politics and Rural Women: Barriers to and Strategies for Enhancing Resiliency

Nikki Gerrard and Alanah Woodland

Despite harsh economic times, brutal weather extremes, and disappearing rural populations that have resulted in loss of community members and greater isolation for others, many farm people continue to survive. The first author, a farm stress specialist (1995, 1998) and community psychologist, wanted to understand more about how they managed to survive under these conditions. 'Resiliency' is a term in the academic literature that seems to apply to these people's survival, but questions remained. What is resiliency, exactly, and what are the barriers to and enhancers of resiliency in rural populations? What strategies can be developed to become more resilient? What role does gender play in resiliency?

Resilience is often thought of as an individual attribute, but we introduce the theoretical framework of determinants of health (Marmot & Wilkenson, 2006; Public Health Agency of Canada, 2010) to provide the perspective and structure to house the emergence of resilience as a community attribute. We explore a definition of resiliency in a broader context wherein the understanding of resilience expands beyond individual behaviours and coping skills and is derived from the larger context (i.e., social environment, physical environment); mediated by a shared social and economic climate, working conditions, and social support networks. Based on a study of rural residents in the Province of Saskatchewan, on stress resiliency, or the ability of people to manage and cope with unusual levels of and/or chronic stress (Gerrard, Kulig, & Nowatzki, 2004), we apply the lens of gender and gender politics to what was learned about rural women and their barriers to and enhancers of resiliency, consider how other determinants of health play a role in rural women's individual and collective resiliency, and recommend health promotion strategies to strengthen rural women's resiliency.

Background

Using qualitative research methods, we interviewed seventeen rural people, nine of whom were women. The ages ranged from the mid-thirties to the mid-seventies. Participants resided in the southern half of Saskatchewan, in every sector: north, south, east, west, and central. All of the participants were or had been farmers, had lived on a farm, or were connected to farming in some direct way. The unstructured interviews explored such things as their definition of resiliency, experiences when they felt they had been resilient and when they felt they had not, what they felt the differences were, what they do to protect themselves from adversity, and what puts them at risk for adversity. Factors such as changing health care and the tensions between a rural and urban culture were also explored. Participants were asked to describe what the barriers to and enhancers of resiliency might be in their lives.

Analysis of transcribed interviews was conducted using a process of coding ideas in the data into categories, organizing subthemes from the categories, and then creating broad themes from subthemes (Cropley, 2002). The written results were sent to participants for their further comments and/or changes, including additions or omissions.

The Role of Gender Politics in Rural Women's Lives

'Gender' refers to a whole array of social constructions associated with biological sex (World Health Organization [WHO], 2010). Access to power and resources, expected roles, rules of behaviour, and expectations about the conduct of such things as care-giving and child-raising are just a few examples of these constructions. 'Politics' refers to access to and relationship with power. 'Gender politics' refers to every aspect of life in which gender plays a role in the power dynamics of events (McLean & McMillan, 2009), and play a critical role in lives of rural women. Women have become more involved in farm operations, but historical gender roles governing the division of labour and decision making still prevail (Martz & Brueckner, 2003). Recent health and agricultural policy changes made without the participation of rural women have contributed to the reduction of their economic, political, and social power alongside the erosion of social supports (Gerrard & Russell, 2000; Gerrard, Thurston, Scott, & Meadows, 2005) and health and women's resources (Leipert, 2006; Leipert & Reutter, 2005; Price, Storey,

& Lake, 2008). As this study participant reported, gender politics are rife in rural communities:

> It's very, very hard to work out gender politics in a rural community. And I think it matters a lot and I think it really makes a big difference to women's lives if their gender stuff was better. They're really restrained a lot, rural women ... they might have better resiliency if left to their own devices, but their partners take away a whole bunch of things that they might be able to do ... You're telling your neighbour about problems that turn out to be your husband's problems – you can't do that. So some of the key things that are, that they [women] might do on their own, they're restrained from doing.

This woman identifies the responsibility of women to protect their husband's and family's confidentiality even if it means not relieving one's own stress in talking to friends. Since the farm is both the workplace and the home, it is more difficult to separate family and work problems, and gender politics affect women in both spheres. As we point out below, gender politics is played out for rural women through sex-role stereotypes, lack of economic opportunities, and familial roles and expectations. These politics create barriers to resiliency for rural women. But what, exactly, is resiliency?

Resiliency Defined

'What doesn't kill you makes you stronger.' This comment, expressed by one of the research participants, captures the essence of resiliency, but it fails to capture the detailed nature or complexity of the definition of resiliency that emerged from this study.

The common thread throughout interviews with both men and women was that resilience involved being able to bounce back from adversity. One woman said:

> I think that's the only thing you've got to look forward to in life is bouncing back cause there's so many, I mean one year we don't have a very good crop and we can't pay some bills and stuff; that's the only thing that's going to keep you on the farm is thinking that we'll bounce back.

However, bouncing back was not generally perceived to be enough to be called resilient. Participants talked about bouncing back to a different point. They talked about gaining capacity to cope from the experience, where, as one participant said, 'Maybe you would be better because of it.'

Coping was identified as an important ingredient in resiliency, but coping was not enough to be called resilient. As this woman said:

> [Resiliency], it's definitely coping but I think it's more than that too because if you just coped, to me, you just get through and you may or may not be resilient when you are through, you may just be there kind of like a blob.

Beyond simply coping, then, one of the most important skills in being resilient was learning. According to one participant, resiliency is about 'What did I learn, what would I not do again, or what would I do differently or what can I learn from this?'

Another way of looking at resiliency is to see it as an interactive endeavour that benefits from input from others. A male participant said his resiliency depended on how he felt after he had interacted with another person. First he had to have some connection with them, and then the resultant feeling he had would determine whether or not he felt resilient. He said, 'Going from a state of not feeling good about something to feeling better about it' would constitute resiliency.

It is important, therefore, to define resiliency as a process, a work in progress, which changes over time and in different circumstances. One woman summed it up:

> If you keep on going back to where you were, you're still going back; it's like going back to when you're eighteen. No, when you go through this adversity and you come out on the other end and you still got all your marbles and you're still able to cope nicely with life, you have added something there to yourself, you've learned lessons hopefully. You should be stronger so that the next time something happens you have a little bit more strength.

Thus resilience was seen as a process of coping that was dependent on the circumstances and the stressors involved, and on the physical and social context surrounding the individual.

This is a very different definition of 'resiliency' than is traditionally presented in the literature. In the past, research focused mostly on children and their ability to cope in the face of adversity or vulnerability. The presence or absence of resiliency was attributed to intrapsychic factors or an individual's 'instrumentality' or skills such as good self-esteem, good decision-making skills, and belief in a higher force (Richardson, Neiger, Jensen, and Kumpfer, 1996). Beardslee (1989), Werner (1990), Flach (1989), and Rutter (1985) all espoused numerous individual attributes as preconditions for resiliency.

The understanding of resilience that emerged from the rural participants in this study is contextualized and collective; such definitions are also emerging in others' research. For example, Leipert (2006) and Leipert & Reutter (2005) examine the development of resilience strategies of rural women that rely upon both environmental and personal factors; earlier work by Breton (2001) identified the role of social and physical capital, active voluntary associations, and stable local organizations in a neighbourhood's resilience; and Ungar (2004, 2005) asserts that resilience is reliant upon structural conditions, relationships, and social justice. In addition to the contextualized and collective definitions, the participants in our research identified that resilience required an interaction with their environment and that environments are constantly changing; hence we define resiliency as a process, interactive in nature, changing over time, and embedded in a context related to economic, political, and social pressures and opportunities. For further discussion about the definition of resiliency, see Gerrard et al. (2004).

Barriers to Resiliency for Rural Women

From the interviews with both women and men, we identified the following gender politics as barriers to resiliency.

Sex-role stereotypes. Some women described the barriers to resiliency as being the result of the things they are expected to do because they are women. They may not be able to take the time to connect that was identified as important to resiliency. These expectations are not always verbalized or made explicit. One woman described it this way:

> I want to get things done quickly and fast and get it all done right now so I can relax. But it never works like that cause you have to take one thing and deal with it and you see that's what I do. I write papers, do laundry, bath a kid, cook supper and I'm doing all that stuff at the same time ... It has a lot to do with gender and the fact that because I'm female those are my jobs ... those are my things that I have to deal with ... I question if [my husband] even realizes it.

Lack of economic opportunities. A male participant talked about the double whammy that rural women face when looking for employment, where 'opportunities are so limited [for] women ... almost impossible to get a job' yet the farm, another business affected by the rural economy, is dependent on her income. When a farm needs two incomes, he said, 'If the woman cannot find employment in the area, it's sort of a double whammy ... we're sort of saddled with double burdens out here in a lot of ways.'

Male-dominated world of business. Being a woman in a business that is viewed as male and is dominated by males in sales and service can be difficult. In the case of farm women the business partner is also her husband. As resiliency is relational, women are excluded from opportunities to build resilience because they are not even seen to exist in their role as business partner. As one woman reported:

> I've had to make lots of adjustments, with some of the realities that are there and they're disappointments ... I've had to compromise a little more than I wanted to but sometimes I felt I didn't have a choice ... In the business, where I deal with a big company that is more male oriented ... when you're a husband-and-wife team and he definitely is [viewed by them as] the head of our business, there is no question [in their mind], but we are an equal partner. But I'm never viewed as that and I feel that has probably caused me more hurt or more distress cause I feel I'm less in control or some of the other things ... whether it's employees who view you as a little less, or the big shots coming down who definitely view you as totally less. You know, decisions that get made that you're not included in.

Being a daughter-in-law on an intergenerational farm. There is, arguably, no more potentially distressing role for a rural woman than to be the daughter-in-law on an intergenerational farm on which you own no property and are not recognized as a legal partner in the farm. One participant captured the essence of this issue:

> For a lot of women there's a lot of gender stuff attached to farm life that's really bad and is hard on them. There's a lot of values in there ... they marry into farm families that are owned by men and there's moms and dads there ... It's hard to get involved in the farm and you're never the expert ... no matter how long you live there you're always the bottom on the totem pole for more than one reason.

Being on the bottom of the totem pole would be another case of not being recognized in one's role as a business partner who might need support for resiliency. This position would also lessen opportunities to gain the assets needed for resiliency in the context of farming and rural communities.

Lack of communication opportunities. The opportunities to talk about significant issues in rural women's lives were reported to be few and far between. With some despair, one participant recalled a time when women had a rare opportunity to talk about farm stress and it did not happen:

> That was the first and only time that women in this community have sat down … to talk about farm stuff and would have had the chance to bridge into a conversation about women and farm stress, and it didn't go … it didn't happen again …

As resiliency is viewed as interactional and dependent on community, this is a barrier to resiliency. The sex-role stereotypes for women, lack of economic opportunities, male-dominated world of business, problems associated with intergenerational farming, and lack of communication opportunities for rural women are thus part of the context for rural women when resiliency is needed. Structural conditions, relationships, and social environments are gendered in ways that present challenges to resilience for women in rural communities. However, many of these women also talked about strategies that enhanced their resiliency.

Rural Women's Strategies for Enhancing Resiliency

The participants in this study employed many strategies for enhancing resiliency. These strategies also enforce the definition of resiliency as interactive in nature, changing, and embedded in context. We focus on examples of challenging sex-role stereotypes and on the importance of support at many different levels. Being an agent in your own life is essential in enhancing resiliency; participants talked about achieving this through learning. Finally, we discuss the connection between control, real or perceived, and resiliency.

Challenging sex-role stereotypes. Many women challenge sex-role stereotypes using different strategies. Some break through employment or educational barriers, others break through relational barriers. One woman illustrated how this took place over time:

> For me, getting married was a real shocker. Which I think is quite surprising, but ... it changed, well, I'm sure it changed my partner's expectations. And it suddenly triggered in everybody this ... expectation that I would be making meals at suppertime. Well, I mean [he's] a [husband's off-farm profession], I'm a teacher, you know, we've got to work this out better. And so it was hard, if I hadn't been just married at the same time as I was doing a profession, at the same time that we were running a farm a distance away ... I actually think now I could probably [have] handled that a lot better. I could deal with those things a lot better, I'd be way better at saying I'm sorry, I'm just going to stay at school till 7:00 every night; you're going to have to handle supper on your own, but then maybe I'll be able to come to the farm most weekends or whatever ... I think I'm more resilient now than I was then; I've learned way more things.

Of necessity, rural women have had to get off-farm employment, and that has been both positive and negative for them. It has been positive in that they have challenged the sex-role stereotype of staying on the farm and doing the childcare and housework, with their husbands earning the income. But it has also had a negative side as there is still farm and house work to be done.

Support at many different levels. Support was extremely important for enhancing resiliency for rural women. In light of the limited opportunities for communication, support is needed when, as one person said:

> You recognize that there is something wrong and you can't cope with it on your own; you need something out there, somebody out there that doesn't know anything about it, to be able to look at it objectively and tell you, or maybe lead you, in the right direction.

People can provide support by acting as a sounding board so that problems can be assessed, but they are very important as a source of information:

> If you have bad days you have supports to help you through those or to bounce ideas around or think of other options, connect or network with someone to help get you networked with others to kind of learn from or with, mentor, whatever.

Seeking out or accepting support requires an awareness that one needs it, and then one needs to open up and, perhaps, take a risk. Being able to identify appropriate networks is a strategy for enhancing resiliency. Speaking from experience, one woman said:

> People have to recognize it early on, and if you're able to talk to somebody that's gone through the same thing, I think that helps a lot. If you're able to surround yourself with people that have gone through similar experiences so that you know that you're not all by yourself out there, I think that helps ... we surrounded ourselves with some people ... that didn't criticize you for the mess you were in. They realize it happens to everybody and you go from there.

Support from family. Encouragement, decision making, sharing the load and coping together, taking turns, and sharing work and resources were all spoken about in relation to supportive family relationships that enhanced resiliency. Skills to maintain a collaborative spousal relationship, given the gendered barriers identified above, are thus a strategy for enhancing resiliency.

Encouragement from a spouse can go a long way in enhancing resiliency, as this woman stated: '[If women] have support from their significant other ... then it's much easier than if their other is saying, "No you just stay home and you don't need to go there or do that."'

A partner can share the burden of decision making, according to some participants:

> The two of us are quite open and talk about situations and what's going on and try and share the management decisions so that you don't feel like you're the only person that, or, so he wouldn't feel like he's the only person that's burdened with them so that once they're made then we both live and try and make them work.

Another participant agreed: 'On the farm, if you're married I think the [female] spouse should be involved in decision making and she should know what's going on ... It's something you work at together.'

Support may mean taking turns with your partner in dealing with adversity, as this woman reported she and her partner did:

> Preserving the other person a wee bit. If you see that they're down and, you know, it's quite true that [my spouse] and I take turns being depressed ... We just literally take turns being depressed and I think that [my friend]

and I do that too ... If you take turns, like once somebody's claimed the 'I'm down' territory, then you can't.

Support from friends. As one participant said, friends are part of her 'resiliency package', and therefore opportunities to build and maintain friendships are an important strategy:

> My friends are part of my resiliency package and if something happened to some of them ... if they left, geographically ... it would definitely interfere with my ability to be resilient ... And my closest friends ... if they weren't available ... like if they died, I think I could even handle some geography if I didn't lose them all, but I think those key relationships that help you be strong, if they go missing then it's harder to do that [be resilient].

Some of the reasons friends are part of her resiliency, she stated, is that close friends 'know a lot about you and they sort of accept the whole package. Which tends to include your weird husband and your rude kids ... they're just very, very accepting.'

One woman talked about how she got support at an organization's board meetings:

> The people that I connect with are my people in [her organization]. You go for a board meeting and you share a room at night and I think I get more of that, 'Lay me on the couch, let me tell you my problems,' type of thing through that group!

Another talked about how her friends support each other:

> Over the years we have found that we get together and we have a bitch session really. When I started experiencing really serious financial problems, do you know what I found was the most helpful? [It] was having a friend of mine who also owned a business say, 'Oh God I know what you're talking about. Don't you hate it when the wholesaler phones and wants money and you haven't got any?' And all of a sudden, I thought, 'I'm not alone.' There is somebody else that is experiencing the same problem that I am experiencing and so it sort of went from there. We would get together and have coffee once in a while and, like, 'How've you been doing?' 'Oh it's been just awful,' and we would tell each other little stories about what was going on. Well, pretty soon there's another gal that comes

into it and, 'Oh my God I could tell you stories,' and the next thing there's five or six of us that would get together.

This does not mean that others can solve your problems. But, as this woman said:

We really couldn't tell each other anything about how to make things better because we were just sort of all in the same boat, but the talking about it. You would be so uptight you'd be sick to your stomach and you'd get together ... Well, the next thing we'd be laughing about our various problems and you'd go back to work and you'd think, it's not that bad. I can cope another day. If you can find a friend that you can sort of cry on their shoulder and get it all out and when it's all out and you look at it and you think, 'What the hell, I can cope with this,' but until you lay it out, it's like running round in your mind like a rat trying to get out. And it just, over and over and over again, and you're not getting anywhere. You have to have somebody to talk it out with, so if you can find a good friend that can keep her mouth shut and listen, that's the best thing that can happen.

Support from community. Community, a group of people who share geography, common services, or a value system or beliefs, was viewed as a strategy for resiliency. As resiliency is defined as related to social pressures and opportunities, building a sense of community can be seen as more critical to resiliency than individual skills. Community provided resources for learning as well as a source of monitoring to identify when resiliency needed to be built. One woman described the commitment she had to her community:

We said ... really publicly to a lot of people in the community, that we were prepared to spend time with people who were going through farm crisis. Just this neighbourhood, we would be prepared to weigh in there with them and in the end we got ourselves quite a few.

She gave an example of how one neighbour was so depleted of resources and how, without support, the speaker felt the neighbour would die, at least emotionally:

I wanted to stand with the neighbours, we wanted to help with this ... it was the farm crisis stuff and ... they were in terrible shape and she'd gone and got a job and then we asked her, 'Well what do you do about this?' and she said, 'I don't do anything about it. I go to work. I come home. I close the blinds. I open a Danielle Steel book and I just close the door. I don't do anything about it.' And, you know, she was making this little place for herself to survive but it was so small and it would have to keep getting tighter and tighter and tighter and it will kill her. It'll kill her to make it that little, to just decide I'm only going to control what I can control inside of this tiny, tiny, tiny cup.

Not surprisingly, this kind of support leads to lasting friendships and, as she related, the gifts of support are a two-way street:

When we started working, when we started doing this thing with these people about farm crisis stuff, I was quite aware ... I really respected all those people when they came and said, 'Can you stand with us' ... I was really impressed that somebody had enough self-preservation to say we don't need a therapist, we don't need the banker there, we just need somebody to stand in there with us for a couple years ... I really liked that ... those friendships ... those people, it's brought us closer to all those people, they were people we didn't know very well and wouldn't have known. And I was really impressed that they'd be prepared to do that and kind of, I felt like it was sort of a gift to us. Although it's really hard on you to do that because you're not a professional, and ... not their therapist ... not their accountant ... not their any of those things and don't want to be. What we were saying was, 'We're fellows, we're neighbours, or we're in this community and you people matter to us and we think that you need somebody just to be there with you, to help you listen to the banker, and to say things, sometimes, you can't say.'

Learning was seen as both protective from stress and proactive in developing resiliency. One participant said, 'The best way to protect myself from it [adversity] is try to keep up with the learning process, in terms of getting comfortable or else, rather than sitting back doing nothing, become proactive.' Another added, 'What doesn't kill you makes you stronger, you learn from it.' Most participants said they learned from stepping back and re-examining some incident or aspect of their lives. For instance, according to one participant, 'You can then look back and try to examine what did I learn, what would I not do again or what would I do differently or what can I learn from this.' Another talked about stepping back and learning to let go: 'If the [job doesn't get done] this week, it's probably not the end of the world, the sun will probably come up tomorrow ... let go of it ... you do things for a while and you learn.'

Learning from a difficult experience gave the experience a more positive meaning for some. This participant explained how this works:

> It's tougher if you're coping and you're getting by, but it's not so easy to go back now because there's more pain and hurt every time you do that. Versus you've been through it, you've tried to deal with it and now you can learn something from it.

Real or perceived control. A sense of being in control of one's life was one of the outcomes of the strategies to enhance resiliency and played a major role in being resilient. When one participant was asked to describe the difference between the two for her, she said:

> Control ... When I'm not resilient, I've lost control and when I'm in control of my thoughts and in control of my physical environment ... when I'm resilient those are the times when I think I have more control over my thoughts and my environment.

Another remarked, 'I can cope with what I can control.'

Perceptions of control are important. As an enhancer to resiliency, a sense of control depends on an internal assessment that presumes control. In other words, anticipating events, taking action, and benefitting from earlier experiences only leads to control if the individual believes she has the ability to be in control. As a piece of conventional wisdom says, 'Whether you believe you can or you believe you can't, you're right.' Control was defined by one person as 'know[ing] what's coming down the road ... I think you know where you are going with the process; it's structured.' Another said:

> You can see a beginning and an end ... If you can see an end then you can probably get through it, you can last, you can put out, you can whatever cause you know it will end, at such and such a time, but otherwise you don't really know.

Again, participants related control not just to their individual experiences, but to resiliency as a process in the interactions in community and political context . Some factors related to having control had to do with taking action at the community or some other collective level. In fact, one participant gave her opinion that being in control was all about being in control *together*, at the community level, which is a powerful concept. She said, 'Just be willing to get out there and be involved in community affairs.' Another expanded on this idea, saying:

> We've got to take charge ... They have to do it on a community level ... There has to be some leadership. There has to be a mindset that will accept that maybe there's different ways of doing things ... has to be the ability to say we need help and the ability to go out and find the help that's needed ... the ability to interpret that help as to whether the solutions that are offered are right or wrong or a mixture and what you can use and what you can't.

Implications

In this chapter we have given numerous examples of how gender politics is played out in rural women's lives and affects their abilities to be individually or collectively resilient. A definition of 'resiliency' emerged that is temporal, relational, and embedded in social, economic, and political contexts. If one examines any 'list' of determinants of health (see, e.g., Hamilton & Bhatti, 1996; Public Health Agency of Canada, 2010), these determinants cut across many of the issues related to gender politics and resiliency that we illustrated in this chapter. For instance, income and social status were identified in the section above on economic opportunities and the male-dominated world of business; social support networks were illustrated in the section on being a daughter-in-law in a patrilinear world of farming and also in the section on communication opportunities. Despite the negative effects of these gendered issues, we also illustrated the 'antidotes' to these barriers to resiliency for rural women, and how these women are navigating the challenging of sex-role stereotypes and are demanding, creating, and sustaining supportive relationships, both within and outside of the family, in order to enhance their resiliency.

Through health promotion, opportunities exist for reducing barriers to and enhancing resiliency for rural women. Health promotion is 'the process of enabling people to increase control over their health and its determinants, and thereby improve their health' (WHO, 2005, p. 1); therefore, our recommendations seek to enhance rural women's resilience using the five action areas of health promotion (WHO, 1986, pp. 2–3).

Promote healthy public policy. As the work of Gerrard and colleagues (2005) outlines, there has been ongoing erosion of women's support programs, affecting not only the social support of women but their opportunity to have a political voice in the decisions being made for them. Adequate funding of gender-specific organizations in conjunction with political will to improve the status of women, especially rural women, needs to be reinstated (Gerrard et al., 2005). It is also critical that policy and funding support the development and implementation of strategies to stop the abuse against rural women and children and provide supports (i.e., economic security, safe houses, counselling, education).

Reorient health services. The goal of all health services should be to envision beyond simply helping people return to the point they were at before adversity struck. The influential role of practitioners make them well positioned to be advocates for the health and well-being of rural women (Leipert & Reutter, 2005); ensuring practitioners are informed, through curriculum inclusion and ongoing continuing education forums, of the situation of rural women will better enable them to fulfill that role. All needs assessments conducted in the health district must insist on a gendered analysis of services to ensure that they are providing adequate health services, especially women's services; innovative health care delivery models can be used to ensure access to services (Gerrard et al., 2004). Lastly, but most importantly, health services must have women involved in the planning, implementation, and evaluation of health care service processes (Leipert & Reutter, 2005).

Strengthen community action. The rural way of life is under duress, which brings stress to individuals, families, and communities. Earlier work by Gerrard et al. (2004) appropriately calls for community-level activities in rural and urban environments to increase rural sustainability and address economic and social issues. We strongly recommend that women be encouraged to become involved at the community level of organizations and in political action (i.e., in public office, community health boards); communities and programs can facilitate this by removing barriers specific to women (i.e., lack of rural childcare). Women's abilities and involvement can directly contribute to strengthening community action and developing innovative community-based economic opportunities (Tesoriero, 2006).

Create supportive environments. Governments, social and health services organizations, and corporations need to ensure the ongoing support and viability of service providers and services such as the Farm Stress Line that employ good listening skills and provide connections to other support services. They must also ensure that opportunities for support are equally available to men and women.

Community organizations, social services organizations, and corporations need to provide forums and opportunities for individuals, families, and communities to discuss and address the issues of gender and discrimination, including intergenerational farm issues that focus on the roles of the daughter-in-law.

Community services and organizations need to create opportunities for women to come together for social support and to share their strategies for enhancing resiliency, for example in discussion groups, educational experiences, art or recreational activities, or even a conference. Providing social support enhances communication, improves relationships, and builds resiliency for rural women and in families and communities.

Develop personal skills. There must be opportunities for women to reflect on learning and education as tools for reducing their adversity and gaining control over their lives. Governments and educational institutions need to provide the means for making or acquiring resources, such as more distance learning courses (online), video and audio tapes, and written material. Learning opportunities enhance a person's sense of control, and we've seen in this chapter how a sense of control enhances resiliency.

Conclusion

Resiliency must be seen as a dynamic process that takes into account both inner and external resources and that changes over time. It is not just a set of attributes that individuals may or may not possess. Resiliency is embedded in economic, social, and political contexts, and so the determinants of health are also determinants of resiliency. Gender and gender politics affect resiliency in a critical way. As long as women as a group face inequities in economic opportunities, for instance, their resiliency will be compromised. The Ottawa Charter for Health Promotion strategies (WHO, 1986), plus working hand in hand with rural women to challenge negative gender politics, are both essential to eliminating barriers to and enhancing resiliency for not only rural women but women everywhere. Finally, it is essential that future research track this work and monitor the effects of ongoing changes in government policies regarding agriculture.

References

Beardslee, W. (1989). The role of self-understanding in resiliency individuals: The development of a perspective. *American Journal of Orthopsychiatry, 50,* 266–78.

Breton, M. (2001). Neighborhood resiliency. *Community Practice, 9,* 21–36.

Cropley, A. (2002). *Qualitative research methods: An introduction for students of psychology and education.* Riga, Latvia: Zinatne.

Flach, F. (1989). Psychobiological resilience. In Flach (Ed.), *Stress and its management* (pp. 1–14). New York: W.W. Norton.

Gerrard, N. (1995). Farm stress: A community development approach to mental health service delivery. In H. McDuffie, J. Dosman, K. Semchuk, S. Olenchock, & A. Senthilselvan (Eds.), *Agricultural health and safety: Workplace, environment, sustainability* (pp. 433–8). Boca Raton, FL: Lewis.

Gerrard, N. (1998). Community development: A new model for dealing with farm stress. In W.E. Thurston, J.D. Sieppert, & V.J. Wiebe (Eds.), *Doing health promotion research: The science of action* (pp. 207–19). Calgary: University of Calgary, Health Promotion Research Group.

Gerrard, N., Kulig, J., & Nowatzki, N. (2004). What doesn't kill you makes you stronger: Determinants of stress resiliency in rural people in Saskatchewan, Canada. *Journal of Rural Health, 20,* 59–66.

Gerrard, N., & Russell, G. (2000). *An exploration of health-related impact of the erosion of agriculturally focused support programs for farm women in Saskatchewan.* Regina: Prairie Women's Health Centre of Excellence.

Gerrard, N., Thurston, W., Scott, C., & Meadows, L. (2005). Silencing women in Canada. *Canadian Women's Studies, 24,* 59–66.

Hamilton, N., & Bhatti, T. (1996). *Population health promotion: An integrated model of population health and health promotion.* Ottawa: Health Canada.

Leipert, B. (2006). Rural and remote women developing resilience to manage vulnerability. In H.J. Lee & C.A. Winters, *Rural nursing: Concepts, theory, and practice* (pp. 79–95). New York: Springer.

Leipert, B.D., & Reutter, L. (2005). Developing resilience: How women maintain their health in northern geographically isolated settings. *Qualitative Health Research, 15,* 49–65.

Marmot, M., & Wilkenson, R. (2006). *Social determinants of health* (2nd ed.). Oxford: Oxford University Press.

Martz, D., & Brueckner, I. (2003). *The Canadian farm family at work: Exploring gender and generation.* Muenster, SK: Center for Rural Studies and Enrichment.

McLean, I., & McMillan, A. (Eds.). (2009). Gender and politics. In *The Concise Oxford Dictionary of Politics.* Oxford Reference Online. Retrieved from

http://www.oxfordreference.com/views/ENTRY.html?subview=
Main&entry=t86.e538.

Price, S.L., Storey, S., & Lake, M. (2008). Menopause experiences of women in
rural areas. *Journal of Advanced Nursing, 61*, 503–11.

Public Health Agency of Canada. (2010). What determines health? Retrieved
from http://www.phac-aspc.gc.ca/ph-sp/determinants/index-eng.php#
determinants.

Richardson, G., Neiger, B., Jensen, S., & Kumpfer, K. (1996). The resiliency
model. *Health and Canadian Society, 4*, 11–26.

Rutter, M. (1985). Resilience in the face of adversity: Protective factors and
resistance to psychiatric disorder. *British Journal of Psychiatry, 147*, 598–611.

Tesoriero, F. (2006). Strengthening communities through women's self help
groups in South India. *Community Development Journal, 41*, 321–33.

Ungar, M. (2004). A constructionist discourse on resilience – Multiple contexts,
multiple realities among at-risk children and youth. *Youth & Society, 35*,
341–65.

Ungar, M. (2005). Resilience among children in child welfare, corrections,
mental health and educational settings: Recommendations for service. *Child
and Youth Care Forum, 34*, 445–64.

Werner, E. (1990). Protective factors and individual resilience. In S. Meisels
(Ed.), *Handbook of early childhood intervention* (pp. 97–116). New York:
Cambridge University Press.

World Health Organization (WHO). (1986). *Ottawa Charter for health promotion.*
Ottawa: Author.

World Health Organization. (2005). *Bangkok Charter for health promotion in a
globalized world.* Bangkok: Author.

World Health Organization. (2010). What do we mean by 'sex' and 'gender'?
Retrieved from http://www.who.int/gender/whatisgender/en/index.html.

15 Defining Health: Perspectives of African Canadian Women Living in Remote and Rural Nova Scotia Communities

Josephine B. Etowa, Wanda Thomas Bernard, Barbara Clow, and Juliana Wiens

In the last decade, rural health has emerged, sometimes sporadically, on research, community, and political agendas (DesMeules, Pong, et al., 2006). Interest in gaining a better understanding of rural women's health has spawned new research (Leipert & George, 2008). While there is recognition that rurality creates health challenges for many women, including compromised health status and restricted access to services, limited attention has been paid to the experiences and needs of ethnically diverse rural women (Kisely, Terashima, & Langille, 2008). Aboriginal women and recent immigrants are sometimes included in research on rural health in Canada (Sutherns, McPhedran, & Haworth-Brockman, 2003), but much of the health research on Aboriginal and immigrant women continues to be shaped by an assumption that members of visible minority groups are found only in cities, and often very large cities such as Toronto (Probst, Moore, Glover, & Samuels, 2004). This chapter challenges this assumption, providing a ground-breaking perspective on the ways in which African Nova Scotian women living in rural and remote communities understand and manage their health and health care.

From 2002 to 2007 the authors and other researchers worked with African Nova Scotian women living in rural and remote communities along the south and west shores of the province to develop and conduct a research project, *On the Margins: Understanding and Improving Black Women's Health in Rural and Remote Nova Scotia Communities*. This mixed-method research is informed by the principles of participatory action research (PAR), which enabled the 237 women who participated in the study to talk about their personal health concerns, the health concerns of their families, their experiences with health care providers, their understandings and experiences of racism and of community, and their ideas of how the health of their families and communities might be improved. The discussion presented in this chapter is derived from statistical analysis of questionnaire-generated data and the thematic analysis of the qualitative data. We first present some background information on African Nova Scotians, followed by a discussion of two key themes from our study and discussion of the implications of these themes. The concluding section highlights some key messages from the study.

Background

Unlike many other parts of the country, where the majority of black people are relatively recent immigrants from African and Caribbean countries, Nova Scotia is home to one of the largest populations of multigeneration African Canadians. People of African descent first arrived in the region in large numbers in the late eighteenth century, as Black Loyalists during the American Revolution and as slaves seeking freedom (Canada's Digital Collections, n.d.). Subsequent waves of immigration in the nineteenth and twentieth centuries swelled the population, and there are currently close to twenty thousand Nova Scotians who self-identify as people of African descent, representing more than half of the visible minority population of the province (Government of Nova Scotia, n.d.). Similarly, while African Canadians elsewhere in the country tend to be urban dwellers, and some African Nova Scotians reside in the capital city of Halifax and other cities in the province, many reside in rural and remote communities. As a result, Nova Scotia represents a rare opportunity to generate new knowledge and new insight about the health of black women living in rural and remote communities.

In many respects, African Nova Scotian women living in rural and remote communities face the same challenges as other rural Canadian women: lack of health and social services, limited or substandard childcare, lack or high cost of transportation, economic insecurity, inadequate housing, limited educational and employment opportunities, and social isolation (Dolan & Thien, 2008). They also enjoy many of the benefits of living rurally, such as strong social capital in the form of extended kinship and friendship networks and calmer, quieter communities in which to build and raise families. However, one of the defining features of the experiences of African Nova Scotians living in rural and remote communities is the origins and ongoing nature of their rurality. Rural living for the majority of African Nova Scotians did not begin as a life or vocational choice, as it did for many pioneer farmers and fishers from European countries, but rather had its origins in a series of racist acts. The Black Loyalists, who were promised land, work, and equality in exchange for their service during the American Revolution, were instead pushed to the margins of social, economic, and political life in Nova Scotia and settled in the communities outside the main towns (Canada's Digital Collections, n.d.). Subsequent waves of immigrants were more likely to settle in Halifax if they could because employment opportunities were more plentiful there, but they often lived in separate, if not segregated, communities within the city. In rural and remote settings, African Nova Scotians were also likely to settle in specific neighbourhoods, as in Yarmouth, or congregate in communities adjacent to existing communities, resulting in a rural landscape dotted with communities that shared boundaries but little else. For instance, the community of Weymouth is populated predominantly by people of European descent while the adjacent community of Weymouth Falls is populated mainly by people who self-identify as African Nova Scotian. As one woman observed:

> When I first got here ... nobody wanted me here. Right, I was the first black person to move up to [name of community]. And that was a no-no. I wasn't told to my face, but I was told by some other adults when I got here, like, that this was not a black community.

Historic and enduring racism has created profound disadvantages for African Nova Scotians, rural as well as urban (Amaratunga, 2002; McGibbon & Etowa, 2009). Although 15% of the women involved in this study were reluctant to discuss their economic situation, those who did described deep poverty, with annual personal incomes and annual household incomes less than fifteen thousand dollars. This is not to suggest that other rural Canadians are wealthy; we know that economic activity in rural and remote communities tends to be precarious, whether it revolves around agriculture, resource extraction, tourism, or other means of generating revenue. But the experiences of poverty among rural African Nova Scotian women are inextricably linked to and exacerbated by racism because prejudice limits their opportunities for housing, employment, and education. One woman recalled: 'I was applying for a ... housing grant and I had somebody come visit me and addressed us as "you people." Well I don't know maybe it was just him but the more he said that the madder I got.' Racism itself is also implicated in health issues for rural African Nova Scotian women. One study participant said:

> Anybody will tell you that they battle with their self-esteem every day. But I think particularly as a black woman, when you get ready for the day and you step outside the door, you never know what you are going to face. And as you walk the streets with your head high, people have certain preconceived ideas about who you are. And some of them are good and some of them aren't. And I guess I struggle with that every day.

Clearly, the experiences of African Nova Scotian women living in rural and remote communities are different from those of many other groups of rural Canadians. Recognizing the specific contexts of their lives is a necessary first step in understanding their views on and experiences of health and care. How people promote, maintain, and manage their health is greatly influenced by contexts, including race, sex and gender, socio-economic status, rurality, and other social determinants. Definitions of health are both a product of and an influence upon such contexts. Thus, understanding the meaning of health for different people in different social and geographical locations is critical to understanding their motivation to engage in health promotion and maintenance, and illness treatment activities.

African Nova Scotian Women Define Health

While many health researchers would agree that contexts, such as rurality and access to social capital, are fundamental to health (Cattell, 2001; Lochner, Kawachi, & Kennedy, 1999; Lomas, 1998), there is a tendency to define both health and care in biomedical terms, ignoring the ways in which diverse populations understand and manage their health and that of their families (Edmonds, 2001; Thomlinson, McDonagh, Baird-Crooks, & Lees, 2004). This is certainly the case for rural African Canadians, as much of the health research on people of African descent originates in the United States or focuses on urban settings (Atwell, 2001; Dana, 2002; Graham, Raines, Andrews, & Mensah, 2001). Our study findings suggest that African Nova Scotians living in rural and remote communities define health in a variety of ways, including functional, behavioural, relational, and economic, as well as biomedical.

When asked 'What does health mean to you?' many participants responded initially by describing physical wellness, including the absence of illness and the absence of pain. Several women associated good health with not having to take medication. These responses fit well with biomedical definitions of health, and they make a great deal of sense given the prevalence of illness among rural women in general (Crosato & Leipert, 2006) and in rural and remote African Nova Scotian communities (Kisely et al., 2008). Of the 237 women interviewed for this study, 48% had high blood pressure, 35% had high cholesterol, and 28% were diabetic (Bernard, Etowa, & Clow, 2007). Studies with African American women likewise demonstrate high rates of illness, including diabetes, high blood pressure leading to stroke and heart disease, obesity, kidney disease, arthritis, lupus, and breast cancer (Graham et al., 2001; Walcott-McQuigg, 2000).

Nonetheless, when interviewers probed further, most of the women participating in our study added mental, psychological, and/or emotional wellness to their definitions of 'health.' One participant described health in holistic terms: 'Health to me means the stability of everything: spiritual, psychological, as well as physical. And if one [of those] is off balance, I think all the rest is off balance.' Some women in our study did not address these aspects explicitly, but many of the definitions they provided revealed an implicit recognition that health means more than simply the absence of illness: 'My definition of health is to be able to get up in the morning and get out of bed and take care of myself, go to work, do things, feel good. Not just survive but to feel great!' Several women also included spirituality in their definitions of health and emphasized the importance of believing in a higher power. This holistic interpretation of health resembles the views of rural women and men in Alberta and Manitoba (Thomlinson et al., 2004). Following these initial discussions, participants were then asked two related questions: 'What does it mean to you personally to be healthy?' and 'What does it mean to you personally to be unhealthy?' Several specific themes emerged from analysis of the answers: health as ability, health as independence, health as activity, and health as access to resources. Each of these themes will be considered in turn.

The first two themes, health as ability and health as independence, are clearly related. Many women in the study defined health in functional terms of ability and evaluated their own health according to their capacity to do the things they needed or wanted to do, such as going to work or on outings. For one woman who suffered from chronic pain, being healthy meant 'being able to do things without having to worry about a sore back.' Women who were care givers included the ability to care in their definitions of health, tending to measure their own health in terms of their ability to care for children, partners, and families. As one woman said, 'Health means to me to be on my feet and to be able to be there for my husband and look out for him because he is not that well, and take care of my house.' In turn, poor health was defined as the inability to fulfil care-giving responsibilities. 'For me,' said one woman, 'being unhealthy would be just not being able to take care of my family or kids ... because I am the mommy and I do everything.' At the same time, some women in the study equated poor health with dependence on others, thereby linking independence with health. According to one participant,

> Health ... [to me] means you feel well enough, and are well enough, to do whatever you have to do for yourself, and not have to have somebody come and do for you, or wait for a family member to come and do it for you.

Another woman defined poor health as the inability to get out of a chair or to use the washroom without assistance.

These functional and relational definitions of health together provide important insight into the roles that black women play within rural African Canadian communities. For these women, health means the ability to look after everyone else (partners, children, relatives) while at the same time not having to depend on anyone to look after them. Such findings are consistent with the overall project findings, which demonstrate that black women see themselves as the 'backbone' of their families and as the ones responsible for looking after the overall well-being of their communities. These definitions are similar to those reported by other rural dwellers. Long's (1993) study with rural women in Montana, for example, revealed a definition of health related to 'role performance,' specifically participants' ability to work and meet family obligations. Contributing to family and community life and care giving, specifically 'taking care of their own,' seem to be features of both rural communities and African Nova Scotian communities (Bernard, 2002).

Taken together, these definitions of health also have implications for the well-being of African Nova Scotian women living in rural and remote communities. Research from the United States suggests that the multiple social roles filled by African American women both sustain and diminish their ability to maintain individual health as well as the health of others (McCallion & Kolomer, 2000; Musil, 2000; Whitley, Kelley, & Sipe, 2001). On the one hand, a commitment to care for others can encourage self-care in the case of acute health concerns and, on the other hand, discourage self-care in situations of chronic illness (e.g., type 2 diabetes) (Samuel-Hodge et al., 2000; Skelly, Samuel-Hodge, Headen, Ammerman, & Keyserling, 1997). Bani's (2001) study with African American women demonstrated that those who identified as 'strong black women' were more likely to report health problems. Clinical psychologists also suggest that the primary themes of the 'strong black woman' iconography – a combination of personal strength, self-reliance, and self-containment with the impulse to nurture and preserve the family – can create physical stress as well as psychological 'defenses' that can lead to negative health effects for self and others (Romero, 2000).

The third theme of health as activity emerged from the research as many study participants linked health with 'healthy' habits or activities. In other words, being healthy meant engaging in a series of health-promoting behaviours, including staying active, getting enough sleep, exercising, maintaining a healthy weight, quitting smoking, visiting a doctor for regular checkups, and eating properly. As one woman said, 'Healthy ... it means to eat good, and do exercise, and keep your body in shape, and don't do anything to damage your body.' Some women consequently assessed their own health in terms of the extent to which they exercised, paid attention to their diets, and visited their doctors for checkups. Some participants also concluded that their health would improve if they participated in health-related activities. Of all the health-related behaviours mentioned, healthy eating and exercise emerged most regularly in the interviews. These findings may point to the success of the dominant public health discourse with its emphasis on healthy eating and active living. But these definitions of health also suggest that the women we interviewed saw themselves as active agents who could exert some control over their health status. Research with rural dwellers in western Canada also revealed a conviction that individuals can take control of their health and well-being (Thomlinson et al., 2004).

The fourth theme was health as access to resources. Although some participants embraced definitions of health that affirmed personal choice and control, others recognized the limits of agency imposed by access to resources. One participant stated:

Health, what's associated with that? I think being able to afford the proper foods, you know, I find some of them are very expensive. You know, they're always saying eat right, eat right. But when you're on a limited budget, you can't always eat right. I think also having the medical structure there, you know, a good medical structure that you can rely on, that you know if you're not feeling well you can go to your family doctor and within a reasonable time have an answer ... It's not like that unfortunately today, but I think that would be part of good health to me.

One woman directly attributed her ill health to limited educational opportunities:

When I look at myself like my health is not that good, but I didn't have the education to actually push myself ... to do things ... So then I put school off and that is not healthy ... In order to live a decent, healthy life to me you need education. Your health could be way up here but if you don't have the education to motivate yourself everyday to get up then you really aren't healthy, in my opinion of healthy.

Women who were already dealing with chronic health conditions likewise understood the economic dimensions of health. One woman, a cancer survivor without private health insurance, told us she was scared because she could not afford to get sick again, nor could she afford to pay for treatments. Health care in Canada is provided on the basic assumption that individuals and families can afford peripheral costs such as transportation, prescription medications, over-the-counter antibiotics and anti-inflammatory drugs, orthopedic braces, time away from work, childcare, and so on. Adequate employment and income are thus essential for both health and care, particularly for rural, remote, and northern Canadians who face higher costs associated with access to treatment. These findings are interesting in that they reflect the barriers to health, particularly poverty, that define the lives of many African Nova Scotian women living in rural and remote communities (Bernard et al., 2007).

Changing Views of Health

Researchers asked participants if and how their understandings of health had changed. Some participants reported no change in their attitudes about health, either because they 'never thought about' their health or because they had always made an effort to be health-conscious. But most participants indicated that their beliefs around the meaning and importance of health had shifted, sometimes dramatically, at critical points in their lives. Aging, major life events, and becoming a parent were identified as pivotal for changing perceptions of health.

Almost all of the women reported that they had not spent very much time thinking about health when they were younger. Many enjoyed good health as teenagers and young adults, and therefore they were unconcerned about eating and exercise habits, or the potential for health problems. As women got older, however, they became less likely to take their health for granted:

> I think as you get older you start thinking about your health. And I think you start thinking of, you know, what things can I do to improve myself, i.e., exercise, proper foods, cutting some habits. If you're a smoker then you know that's impeding your breathing, so you quit that; if you're a drinker, you think, oh well, you know. So, I think you get a little bit wiser, you start being more interested in what is in your food, where is it coming from.

As women in the study aged, some began to pay more attention to their health in response to physical changes. One woman observed that her body started feeling 'different' when she began menopause at age forty-five, and these changes prompted her to pay closer attention to her overall wellness. Some participants were distressed by age-related changes to their bodies. As one woman stated:

> I am older, and I don't feel the same, my body is not giving me the energy that I had a few years back when I could just – oh I was just able to do so much exercising then and now it is gone.

Even without specific physical changes to prompt new interest in health, some women became increasingly concerned about negative consequences in the future if they were not more intentional in their efforts to maintain good health. As one participant said:

> When I was younger, it wasn't a big deal because you are not really told ... that you should watch what you eat and stuff like that. But as I got older, it's something that you have to really watch because if you are eating all the wrong things, it will come out ... You will feel it after a while ... [I]f you take in too much sugar, you get high blood pressure.

Some participants were able to see bodily changes and a resulting increase in health consciousness as positive. One woman reported that she felt much better once she started to take more of an interest in eating healthy foods.

Major life events also caused women's understandings of health to shift. In some cases, these events were positive. One participant spoke about a new relationship that prompted her to pay closer attention to her health. Another became more interested in preventive health care when she started working in a nursing home, while a young woman became more health-conscious when she moved out on her own and started making her own food. But negative life changes also led to shifts in perception of health. Illness diagnosis was sometimes responsible for a new view of health. For example, one participant said she had never thought about her health or took medication until she had a sudden stroke. In some case, these diagnoses served as 'wake-up calls.' One woman began researching information on exercise and healthy eating after she developed diabetes. Another participant felt that her diagnosis of fibromyalgia helped her redefine her priorities, including better health. She said:

> People who do not suffer from illness or chronic pain tend to waste themselves. I am thinking about things that are not important. But once you get a chronic illness you start to realize what is important and start to pare down everything. I don't need the fancy cars, and I don't need the fancy house, and just focus on yourself, gain your rest and eating right, and trying to take care of yourself.

Traumatic events such as the illness or death of a family member, friend, or acquaintance also caused some women to reflect more seriously on their own health status. One woman talked about the death of her mother: 'I didn't really think about being healthy. And then I lost my mother two years ago with heart disease. So that is when ... the light bulb just came on. I'm obese, which is not good for your heart.' Similarly, participants became more aware of their own health when they learned about health issues within their communities. As one woman explained:

> When you think with all the people dying this year and last year and like the year before it means a lot like for me to be healthy so I am, this year I can say I'm trying, I rest and I'm eating healthier. And I'm trying to make

sure that I have three meals a day and I drink water, that's good for you. But like this year, with everybody like being sick and just not even people that are being sick and they just die all of a sudden so it kind of scares me and like I'm trying to keep going. Be healthy, now that I'm young, and try to keep up.

Significant life events, both positive and negative, thus contributed to heightened awareness of and attention to health.

Many of the participants in this study were parents, and it was evident that these women constructed, re-evaluated, and transformed their ideas about health in relation to their experiences of parenthood. Women not only focused on the health of their children, but also became more cognizant of their own health. In some cases, increased personal health consciousness began during pregnancy. One participant described how she had to quit drinking, quit smoking, and 'smarten up' after she became pregnant with her first child. Women were also more likely to attend to their own health when they realized that they were responsible for looking after these young lives. As one woman said:

I really never thought about health – 'cause I was never sick – until after I had my family and then you start thinking about your health. What if my health gets bad, or something happens and [I've] got a family of little ones? Who would take care of them if something happened to me? … So that really started me thinking of my health. I made sure that I would go for my regular checkups with the doctor. And if I had pain … or whatever I always went and seen someone. I still do today.

This perception appeared especially strong among mothers who were the main financial providers for the family or who were parenting children on their own.

Mothers also became more health conscious when they thought about their children's future. 'Someday I would like to see my kids get married,' observed one participant, 'and I don't want to be somebody that is sick. You know … you would like to have your grandkids and take care of them or spend the day with them or whatever.' Women who were mothers wanted to be healthy enough to enjoy their families at all different life stages. This point is echoed by Novik (chapter 16), who found that Ukrainian women in rural Saskatchewan described family and community relationships as essential for good quality of life, and had a great sense of pride in their roles as grandparents.

Women who became more health conscious as a result of aging, major life events, and parenting incorporated these shifts into their lives in a number of ways. In some cases, women changed their behaviours. They not only became more attentive to their health, but also took concrete steps to improve their health, including changing diets, increasing exercise, instituting regular health checkups, and quitting smoking. For some participants, this increased health consciousness also prompted changes in their thinking about health, leading them to be much more anxious and worried about staying healthy. Women who had lost friends and loved ones, for instance, feared that they would also become ill. Many of these participants were caring for children and/or family members at the time of the interviews, and they worried about who would take over their responsibilities if their health suffered. As one participant explained:

> I overwhelmingly think of constantly dying suddenly and leaving my kids, and what are they going to do? I have a major fear of that ... And the older I get, the worse it is ... I don't know if it's because I'm getting older and the kids are a certain age, or whatever. And [mother] is at a stage and age that she ... is so dependent on me. And I want to be there for her. And I keep thinking the craziest thing. Like sometimes I think I'm not even going to wake up in the morning. And I know I take care of myself but the stuff that has been happening in the last five years to different people that I know, it's like, am I going to wake up tomorrow?

In a study with rural women and men in Alberta and Manitoba, Thomlinson et al. (2004) found that approximately 10% of participants felt that health 'means different things at different times in your life' (p. 261). Rural African Nova Scotian women involved in our study echoed this interpretation. They told us that aging, major life events, and parenting not only made them more health conscious but also led them to redefine what it means to be healthy. Many found that their definitions of health became much broader, encompassing physical and mental health and an overall sense of well-being as well as the absence of pain and illness.

Implications

This research gives us a first glimpse of the definitions and perceptions of health held by rural African Nova Scotian women and, in doing so, it raises as many questions as it answers. Some of the definitions of health proffered by participants in the *On the Margins* project mirrored those of rural dwellers elsewhere in Canada and the United States. The ability to care for self and others, in particular, was paramount for those rural African Nova Scotian women as it is for other women and men living in rural communities. Similarly, the women in Heather et al.'s study outlined in chapter 13 of this book described 'health as having the support of family and friends or as ... helping, contributing to the community' (p. 257). An emphasis on functional and relational definitions of health may be related to geography: in isolated settings, self-reliance is not merely a desirable trait, it may well be critical to survival, economic and otherwise.

Certainly the research conducted by Thomlinson et al. (2004) indicates that rural women and men in Alberta and Manitoba regarded rurality as a significant component of health as well as a feature of their identities and lives. But the myth of the 'strong black woman' and local studies with African Nova Scotian women also suggest that functional and relational definitions of health are not necessarily or solely tied to rurality. Bernard (2002) has highlighted 'the legacy of African Nova Scotians taking care of their own' (p. 153), and participants in our study also spoke about the role of black women as care givers in their families and communities. African Nova Scotian women residing in rural communities are not just isolated by geography but by discrimination and marginalization, and therefore are somewhat forced to be independent and 'take care of their own.' Definitions of health that emphasize ability and independence may thus be a product of diverse forms of discrimination and marginalization, including cultural and historic as well as geographic isolation. This is congruent with Gerrard and Woodland's definition of resilience as 'What doesn't kill you makes you stronger' (chapter 14 of this volume, p. 271). More research is needed to tease out the intersections of these determinants (i.e., discrimination, cultural barriers, and geographical location) as they shape understanding of health in different communities.

Other definitions of health, those that emphasized activity and resources, did not appear in the limited body of research on perceptions of health in rural and/or visible minority communities. Some of the women who participated in the study defined health as participation in 'healthy' activities. For some women in the study, being healthy meant engaging in a series of health promotion activities or behaviors, including staying active, getting enough sleep, exercising, maintaining a healthy weight, quitting smoking, visiting a doctor for regular check-ups, and eating properly. For example, one woman, quoted above, said that being healthy 'means to eat good, and do exercise, and keep your body in shape, and don't do anything to damage your body,', and another women defined health as 'taking care of your body and your lifestyle. Eating healthy, exercising, yearly checkups and visits to the doctor ...' Overall, participants equated poor health with the inability, failure, or unwillingness to participate in health-related activities. The lack of focus on economic resources is likely not explained by other rural communities being wealthy, but it may reflect the relative poverty of African Nova Scotians living in rural and remote settings.

Conclusions

Our study indicates that rural African Nova Scotian women are living in profound poverty by federal and provincial standards, but we do not currently have studies comparing levels of poverty among visible minorities in rural versus urban communities, nor do we have research on the economic health of diverse rural communities. Further study of the relationship between rurality, poverty, race, and sex is warranted to illuminate their impact on definitions of health. Bernard and colleagues have written extensively about the 'triple jeopardy' experienced by women of colour who suffer gender and racial discrimination combined with economic privation (Bernard, 2002; Bernard & Bernard, 1998; Bernard & Hamilton-Hinch, 2006; Etowa, Bernard, Clow, & Oyinsan, 2007; Etowa, Weins, Bernard, & Clow, 2007). The noxious mix of racism, sexism, and poverty has predictable consequences for the health and well-being of women of colour. Our research suggests that rural African Nova Scotian women may be subject to 'quadruple jeopardy' as geographic isolation further compounds the inequities fostered by racism, sexism, and poverty (Etowa, Bernard, et al., 2007; Etowa, Weins, et al., 2007). Comparative studies of African Canadians in rural and urban settings and comparative studies of ethnicity and rurality could shed light on the nature of intersecting disadvantages and provide direction for remediation.

References

Amaratunga, C. (Ed.). (2002). *Race, ethnicity and women's health*. Halifax: Atlantic Centre of Excellence for Women's Health.

Atwell, Y. (2001). *Finding the way: Establishing a dialogue with rural African Canadian communities in the Prestons*. Halifax: Author

Bani, C.P. (2001). *Exploring the 'strong Black woman' motif: Implications for health promotion and disease prevention among African-American women*. Paper presented at the American Public Health Association Annual Meeting, Atlanta, GA, 21–25 October.

Bernard, W.T. (2002). Including Black women in health and social policy development: Winning over addictions.In C. Amaratunga, J. Stanton, & B. Clow (Eds.), *Race, ethnicity and women's health* (pp. 153–82). Halifax: Atlantic Centre of Excellence for Women's Health.

Bernard, W.T., and Bernard, C. (1998). Passing the torch: A mother and daughter reflect on their experiences across generations. *Canadian Women's Studies Journal, 18*(2–3), 46–51.

Bernard, W.T., Etowa, J., & Clow, B. (2007). *On the margins: Understanding and improving Black women's health in rural and remote Nova Scotia communities*. Research Project report. Halifax: Authors.

Bernard, W.T., & Hamilton-Hinch, B. (2006). Four journeys – One vision: ABSW comes to Halifax. In W.T. Bernard (Ed.), Fighting for change: Black social workers in Nova Scotia (pp. 18–26). Lawrencetown, NS: Pottersfield Press.

Canada's Digital Collections. (n.d.). *Black loyalists: Our history, our people*. Retrieved from http://epe.lac-bac.gc.ca/100/205/301/ic/cdc/blackloyalists/index.htm.

Cattell, V. (2001). Poor people, poor places, and poor health: The mediating role of social networks and social capital. *Social Science and Medicine, 10*, 1501–16.

Crosato, K.E., & Leipert, B. (2006). Rural women caregivers in Canada. *Rural and Remote Health, 6*(520) (online), 1–11.

Dana, R.H. (2002). Mental health services for African Americans: A cultural/racial perspective. *Cultural Diversity & Ethnic Minority Psychology, 8*(1), 3–18.

DesMeules, M., Pong, R.W., et al. (2006). How healthy are rural Canadians?: An assessment of their health status and health determinants. Ottawa: Canadian Institute for Health Information.

Dolan, H., &Thien, D. (2008). Relations of care: A framework for placing women and health in rural communities. *Canadian Journal of Public Health, 99* (Supplement 2), S38–42.

Edmonds, S. (2001). *Racism as a determinant of women's health*. Toronto: National Network on Environments and Women's Health.

Etowa, J., Thomas-Bernard, W., Clow, B., & Oyinsan, B. (2007). Participatory action research (PAR): An approach for improving Black women's health in rural and remote Communities. *International Journal of Transcultural Nursing, 18*(6), 349–57.

Etowa, J., Weins, J., Thomas-Bernard, W., & Clow, B. (2007). Determinants of Black women's health in rural and remote communities. *Canadian Journal of Nursing Research, 30*(3), 56–76.

Government of Nova Scotia. (n.d.). *Nova Scotia community counts.* Retrieved from http://www.gov.ns.ca/finance/communitycounts.

Graham, G.J., Raines, T.L., Andrews, J.O., & Mensah, G.A. (2001). Race, ethnicity, and geography: Disparities in heart disease in women of color. *Journal of Transcultural Nursing, 12*(1), 56–67.

Kisely, S, Terashima, M., & Langille, D. (2008)..A population-based analysis of the health experience of African Nova Scotians. *Canadian Medical Association Journal, 179*(1), 653–8.

Leipert, B., & George, J. (2008). Determinants of rural women's health: A qualitative study in southwest Ontario. *Journal of Rural Health, 24*(2), 210–18.

Lochner, K., Kawachi, I., & Kennedy, B.P. (1999). Social capital: A guide to its measurement. *Health and Place, 5*, 259–70.

Lomas, J. (1998). Social capital and health: Implications for public health and epidemiology. *Social Science and Medicine, 47*, 1181–8.

Long, K.A. (1993). The concept of health: Rural perspectives. *Nursing Clinics of North America, 28*, 123–30.

McCallion, P., & Kolomer, S.R. (2000). Depressive symptoms among African American caregiving grandmothers: The factor structure of the CES-D. *Journal of Mental Health & Aging, 6*(4), 325–38.

McGibbon, E., & Etowa, J. (2009). *Anti-racist health practice.* Toronto: Canadian Scholars Press.

Musil, C.M. (2000). Health of grandmothers as caregivers: A ten month follow-up. *Journal of Women & Aging, 12*(1–2), 129–45.

Probst, J.C., Moore, C.G., Glover, S.H., & Samuels, M.E. (2004). Person and place: The compounding effects of race/ethnicity and rurality on health. *American Journal of Public Health, 94*(10), 1695–1703.

Romero, R.E. (2000). The icon of the strong Black woman: The paradox of strength. In L.C. Jackson & B. Greene (Eds.), *Psychotherapy with African American women: Innovations in psychodynamic perspective and practice* (pp. 225–38). New York: Guilford Press.

Samuel-Hodge, C.D., Headen, S.W., Skelly, A.H., Ingram, A.F., Keyserling, T.C., Jackson, E.J., Ammerman, A.S., & Elasy, T.A. (2000). Influences on day-to-day self-management of type 2 diabetes among African-American women: Spirituality, the multi-caregiver role, and other social context factors. *Diabetes Care, 23*(7), 928–33.

Sharif, N.R., Dar, A.A., & Amaratunga, C. (2000). *Ethnicity, income and access to health care in the Atlantic region: A synthesis of the literature.* Halifax: Maritime Centre of Excellence for Women's Health.

Skelly, A., Samuel-Hodge C., Headen, S., Ammerman, A, & Keyserling T. (1997). Life stress and the multicaregiver role of African American women with NIDDM: Influences on self-care practices. *Diabetes, 46,* 1041.

Sutherns, R., McPhedran, M., & Haworth-Brockman, M. (2003). *Rural, remote, and northern women's health: Policy and research directions final summary report.* Ottawa: Centres of Excellence for Women's Health. Available at www .pwhce.ca (accessed 19 April 2012).

Thomlinson, E., McDonagh, M.K., Baird-Crooks, K., & Lees, M. (2004). Health beliefs of rural Canadians: Implications for practice. *Australian Journal of Rural Health, 12,* 258–63.

Walcott-McQuigg, J.A. (2000). Psychological factors influencing cardiovascular risk reduction behavior in low and middle income African-American women. *Journal of National Black Nurses' Association, 11*(1), 27–35.

Whitley, D.M., Kelley, S.J., & Sipe, T.A. (2001). Grandmothers raising grandchildren: Are they at increased risk of health problems? *Health and Social Work, 26*(2), 105–14.

16 The Quality of Life of Elderly Ukrainian Women in Rural Saskatchewan

Nuelle Novik

Small-town and rural Saskatchewan looks different today than it did as recently as fifty years ago (Butala, 2003; Gerrard, Kulig, & Nowatzki, 2004). At one time, every small town boasted any amenity that one could possibly want, and agriculture still formed the primary economic base in the province (Butala, 2003). Farms were single-family operations, most of which did not exceed a section[1] in size. Today, however, farms are much larger and, out of necessity, are run much like corporations (Cushon, 2003; Warnock, 2003). The authors of chapter 13 in this book discuss similar changes occurring in rural Alberta.

Many rural areas and small towns in Saskatchewan have experienced notable population declines (Butala, 2003; Kubik & Moore, 2003). The remaining rural residents must travel long distances for goods and services, and health and educational needs are now met in more populated and centralized locations (Widdis, 2006). Demographic and economic shifts have resulted in high numbers of young people choosing to abandon rural life in order to move to urban locations in search of employment and to further their education (Butala, 2003; Kubik & Moore, 2003). As young people move out of rural Saskatchewan, many of those aged sixty-five and older have remained. As such, rural residents in the province have essentially become an aging population (Statistics Canada, 2007; Widdis, 2006). In general, rural areas within Canada identify more residents aged sixty-five and over than metropolitan areas. In 2006 the proportion of rural elderly had increased by 1.1%, while metropolitan areas saw a 0.7% increase in elderly individuals overall (Statistics Canada, 2007). The Province of Saskatchewan has the highest percentage of elderly people in Canada, with 15.4% of its total population aged sixty-five and older (Statistics Canada, 2007).

Within social science research, terms referring to older members of society remain loosely defined (Cheal & Kampen, 1998). The term 'seniors' most often refers to people aged fifty-five to sixty-four, and 'elderly' refers to those sixty-five and older (Hilleras, Pollitt, Medway, & Ericsson, 2000). Within this chapter, the term most often used will be 'elderly'. The total Canadian population over the age of sixty-five years also has a very high immigrant composition; it is estimated that one in every four elderly Canadians was born outside of Canada (Ujimoto, 1995). Of these immigrant-based groups, Ukrainian Canadians in particular have a unique history. As one of the largest ethnic groups that came to Canada through planned immigration and nation-building policies, Ukrainian Canadians have lived in this country for more than four generations (Luciuk, 2000). Within this chapter, the term 'first generation' refers to those foreign-born individuals who immigrated to Canada, 'second generation' refers to Canadian-born participants with at least one foreign-born parent, and 'third generation' refers to Canadian-born individuals with Canadian-born parents (Hansen & Kucera, 2004). The population of the world is aging, and the United Nations (2006) estimates that by the year 2050 one in every five persons will be sixty years or older. Women have always outnumbered men in all age categories. As women have continued to live longer, they have also continued to outnumber men as populations have aged (Cheal & Kampen, 1998; McDonough & Strohschein, 2003). Fifty-five percent of elderly people in the world currently are women (United Nations, 2006). Although this sex-based gap diminished slightly in Canada between 2001 and 2006, the majority of the population of elderly Canadians continues to be women (Statistics Canada, 2007).

In the Canadian Prairie provinces, where the initial settlement of Ukrainian immigrants came in three waves beginning in 1890 and ending in 1954, the current population continues to reflect a Ukrainian Canadian ethnicity. This is especially the case in rural areas (Swyripa, 1993). As such, in the Province of Saskatchewan, there are many elderly and widowed Ukrainian women residing alone in rural areas and small towns.

This chapter focuses on a research study that examined the lived experiences of elderly Ukrainian women in the Province of Saskatchewan. A brief history of Ukrainian immigration is provided, with an emphasis upon the experiences of Ukrainian women. The results of this study highlight the views of these elderly Ukrainian Canadian women in regard to their current quality of life. The results also emphasize the importance of relationships as they affect the quality of life of these women, as study participants specifically identified marital, familial, and community relationships as being of primary importance.

Background

The Canadian government first began to institute agricultural settlement policies in the area now known as Saskatchewan in the late 1880s (Scholz & Derbawka, 2002). By 1896, these policies were focused primarily on encouraging settlers from northern and central Europe (Scholz & Derbawka, 2002). Amongst these settlers were large numbers of Ukrainians.

There were three main waves of Ukrainian immigration to Canada. The first wave occurred between 1890 and 1914, prior to the First World War (Barlow & Barlow, 2003). Ukrainian immigrants during this first wave numbered approximately 170,000 (Barlow & Barlow, 2003; Ostryzniuk, 2002). While families were encouraged to move together, men far outnumbered women at that time. This resulted in the ongoing male domination of community life (Swyripa, 1993). The second wave of Ukrainian immigration to Canada occurred during the interwar period, 1919 to 1939 (Barlow & Barlow, 2003). This wave brought in approximately 68,000 Ukrainian settlers (Barlow & Barlow, 2003). The period between 1947 and 1954, the third wave of Ukrainian immigration to Canada, brought approximately 34,000 Ukrainian refugees from camps across Europe following the Second World War (Cipko, 1991).

In terms of a gender breakdown, the first wave of Ukrainian immigration brought approximately 41,000 females to Canada, the second wave brought 21,000, and the third wave brought 13,000 (Petryshyn, 1980). The dependent and minority status of most Ukrainian women kept them isolated and hidden from active participation in Canadian society for many years (Swyripa, 1993). While economic conditions forced Ukrainian men to leave and seek work across the country for months at a time, the women were left to maintain the homestead on their own (Luciuk, 2000; Swyripa, 1993). Although they received little recognition, these women carried out all of the necessary work on the homestead in the absence of their husbands. However, patriarchy continued to be the norm within these families (Swyripa, 1993). In examining the historical roles of women, Ostryzniuk (1997) states that 'the Ukrainian woman's role was a traditional one of dependence and subordination in a patriarchal society, and this cultural baggage was brought to Canada' (p. 24).

Although there remain gaps in the study of rural older women in general terms, the challenges that they face have been well documented (Kenkel, 2003). These women often report high rates of isolation and loneliness, both of which are seen as being detrimental to good health, successful aging, and the maintenance of a good quality of life (Kenkel, 2003; Stevens, 2001). As noted above, women live longer than men (McDonough & Strohschein, 2003). This reality has often dictated that women are left behind to carry on alone long after their husbands have died (Health Canada, 2002; Kenkel, 2003).

Research has shown that approximately 80% of older women in North America have living children and approximately 94% have grandchildren (Roberto, Allen, & Blieszner, 1999). Most of these women report having frequent contact with both their children and grand-children, regardless of their geographic proximity, and this is seen as contributing to a sense of well-being and success in their lives. Many elderly Ukrainian Canadian women had large families and have large numbers of grandchildren and great-grandchildren.

Religion and spirituality hold significance in the lives of Ukrainian Canadian immigrant women, regardless of their geographic location, and their roles and work within the church are highly valued. Many elderly women continue to be active in their church congregations and associated women's organizations and, in many cases, are the ones that continue to ensure the survival of the church in diminishing rural com-munities (Ostryzniuk, 2002; Swyripa, 1993). These involvements are seen to provide important mutual support and a sense of personal belonging (Kestin van den Hoonard, 2003; Mitchell & Weatherly, 2000).

Regardless of age or ethnicity, relationships are an important aspect of women's lives (Barnes & Parry, 2004). Of importance, as noted in the literature, are family and marital relationships (Roberto et al., 1999). In particular, older women are most embedded in family and community and the relationships found within (Markson & Hess, 1997). Central to these relationships are the roles played by the women themselves and the changing and fluctuating nature of those roles. It is not uncommon for women to talk about how they have come to know themselves as they are known through their relationships with others (Roberto et al., 1999). The authors of chapter 18 in this book also discuss the fact that rural community identity plays a very important role in the health of rural women.

The life experiences of rural elderly Ukrainian Canadian women have had a direct impact upon their overall current quality of life. Life experiences include the experience of immigration. The research suggests that this is generally the case with members of ethnic elderly populations in North America (O'Connor, 2003).

This exploratory research study examined the factors that affect the quality of life of rural elderly Ukrainian Canadian first-generation immigrant women from their own perspectives, as well as from the perspectives of daughters and granddaughters. This multigenerational approach to research, which draws upon three generations of life experience, is unusual in the literature and served to enhance the depth and richness of data.

This study utilized a 'reminiscence' or life review approach (de Vries, Blando, Southard, & Bubeck, 2001), a technique that involves the creation of a forum for a person to share personal meanings of life experiences and that can be conducted through the use of either structured or unstructured interview questions (Sheridan & Kisor, 2000). Qualitative in-depth interviews were conducted with twenty women representing three generations of seven distinct family units. First-generation participants were drawn through a process of purposeful sampling. It was also required that each of these elderly women have daughters and granddaughters who were willing to participate in the research.

Initial data analysis involved engaging in first-level coding. Meaning units were identified and fit into categories, and codes were assigned to the categories (Coleman & Unrau, 2005). The constant comparison method, a procedure in which meaning units are grouped together with other meaning units that are perceived to be related (Coleman & Unrau, 2005), was utilized throughout this phase of the coding process. Consequently, consistent themes were identified.

What evolved from the analysis was a picture of the current quality of life of the seven first-generation participants, that is, rural elderly Ukrainian Canadian immigrant women living in Saskatchewan. The data revealed three categories that these women use to define quality of life and ways to maintain it: marital relationships, family relationships, and community relationships.

The first-generation participants ranged in age from seventy-two to eighty-eight years at the time of interview. Each of them had come to Canada as a child or young adult. Their ages at the time of immigration ranged from one to twenty-one years, and they had been living in Canada an average of seventy-three years.

Following immigration, six of the first-generation participants originally lived on farms in rural Saskatchewan, and one initially settled in a small Saskatchewan urban area. Three of the women eventually moved to small towns, and one of the women moved to an urban location. At the time of the study, only two of the women lived in an urban setting; the remaining five all lived in small towns or on farms. One woman resided with her husband in their family home in a small rural town. Of the remaining women, all widows, one lived in a personal care home, three lived in semi-supported individual residences, and two continued to live in their own homes with no formal supports.

All of the first-generation participants maintained active membership in their churches. Their ability to attend services or to actively participate in different types of volunteer or committee work varied between women. Three of the women continued to drive on a regular basis. All of the women reported fairly good levels and ranges of health condition.

Quality of Life

The standard definition of 'quality of life' found in the literature usually incorporates criteria that include a sense of well-being, meaning, and value (Johansson, Ek, & Bachrach-Lindstrom, 2007). Researchers have identified a number of subjective states that are often considered when assessing quality of life, among them psychological well-being, perceptions of general health, level of pain, energy level, self-esteem, control, functional ability, autonomy, and independence (Higgs, Hyde, Wiggins, & Blane, 2003). The first-generation participants in this study identified similar criteria when talking about their perceptions of what factors contribute to quality of life. However, research has also suggested that social supports and a sense of individual spirituality directly affect health and well-being as factors identified in a good quality of life (Johansson et al., 2007; Musil & Ahmad, 2002). Therefore, these factors can also be considered as criteria worthy of consideration in an assessment of life quality. The first-generation participants interviewed for this study identified elements that they perceived as affecting quality of life, and these same elements were also identified by their daughters and granddaughters. In no particular order, these elements may include: a home, money, health, pain management, mobility, formal and informal supports, faith, security, independence, ability to keep a garden, busy work, opportunity to volunteer, a partner/husband, emotional strength, attitude, friendship of neighbours, children, and grandchildren. During the process of data analysis, there were primarily three relationships consistently identified by all three generations of women as having significant impact upon the quality of life of the elderly Ukrainian immigrant women who were the focus of this study: marital relationships, family relationships, and community relationships.

One first-generation participant summed up a variety of factors that she felt directly affected her personal quality of life:

> Well, as long as your health is okay ... the quality of life is fine. If you have enough money to live on, you have enough to eat, and if you want to go out you go out, if you don't want to you don't ... you know. (Baba B1)

The first-generation women all described various states of independence as being important to them. They also identified both the opportunity and the ability to stay busy in various ways as being essential to a good quality of life.

> I love gardening ... oh ... it's so nice. I don't need that much stuff, but I like to watch it grow ... oh ... it's so comfortable and peaceful. (Baba F1)

> I go to church ... all over ... I've got neighbours here ... they're so nice. They pick me up and they take me. I appreciate it so much. I like to go to church ... it's nice. You go and somehow you feel so relaxed. (Baba C1)

> I volunteer here at the Lodge ... we make peroghy ... sometimes we make pies...and some other things there is. And I go singing ... I joined a group ... I love it. We go sing at the Lodge ... at the hospital ... yeah ... I enjoy that very much. (Baba F1)

The daughters and granddaughters confirmed the types of activities that the majority of the first-generation women continued to be involved in. They also discussed the ways in which they saw these activities as positively affecting the life of their mother or baba. ('Baba' is a Ukrainian word meaning 'grandmother' and is commonly used in Canada.)

As should be no surprise, there were differences between rural and urban locations in terms of social and recreational opportunities. The decline of economies and populations in rural and smaller communities has resulted in a lack of social opportunities and formal supports for elderly residents (Johnson, 2005). Many of the first-generation participants who had moved into towns or the city, as they aged and retired, talked about how much they enjoyed the opportunity to be more easily involved in activities outside of their homes after they moved off of the farm. One woman talked about the difficulties that she and many other older women experienced in trying to get to church while living in a rural area. She also talked about how much easier it was to be involved now that she lived in a seniors' housing facility in an urban setting.

One seventy-nine-year-old baba who still lived on the farm discussed the fact that she was completely dependent upon her son to take her where she needed to go:

I wouldn't be still here on the farm if it wasn't for my son living here. Sometimes we get on each other's nerves, but he's okay. He helps me a lot ... and he will take me where I want to go. The only place he won't take me is to church. He won't go to church. And weddings ... he doesn't like to go to weddings. (Baba E1)

This eighty-one-year-old baba had only moved into town from the farm a few months prior to being interviewed. Even though she still felt a desire to go out to the farm where she had lived all of her adult life with her husband, she was no longer feeling able to do so: 'I don't like driving very much anymore ... on the gravel roads ... so I don't go very much to the farm anymore' (Baba F1).

One eighty-eight-year-old baba spoke specifically about the importance of a variety of supports necessary in order to continue to live with some level of independence:

What makes [my life] good is because God gave for me a nice place and nice people to be with. It's no good when you're by yourself, it's no good ... I was for twenty-five years [by] myself. Look, I have homecare. Sure, I pay, but I got enough to pay. I've got enough pension. I get Meals on Wheels five days a week. Sometimes it's perfect. And then I have two times, twice a month people come, she comes to change my bed and wash the clothes and vacuum, wash the floors. Then every week, on Fridays, the girl comes to help me with my bath. (Baba A1)

A number of the daughters and granddaughters spoke about some aspects of aging that they perceived as having had a more negative impact upon life quality for their mother or baba. In particular, they spoke about the loss of ability, independence, and motivation. This daughter described the negative changes that she has seen in her mother:

> My mom has just moved into the care home ... not quite a year ago. I think her quality of life today is way different than it was ... even two years ago. It's not as good ... and she hates that. She hated getting old, she hated getting restricted. She hated not being able to drive. She was so ... she baked ... she never sat idle ... even after my dad died ... you know ... like ... all of that stuff ... and my mom hasn't been able to do that ... physically she hasn't been able to do that. She also used to embroider years ago ... there are a lot of things that she simply can't do anymore. Her quality of her life today is not as good as what it was. (Daughter G2)

The first-generation women all talked about the physical challenges that they have experienced as they aged.

> I would like if I didn't have to be in pain like this, I could go to see my grandkids whenever I want ... which I could do before. This has taken away some of my independence. But, I look at it this way, I am getting old and this is what happens when you get old. (Baba E1)

> Oh ... I don't feel too bad. It could be worse. Sure I have aches and pains ... why not? It comes with the territory. Growing up we didn't have proper clothes ... wearing dresses and the snow was up to the waist ... working ... now we all have arthritis. (Baba F1)

One eighty-four-year-old baba, who still continues to live in her own home in rural Saskatchewan, spoke about some of the adjustments that she has had to make due to the physical changes that she has experienced.

> I do my work and everything, but now I go downstairs and already I'm out of breath. No breath! I'm so upset with myself (laughter) ... I'm not used to that. I just have to be careful. I don't cut grass no more with the push mower like I used to ... so I got a riding mower, and I cut it now with the riding mower (laughter) and I got a self-propelled tiller for the garden (laughter). (Baba C1)

The interviews revealed consistency between the generations in terms of perceptions of the quality of life of the first-generation participants. An eighty-eight-year-old baba described her quality of life as being quite good, and both her daughter and granddaughter appeared to share this perception. The daughter stated: 'My mother's quality of life before probably was harder than it was for me. Her quality of life now … considering how old she is … maybe it's okay. I know that she probably would have liked to be feeling better' (Daughter A2). The granddaughter discussed factors that she identified as having improved her baba's quality of life:

My baba has been alone for a long time … so she's probably quite independent. Men from her generation were very controlling, but I don't think that she lived in that kind of a situation. But … she depends on my mom and dad for lots now … but I don't know that, in her eyes, she sees that. Now that she's living where she is, she's a little more independent. She's definitely happier since she moved out of her house and is living there. (Granddaughter A3)

Similar descriptions of factors related to quality of life were also identified by other families.

Mom's a strong woman … and she's doing okay for herself. She goes to church, she plays cards, she goes to bingo … she keeps going. So … I'm not worried. It's not like she's boxed in, she goes for herself, you know. So, I think it's good for her. And, she says she's happy. (Daughter C2)

One daughter, who lived out of province, talked about some of the recent changes that she believed contributed to an improved quality of life for her elderly mother.

I think that mom, now has tremendous self-realization. Like … even each time I visit … it's a big change. So many years of her life were spent so busy raising a family and helping on the farm … that she didn't have time for reflection. So I think it is important that people do make sure that they take time for themselves to reflect … just to not have every minute of every waking day that you're not having to think of the next meal, the next routine, the next task. And the worry too … I mean … the money wasn't there, and mom tended to be the worrywart more than dad. I think she doubted that things would be alright. I think that, right now, mom has a good quality of life. I mean … other than, as you age, you have health issues. (Daughter B2)

Relationships

All of the first-generation women identified the relationships with their children and grandchildren as contributing to their quality of life in positive ways.

> I'm happy about my kids … seeing the grandchildren. Now it's getting that we can't travel too much … because it's getting to the point that it's too hard. (Baba B1)

> My daughter takes me all the time. She takes me all the time to the doctor. It is good to have kids that close. (Baba C1)

> I'm happy … to me … I have my children and my grandchildren … I'm happy. (Baba D1)

A number of specific elements related to family relationships were discussed by the participants. First, the first-generation women exhibited a great deal of pride in their role as baba. This pride has impacts upon self-esteem and self-identity and directly influences quality of life. The responsibilities and joys associated with storytelling, and the passing on of culture and family ritual, accompany the role of baba. Most of the elderly women identified themselves as family caregivers. This role also appeared to instill a general sense of pride, responsibility, and belonging. All of these women have provided care to immediate and extended family members. However, they now find themselves in the position of having to accept care from their daughters. While these gender-based caring roles can serve to strengthen intergenerational relationships, they can also cause strain between the generations. Regardless, the women identified these relationships as among the most influential factors in assessing their personal quality of life.

Implications

This study has resulted in two main contributions to the existing literature: the production of applied knowledge and the production of process knowledge. Applied knowledge is context specific and is useful for the solution of practical problems. 'Process knowledge' is a relatively new term that refers to the development of knowledge that focuses upon the processes by which judgments are made in both practice and research (Sheppard & Ryan, 2003). The core of process knowledge is found within the concept of reflexivity (Sheppard & Ryan, 2003). As utilized in this particular research, reflexivity is defined as a self-critical approach that questions how knowledge is generated (Sheppard, Newstead, Caccavo, & Ryan, 2000). This study creates process knowledge in terms of the process involved in interviewing elderly Ukrainian immigrant women. What has been demonstrated is the value of an interview approach that encourages narrative and is more unstructured, utilizing open-ended questions and a laddering technique of inquiry. This approach created an environment in which the babas felt comfortable discussing and sharing deeper layers of personal information. This approach also created an opportunity for reflexivity on the part of the research participants themselves. Although this study has focused upon elderly Ukrainian Canadian immigrant women, the factors identified as being important to health status and quality of life may also be applied to other older ethnic women who are Canadian immigrants.

In regard to applied knowledge, this research study offers information that will be helpful in terms of direct practice with elderly ethnic women. Previous research, although limited, has focused on specific roles for health and social service practitioners when working with elderly ethnic immigrant women, and specifically intervention strategies for helping newcomers make the transition into Canadian society (Barlow & Barlow, 2003). While it is commonly perceived that, as a cultural group, Ukrainians were successful in both the immigration and assimilation processes involved with their settlement in Canada, there are specific issues that must still be considered and understood by those who work with members of this population. First, it is essential to understand the issues related to the religious, spatial, and ethnic diversity amongst members of this group. It is also critical to understand the impact of the time of arrival and place of settlement (Barlow & Barlow, 2003). This study draws attention to the importance of marital, family, and community relationships in the lives of elderly Ukrainian Canadian immigrant women, and suggests these as focus areas that also need to be understood.

There continue to be gaps in the general knowledge base specific to elderly Ukrainian Canadian women, as well as other older women of ethnic background. Matsuoka (1993) calls for more focused and targeted studies that will help to build an understanding of the needs of the elderly that arise from ethnic differences. This study has the potential to add to this body of work.

Conclusion

Health and social service practitioners must listen to the stories of elderly ethnic women and familiarize themselves with the information that is most significant to such individuals, and the information that is most significant about such individuals. For example, even though each of the first-generation women interviewed for this study has lived in Canada for more than sixty years, the experiences of immigration and settlement remain a predominant part of their storytelling.

The literature is replete with studies examining the impacts of culture, ethnicity, and immigration upon various aspects of old age (Durst, 2005; Matsuoka, 1993; Mehta, 1997). However, previous research has not focused as much upon the impacts of early-life immigration on the lives of the elderly (Durst, 2005). Again, the cumulative impact of unresolved trauma over long periods of time can be significant. This study suggests that immigration continues to have some impact upon quality of life for women who immigrated when they were young and then aged in place. Finally, all of the babas described multiple roles within their marital, family, and community relationships, and each demonstrated the changing nature of these roles as they are negotiated and re-negotiated based upon life experience and context. It is important to acknowledge this role of multiplicity.

Notes

1   A section is one square mile or 640 acres.

References

Barlow, C., & Barlow, A. (2003). Social work with Canadians of Ukrainian background: History, direct practice, current realities. In A. Al-Krenawi & J. R. Graham (Eds). *Multicultural social work in Canada: Working with diverse ethno-racial communities* (pp. 228–50). Toronto: Oxford University Press.

Barnes, H., & Parry, J. (2004). Renegotiating identity and relationships: Men and women's adjustments to retirement. *Ageing & Society, 24,* 213–33.

Butala, S. (2003). The myth of the family farm. In H.P. Diaz, J. Jaffe, & R. Stirling (Eds.), *Farm communities at the crossroads: Challenge and resistance* (pp. 67–75). Regina: Canadian Plains Research Centre.

Cheal, D., & Kampen, K. (1998). Poor and dependent seniors in Canada. *Aging and Society,18*, 147–66.

Cipko, S. (1991). In search of a new home: Ukrainian emigration patterns between the two world wars. *Journal of Ukrainian studies,16*(1–2), 3–28.

Coleman, H., & Unrau, Y.A. (2005). Analyzing qualitative data. In R.M. Grinnell, Jr., and Y.A. Unrau (Eds.), *Social work research and evaluation: Quantitative and qualitative approaches* (pp. 404–20). Oxford: Oxford University Press.

Cushon, I. (2003). Sustainable alternatives for Saskatchewan agriculture: A farmer's perspective. In H. P. Diaz, J. Jaffe, & R. Stirling (Eds.), *Farm communities at the crossroads: Challenge and resistance* (pp. 223–35). Regina: Canadian Plains Research Centre.

de Vries, B., Blando, J., Southard, P., & Bubeck, C. (2001). The times of our lives. In G. Kenyon, P. Clark, & B. de Vries (Eds.), *Narrative gerontology: Theory, research and practice* (pp. 137–58). New York: Springer.

Durst, D. (2005). Aging amongst immigrants in Canada: Policy and planning implications. In *Proceedings of the 12th Biennial Canadian Social Welfare Policy Conference: 'Forging Social Futures'* (pp. 1–11). Available at http://www.ccsd.ca/cswp/2005/durst.pdf.

Gerrard, N., Kulig, J., & Nowatzki, N. (2004). What doesn't kill you makes you stronger: Determinants of stress resiliency in rural people of Saskatchewan, Canada. *Journal of Rural Health, 20*(1), 59–66.

Hansen, J., & Kucera, M. (2004). *The educational attainment of second generation immigrants in Canada: Evidence from SLID*. Retrieved from http://www.iza.org/en/webcontent/teaching/summerschool/7thsummer_school_files/ss2004_kucera.

Health Canada. (2002). *Canada's aging population*. Ottawa: Health Canada.

Hilleras, P.K., Pollitt, P., Medway, J., & Ericsson, K. (2000). Nonagenarians: A qualitative exploration of individual differences in wellbeing. *Aging and Society, 20*, 673–97.

Higgs, P., Hyde, M., Wiggins, R., & Blane, D. (2003). Researching quality of life in early old age: The importance of sociological dimension. *Social Policy and Administration, 37*(3), 239–52.

Johansson, Y., Ek, A.C., & Bachrach-Lindstrom, M. (2007). Self-perceived health among older women living in their own residence. *International Journal of Older People Nursing, 2*, 111–18.

Johnson, C. (2005). Demographic characteristics of the rural elderly. In N. Lohman & R.A. Lohman (Eds.), *Rural social work practice* (pp. 271–90). New York: Columbia University Press.

Kenkel, M.B. (2003). Rural women: Strategies and resources for meeting their behavioral health needs. In B. Hudnall Stamm (Ed.), *Rural behavioral health* care: An interdisciplinary guide. (pp. 181–92). Washington, DC: American Psychological Association.

Kestin van den Hoonard, D. (2003). Expectations and experiences of widowhood. In J.F. Gubrium & J.A. Holstein (Eds.), Ways of aging (pp. 182–99). Malden, MA: Blackwell.

Kubik, W., & Moore, R. (2003). Farming in Saskatchewan in the 1990s: Stress and coping. In H.P. Diaz, J. Jaffe, & R. Stirling (Eds.), Farm communities at the crossroads: Challenge and resistance (pp. 119–33). Regina: Canadian Plains Research Centre.

Luciuk, L. (2000). Searching for place: Ukrainian displaced persons, Canada, and the migration of memory. Toronto: University of Toronto Press.

Markson, E.W., & Hess, B.B. (1997). Older women in the city. In M. Pearsall (Ed.), The other within us: Feminist explorations of women and aging. (pp. 57–70). Oxford: Westview.

Matsuoka, A. (1993). Collecting qualitative data through interviews with ethnic older people. Canadian Journal on Aging, 12(2), 216–32.

Mehta, K. (1997). Cultural scripts and the social integration of older people. Aging and Society, 17, 253–75.

McDonough, P., & Strohschein, L. (2003). Age and the gender gap in distress. Women & Health, 38(1), 1–20.

Mitchell, J., & Weatherly, D. (2000). Beyond church attendance: Religiosity and mental health among rural older adults. Journal of Cross-Cultural Gerontology, 15(1), 37–54.

Musil, C.M., & Ahmad, M. (2002). Health of grandmothers: A comparison of caregiver status. Journal of Aging and Health, 14(1), 96–121.

O'Connor, D. (2003). Anti-oppressive practice with older adults: A feminist post-structural perspective. In W. Shera (Ed.), Emerging perspectives on anti-oppressive practice (pp. 183–99). Toronto: Canadian Scholar's Press.

Ostryzniuk, N. (1997). Savella Stechishin: A case study of Ukrainian-Canadian women activism in Saskatchewan, 1920-1945. Master's thesis, University of Saskatchewan.

Ostryzniuk, N. (2002). 75 years of service, friendship and commitment, 1927-2002. Regina: Ukrainian Women's Association of Canada, Daughters of Ukraine Branch.

Petryshyn, M.K. (1980). The changing status of Ukrainian women in Canada, 1921–1971. In W. R. Petryshyn (Ed.), Changing realities: Social trends among Ukrainian Canadians. (pp. 189–209). Edmonton: Canadian Institute of Ukrainian Studies.

Roberto, K.A., Allen, K.R., & Blieszner, R. (1999). Older women, their children, and grandchildren: A feminist perspective on family relationships.

In J.D. Garner (Ed.), *Fundamentals of feminist gerontology* (pp. 67–84). Binghamton, NY: Haworth Press.

Scholz, A., & Derbawka, P.T. (2002). *The new pioneers. Saskatchewan: The history of agriculture*. Saskatoon: Saskatchewan Agrivision Corporation.

Sheppard, M., Newstead, S., Caccavo, A.D., & Ryan, K. (2000). Reflexivity and the development of process knowledge in social work: A classification and empirical study. *British Journal of Social Work, 30*, 465–88.

Sheppard, M., & Ryan, K. (2003). Practitioners as rule using analysts: A further development of process knowledge in social work. *British Journal of Social Work, 33*(2), 157–76.

Sheridan, M.J., & Kisor, A.J. (2000). The research process and the elderly. In R.L. Schneider, N.P. Kropf, & A.J. Kisor (Eds.), *Gerontological social work: Knowledge, service settings, and special populations* (2nd ed., pp. 97–135). Belmont, CA: Wadsworth/Thomson Learning.

Statistics Canada. (2007). *2006 Census*. No. 97-551-XWE20060010. Ottawa: Government of Canada.

Stevens, N. (2001). Combating loneliness: A friendship enrichment programme for older women. *Aging and Society, 21*, 183–202.

Swyripa, F. (1993). *Wedded to the cause: Ukrainian-Canadian women and ethnic identity 1891-1991*. Toronto: University of Toronto Press.

Ujimoto, K.V. (1995). The ethnic dimension of aging in Canada. In R. Neugebauer-Visano, *Aging and inequality: Cultural constructions of differences* (pp. 3–29). Toronto: Canadian Scholars' Press.

United Nations. (2006). *The aging of the world's population*. Retrieved from www .un.org/esa/socdev/aging/popaging.html.

Warnock, J.W. (2003). Industrial agriculture comes to Saskatchewan. In H. P. Diaz, J. Jaffe,& R. Stirling (Eds.), *Farm communities at the crossroads: Challenge and resistance* (pp. 303–22). Regina: Canadian Plains Research Centre.

Widdis, R.W. (2006). *Voices from next year country: An oral history of rural Saskatchewan*. Regina: Canadian Plains Research Center.

17 In the Dark:
Uncovering Influences
on Pregnant Women's Health
in the Northwest Territories

Pertice M. Moffitt

The health of pregnant women and their unborn babies is pivotal to community vitality and to the health of future societies. The Northwest Territories (NWT) is home to a diverse population of Aboriginal, immigrant, and non-Aboriginal northern women who share the land and the experience of pregnancy in the Arctic and sub-Arctic. Little has been written of the contexts and the lifeways of pregnant northern women and the way these influence their health and well-being. This chapter will enhance our understanding about the complexity of circumstances surrounding the experience of pregnancy and childbirth for northern women and provide considerations for future directions.

Furthermore, this chapter describes the health of pregnant northern women through a holistic perspective that includes salient historical influences, present-day system indicators of health status, and social determinants that must be tackled to improve the overall health of pregnant northern women. I begin by providing the location and ethnic composition of women who call the NWT their home.

Background and Context

The NWT is located north of the sixtieth parallel, above the western provinces of Canada, between the Yukon Territory to the west and Nunavut to the east. The population of the territory is 41,464 (NWT Bureau of Statistics, 2006a), residing on a land mass of 1.17 million square kilometres. Almost one-half of the population, 18,700 people, reside in Yellowknife, the capital of the territory; the other half live in smaller communities, hamlets, or villages scattered across a remote wilderness. Childbearing women (age fifteen to forty-four years) total 9,950, approximately one quarter of the population of the territory.

The NWT is rich in cultural diversity. Approximately 50% (NWT Bureau of Statistics, 2006a) of the population are Aboriginal[1] people, comprised of Dene, Métis, and Inuvialuit. The Dene consist of further distinct peoples that include the Chipewyan, G'wichin, North Slavey, South Slavey, Tlicho, and Cree. Visible minorities (defined as 'persons other than Aboriginal peoples who are non-Caucasian in race or non-white in colour') accounted for 5.5% of the total NWT population (NWT Bureau of Statistics, 2006a)[2].

History of Childbirth in the Northwest Territories

Since time immemorial, Aboriginal women in the Northwest Territories lived on the land, guided by the cultural beliefs, practices, and knowledge of their mothers and elders (Moffitt, 2004, 2008; Paulette, 1989). Pregnant women ate a traditional diet of plants, berries, fish, and animals from the land and led an active lifestyle that was nomadic in response to the seasons and the availability of food. Women and men assisted at the birth of the babies, and traditional medicines were used based on the knowledge of lay midwives and local people. The birth of a baby was a time of celebration, ceremony, and joy. Sometimes the winters in the Arctic were formidable, food was scarce, and warmth and shelter were difficult. Elders recall that those times were harsh. People, including mothers and babies, starved to death, and life expectancy was much shorter than it is today.

The NWT in the early days encompassed a much larger land mass, including what today is known as Nunavut.[3] Early explorers were searching for a Northwest Passage, and with their exploration, they discovered the great resources of fur from land animals and whale and seal from the oceans (Outcrop, 1990). The Hudson's Bay Company was established in 1668 and, as well as administering the land, for many years managed a lucrative fur trade with the Aboriginal peoples of the NWT. Trading posts were set up across the territory at which Aboriginal hunters would trade resources from the land for materials from the South.

With the establishment of the trading posts, the nomadic lifeways of the Aboriginal people were replaced with settlement living. The population of women expanded to include wives of missionaries and explorers, Grey Nuns, and other settlers who were lured to the North by an evangelic mission or the rich resources. Early physicians were recruited by the Hudson's Bay Company as traders and received extra money by providing medical care to the local people (Spady, 1982). In those early days, all pregnant women continued to be cared for by their families and communities. In some cases, missionaries, fur traders, and policemen were called to assist with health and illness matters (Sperry, 2001).

As mission schools were developed in central locations, children were sent from their homes to be indoctrinated into the religious beliefs and practices of Western societies and educated to conform to Western norms, rules, expectations, and ways of living (Fumoleau, 1984; Legacy of Hope Foundation, 2009; Moffitt, 2004; Royal Commission on Aboriginal Peoples [RCAP], 2006). There were fifteen residential schools[4] scattered across the NWT, and some communities had two schools of differing religious order, often either Anglican or Roman Catholic. Residential schools prevailed well into the twentieth century until the closure of the last school in Inuvik in 1985 (Aboriginal Healing Foundation, 2007). Today, as legal settlements for residential school abuses are received, formal apologies accepted, and healing centres established, survivors are sharing their ordeals through stories and song (Kakfwi, 2006; Legacy of Hope Foundation, 2009). In a song he wrote entitled 'In the Walls of His Mind,' former NWT premier Stephen Kakfwi (2006) shared the suffering with these words 'He tries to be a father for his wife and his children / And he hides the pain that will drive him insane / And that voice each night that is quietly crying / Somewhere in the walls and the halls of his mind.'

The intergenerational impact of residential schools on Aboriginal peoples is well documented in Canada (Aboriginal Healing Foundation, n.d.; RCAP, 2006). The legacy of suffering and pain is felt and experienced by Aboriginal families today (Moffitt, 2004, 2008; Smith, Varcoe, & Edwards, 2005), since the separation of children from their families meant that Aboriginal language and cultural practices and knowledge were lost. Children endured abusive conditions that haunt survivors to this day. Along with these painful encounters is the burden of living with such a legacy, so family violence, substance use and abuse, and suicide are expressions of the physical, emotional, and psychological toll that has accompanied residential schooling experiences. The colonization that enabled the residential school system in the North also fuelled health care provision that was based on southern biomedical norms with little regard for Aboriginal worldviews surrounding pregnancy and childbirth (Moffitt & Vollman, 2006).

The first hospital in the NWT was established by the Order of Grey Nuns in 1867, and this was followed by fifteen other hospitals, most of which were established as religious mission sites, between 1867 and 1953 (Brett, 1969; Spady, 1982). It was representatives from religious organizations that ran the hospitals that petitioned the federal government for physicians to staff six of their hospitals, which were mostly run by Oblate nuns or missionaries' wives who were nurses. In the 1930s, there were six medical officers under the direction of the federal government. In 1939, the government began to build health facilities, and by 1972, thirty-five nursing stations and two government run hospitals in Inuvik and Iqaluit were built. The hospital in Yellowknife was built mostly on government funds but operated on municipal funds. The Northern Health Service was initiated in 1954 with a mandate of treatment and public health programs (Spady, 1982).

With the establishment of government services, Aboriginal people began to stay for longer periods of the year in the newly established communities. Aboriginal women were introduced to Western practices. Bottle feeding was encouraged in the discourse of the day as a means to provide babies with the best nourishment. As well, bottle-feeding was touted because it could be provided by anyone, thus easing the situation of lactating women, freeing them from the physical demands and time commitments required for feeding. Historically, however, breast-feeding had been a natural birth control method that functioned to space out pregnancies. Because breast-feeding was now discouraged and no longer served as a method of birth control, and settlement living with a much larger concentration of people was encouraged, the birth rate increased substantially (Douglas, 2006). The death rate among mothers and babies was high, so reducing infant and maternal morbidity and mortality became a priority for Western medicine and a measure of improved health for Arctic women (Lessard, 1990; Spady, 1982).

With the expansion of northern health care services by southerners, birthing became medicalized (Daviss, 1997; Kaufert & O'Neil, 1990; Moffitt, 2004). Primary care was provided at the local level by registered nurses and local people, with evacuation to a tertiary centre when more specialized care was required. Nursing stations were staffed with nurse midwives, many of whom were recruited from the British Commonwealth. A criterion of low/high risk was established whereby some women had the option to stay in their community to have their babies. This was abolished in the 1980s: immigration laws changed and British midwives could no longer be employed in the North; there was concern about the lack of midwifery legislation in Canada so the practice of midwifery was considered illegal; and there was a prevailing discourse that the safest birth was provided by a physician in a hospital (Douglas, 2006; Moffitt, 2004).

This brings us to the twenty-first century, where the policy of evacuation for birth continues to prevail in most communities in the territory (Moffitt & Vollman, 2006). With medicalization, childbirth has become a condition requiring medical intervention. Perinatal travel to a regional centre where hospital facilities exist is one such intervention that is endorsed as best practice for safe birth. With this way of thinking, health or healthy practice is viewed as compliance with policies and procedures that standardize care for childbirth as a clinical condition.

Birth Statistics

Today, the birth rate in the NWT is decreasing. In 1995 there were 868 reported births while in 2005 there were 712 births (NWT Bureau of Statistics, 2006b). The mean annual birth rate in a ten-year period was 690 (see Table 17.1). Analysing the numbers of births reported in vital statistics records (NWT Bureau of Statistics, 2006b) provides some discussion points. Mother's residence identified by community is on the vital statistics form rather than the place of birth. This captures somewhat the number of pregnant women in the community or at least the number of pregnant women who experienced a live birth and registered their newborn. It becomes quite apparent that in some communities there were very small numbers of births. Of the thirty-six communities listed, the majority have fewer than twenty babies born each year: eighteen communities had fewer than ten reported births averaged over ten years from 1996 to 2005, twelve communities fell within a range from ten to twenty births, and only six communities had more than twenty births. With the low number of births, there is little deliberation on the practicality of providing birthing services in the remote communities. In fact, the recruitment and retention of nurses and midwives, with the specialized knowledge and skills required to provide the service, is a challenge. Therefore, pregnant women in the remote communities have fewer opportunities to access resources from specialized health care professionals. The declining numbers of births affect the feasibility of developing and sustaining formal health programs. It would seem that what remains for pregnant women is to rely on the advice of family and friends.

Maternal Child Health Care

Primary prenatal and postpartum maternity services are provided in the remote communities by community health nurses working in advanced

Table 17.1 Total NWT Births, 1996–2005

Year	2005	2004	2003	2002	2001	2000	1999	1998	1997	1996
No. of Births	712	698	701	635	613	673	659	678	722	814

Source: NWT Bureau of Statistics, 2006b

practice, nurse practitioners, and community health representatives[5] from the local communities. There are nineteen community health centres in the NWT providing care to 30% of the territorial population (Government of the Northwest Territories [GNWT], 2008b). In the larger centres of Inuvik, Fort Simpson, Hay River, and Yellowknife, family practice physicians and nurse practitioners provide the bulk of maternal child health services. There are three midwives practicing in the NWT, two located in Fort Smith and the other in Yellowknife. Yellowknife Territorial Hospital has expanded services that include general surgeons, anaesthetists, obstetricians, and paediatricians.

Maternal health care programs are provided by federal, territorial, and local governments and include, for example, the Canadian Prenatal Nutrition Program (CPNP), Aboriginal Head Start, and Fetal Alcohol Spectrum Disorder Prevention (GNWT, 2006). Mothers and young children do benefit from these federally funded programs that are often coordinated and delivered by local community people. Because they hire local people, the programs are delivered in the local language, and cultural beliefs and traditions are included in plans. For example, through the CPNP, pregnant women come together for cooking classes, sewing circles, and talks with Elders (GNWT, 2009). However, as noted by Smith, Varcoe, and Edwards (2005), these programs are administered and implemented throughout Canada in silos, rather than with the coordination or integration of an overall maternal child health program.

Women living in all communities with the exception of Inuvik, Fort Smith, and Yellowknife are evacuated for birth under the auspices of the Medical Travel Policy[6]. As a result, there is little continuity or personalized care for many women. Depersonalized care is further compounded by the high turnover of staff in the communities, lack of maternal child expertise in remote areas, and the disjointed service provided. As well, family-centred care is nonexistent in the hospitals for most evacuated women since family members are not financially supported to escort pregnant women and many do not have the resources required to cover the childcare and household costs at home and the expenses incurred while away at the hospital.

There has been an attempt to address gaps in the maternal child health service with the creation of the Northern Women's Health Program (Stanton Territorial Health Authority, 2004). This is a centralized service for women in the southern part of the territory and women being evacuated from the Kitikmeot Region of Nunavut. The program provides a 'single point of reference' (Stanton Territorial Health Authority, 2004, p. 12) for all prenatal women and includes coordination of physician appointments and ultrasound, health information, and support.

Midwifery was legislated in the NWT in 2005, largely as a result of lobbying by northern women and midwife activists Lesley Paulette and Gisela Becker. Midwifery services have been integrated into the health centre programming by the Fort Smith Health and Social Services Authority (Paulette, 2007). Women are given options of maternity care through the midwifery program or from physicians in the medical clinic. To help women make this decision, a health information booklet describes the two services. The programs operate under the principle of informed choice. Women may also choose between birth in the health centre and a home birth; the health centre has a birthing room that provides family-centred care. In 2007, 90% of maternal care was provided by midwives in Fort Smith.

Childbirth for pregnant women in other parts of the NWT occurs mostly in hospital in either Yellowknife or Inuvik. The hospital in Yellowknife is a regional centre that is a catchment area for women from the southern part of the NWT and the Kitikmeot region of Nunavut. The Inuvik General Hospital provides childbirth services for women who reside in the Beaufort Delta area.

Missing and Reported Indicators of Maternal Health

There is limited maternal health statistical data available in the NWT. Researchers are recognizing this void and have taken steps to include the territories in national surveys like the Canadian Maternity Experiences Survey (MES) conducted by the Public Health Agency of Canada (PHAC, 2009). There is no perinatal database for the territory (PHAC, 2000), although research investigating the need for a perinatal surveillance system was recently conducted and identified the need for a flexible database that would include a possible four hundred variables relevant for maternal and infant health particular to the unique population and including such variables as transfers for birth (Machalek,

Chatwood, Paulette, & Becker, 2009). The purpose of collecting data and monitoring health through statistics is to identify patterns and trends in the population so that action can be taken to improve health outcomes (PHAC, 2009).

The difficulties in finding usable statistical perinatal data in the NWT can be illustrated in my attempt to identify the number of pregnant women who were transferred south to Alberta and the reason for this medical evacuation (medevac). My thoughts were that since this was one variable being considered in a future surveillance system, I should see what data were currently available and expected that transfer for birth data would provide some indication of health/ill health during pregnancy.

A Department of Health and Social Services health analyst retrieved data for me from the hospital discharge abstract data that includes data from the Capital Health Region in Alberta, where women are sometimes admitted. The hospital discharge database provides a summary of hospital admissions for individuals with NWT health care cards and NWT postal codes in hospitals outside of the territory. The database does not address medevac explicitly because data were missing that identified how the hospitalization occurred, for example, whether the patient was transported by air from the NWT, planned to be hospitalized outside the territory, or just happened to be outside of the territory and required hospitalization. ICD-10 codes, which correlated with the time frame of the hospitalizations selected, were used to identify diagnoses of hospitalized pregnant women. The diagnostic code represents the main reason for the hospitalization or a significant pre-admission co-morbidity. Sometimes up to twenty-five diagnostic codes can be recorded per admission (A. Leamon, personal communication, 11 August 2009).The data represent the number of hospital admissions and not the number of women; a number of women could have had more than one admission within any one year.

The hospital discharge data I received provided forty codes that matched 310 admissions of pregnant NWT women in the Capital Health Authority area in Alberta, our usual transfer location, between 2003 and 2007. I identified assigned codes for hospitalization of pregnant women and, from this data, developed Table 17.2, which indicates the number of hospitalizations for the specific diagnoses that occurred ten or more times over this five-year period.

The hospital discharge data provide an account of medical diagnoses requiring hospitalization in a southern facility. While the data do not explicitly capture medevac data, some of the diagnoses listed are

Table 17.2 Hospitalizations of pregnant women from hospital discharge data 2003–2007

ICD Code*	013	014	024	032	033	036	042	044	047	048	060	070	Other
n	17	11	10	10	28	13	47	15	22	10	16	12	19

* The following diagnoses correspond to the ICD code: *013*, gestational pregnancy-induced hypertension without significant proteinuria; *014*, gestational pregnancy-induced hypertension with significant proteinuria; *024*, diabetes mellitus with pregnancy; *032*, maternal care for known or suspected malpresentation of the fetus; *033*, maternal care for known or suspected disproportion; *036*, maternal care for other known or suspected fetal problems; *042*, premature rupture of membranes; *044*, placenta previa; *047*, false labour, excludes preterm labour; *048*, prolonged pregnancy; *060*, preterm labour; *070*, perineal laceration during delivery; *Other*, complications during labour and delivery, not elsewhere classified (such descriptors, for example, as maternal distress during labour and delivery, shock during or following labour and delivery, pyrexia).

recognized as substantiation to transport pregnant women to a tertiary centre in the south; for example, premature labour (ICD # 42) and complications during pregnancy (ICD #070) are considered to require care above what can be provided by health services in the NWT. The risk to the health of the mother or newborn is considered justification for the evacuation. Hopefully, data such as this will be captured through a NWT perinatal surveillance system. If it is known why pregnant women require medevac to a large centre in the South, health promotion and prevention measures can be instituted at home in the NWT.

Birth weight is considered an indicator of health of the mother and newborn (GNWT, 2005a; Spady, 1982). The healthy-birth-weight babies in the NWT from 2001 to 2005 were 81.38% of all live births, with a range of 80.8% (2001) to 82.0% (2005). This means that approximately 19% of the babies born are of unhealthy weight. According to the NWT Early Childhood Development Report for 2004/05 (GNWT, 2006), babies born in the territory had a higher incidence of high birth weight (HBW), greater than 4000 grams, than incidence of low birth rate (LBW), less than 2500 grams. Table 17.3 shows how the incidence of HBW babies far exceeds the incidence of LBW babies in the NWT and is much greater than the national incidence of HBW babies.

Interpretation of birth weight as an indicator of health must be considered with caution since norms are based on data from non-Aboriginal babies (Smylie, 2001). A 1973–74 perinatal and infant mortality and morbidity study reported that 'native infants were significantly lighter

Table 17.3 Birth weight: NWT vs. Canadian

Year	2001		2002		2003		2004		2005	
Indicator	NWT	Can	NWT	Can	NWT	Can	NWT	Can	NWT	Can
Incidence of Low Birth Weight (%)	3.3	5.5	4.9	5.7	5.9	5.9	5.6	5.9	5.1	6.0
Incidence of High Birth Weight (%)	20.7	13.6	17.8	13.2	20.5	12.8	19.0	12.3	18.5	12.0

* Incidence is presented as percentage of live births
Source: NWT Bureau of Statistics, 2006b

in mean birth weight than White infants'; there was no report of HBW babies (Spady, 1982, p. xxvii). Spady considered both genetics and environment as rationale for LBW and suggested that factors such as maternal smoking, maternal pre-pregnancy weight, and maternal weight gain were important. Today's HBW marks a shift from the LBW four decades ago.

There is reason to be concerned about the increasing weight of newborns since there is increased risk of poor outcome for both the mother and child during childbirth. According to Watts (2010), HBW is the result of uncontrolled diabetes, genetics, multiparity, or a combination of these factors, and it can cause difficulty for the mother and injuries to the baby in childbirth because of the size of the baby. The increased rate of HBW babies in the NWT requires further investigation into factors related to HBW, health outcomes linked with HBW, and health promotion strategies to maintain healthy weight of the growing fetus.

Although Aboriginal babies are not identified as being HBW, other studies in Canada report HBW or macrosomia in First Nations newborns (Caulfield, Harris, Whalen, & Sugamori, 1998; Smylie, 2001; Thomson, 1990; Wenman, Joffres, Tataryn, & Edmonton Perinatal Infections Group, 2004). There is an epidemic of Type 2 diabetes in Aboriginal populations that is continuing to grow and with a trend of earlier onset (Young, Reading, Elias, & O'Neil, 2000). Obesity in NWT children is also increasing and may be linked to HBW (Raves, 2006).

Fatty food in the diet of pregnant women and pre-pregnancy weights are contributing factors to the HBW of newborns (Daniel, 2009). Food security/insecurity is an issue in the small communities of the territory, where traditional food remains salient to northern peoples (Berti, Soueida, & Kuhnlein, 2008; Lambden, Receveur, & Kuhnlein, 2007).

There is a change in dietary intake that may be related to access to traditional foods, climate change, and socio-economic factors in the lives of pregnant women (Berti et al., 2008). The supply of fresh fruit and vegetables is often limited and the cost prohibitive to many northerners. Preserved and processed foods are readily available and less expensive. In a dietary assessment of pregnant Canadian Arctic women, there was a moderate concern regarding low intakes of vitamins A, C, E, and folate that could be addressed through availability of traditional foods and quality fresh produce (Berti et al., 2008).

Risky Behaviours

The rates of alcohol, street drug, and tobacco use in the NWT are considerably higher than the national average (GNWT, 2008a). Substance use by child-bearing women in the territory has been reported locally in survey reports (GNWT, 2003, 2008a), in the government newsletter, *EpiNorth* (Mazan, 2007), and in the MES (PHAC, 2009).

From the *2006 NWT Addictions Report*, self-reported drinking during pregnancy was 15% in the twenty-to-forty-four age group (GNWT, 2008a). Another source of data for alcohol use is the prenatal record form. Health practitioners in the NWT use the T-ACE (tolerance, annoyed, cut-down, eye-opener) as the screening tool to identify alcohol-exposed pregnancies (Kandola, 2006). Used during their prenatal care, the T-ACE involves asking pregnant women questions about alcohol consumption practices. A criticism from one nurse practitioner is that this screening tool does not take into consideration the binge drinking that is a known pattern in the territory, and the questions do not make sense to the local women (J. Buck, personal communication, June 2009). As well, a Canadian review of the prenatal record form pointed out that there was no indication of follow-up or referral of pregnant women who reported high-risk alcohol consumption (Premji & Semenic, 2009).

The *2006 NWT Addictions Report* showed the prevalence of smoking during pregnancy decreased from 59% in 1996 to 10% in 2006 (GNWT, 2008a). This rate differs from that reported by the MES, which found that 24.9% of the women who participated in the study smoked during pregnancy (PHAC, 2009). Also from the MES, 10.5% of women reported using street drugs during their pregnancy (PHAC, 2009).

All of these substances have deleterious effects on the mother and her unborn child. Alcohol consumption is a grave concern for pregnant women because of the devastating effects on the developing fetus, effects that last a lifetime; these children suffer from the cognitive, phys-iological, behavioural, and neurological impairments of fetal alcohol spectrum disorder (Dell & Roberts, 2005; Wilhelm & Hegeman, 2004). Smoking during pregnancy causes many poor maternal and infant out-comes, among them such conditions as intrauterine growth restriction, prematurity, spontaneous abortion, placental complications, and sudden infant death syndrome (Cnattinguis, 2004; Heaman & Chalmers, 2005; PHAC, 2009). Using street drugs also affects pregnancy outcomes, being associated with such issues as low birth weight, preterm birth, and child-hood developmental and behavioural problems (PHAC, 2009).

Sexually transmitted infection is much higher in the NWT than in the rest of Canada (GNWT, 2005b). Chlamydia infection incidence in-creased from 91.7 cases per 10,000 population in the 1990s to 134.6 cases per 10,000 in 2003. Gonorrhea increased from 8.1 per 10,000 in 1996 to 49.5 per 10,000 in 2003. The most at risk were individuals between the age of fifteen and twenty-four living in the smaller communities. As well, there was a syphilis outbreak reported in 2008 that spread from six to thirty-three cases in three months and affected people from the Sahtu, Tlicho, Yellowknife, and Fort Smith regions (CBC News, 2008). With the steady increases of STIs, health care professionals worry that present-day programming is not influencing healthy sexuality. Local researchers are investigating sexual health practices to explicate sexual health attitudes and behaviours (Daniels, Drybones, Lafferty, Moore, & Naedzo, 2009) and the barriers and facilitators of positive health out-comes (Lys, 2009). From these investigations, we will be able to develop better evidence-based sexual health education strategies.

Determinants of Health for Pregnant Women

Culture and Identity

Our sense of identity is established through meaningful social connec-tions that are formed through our relationships with friends and family, promoting self-esteem through feelings of love and belonging (Stryker & Burke, 2000). One study reported that in the Inuit population (includ-ing the Inuvialuit), segments of the population that were unmarried reported lower levels of social support; higher levels of social support (assessed through positive interaction, emotional support, tangible support, affection, and intimacy) were reported in the young, married, and female gender (Richmond, 2009).

In a 1970s perinatal infant mortality and morbidity study, the micro-environment for infants was described as 'between worlds,' that is, not similar to either a traditional environment or the environment of southern Canada (Spady, 1982). It was suggested that this environment of 'between worlds' was a determinant of health for Aboriginal infants and their mothers.

Cultural identity is an important aspect of health that begins to be developed at birth, continues throughout life, and relates to practices expressed through death and dying. For the mother, cultural identity may be linked to the conception and lifecycle of her child. For example, Aboriginal mothers recognize the significance of place of birth to their identity as a people. Territorial Aboriginal mothers who birth their babies in southern Canada worry about their children's status as Dene or Inuit, since land entitlement and status are politically examined with land claim settlements, and birth outside of the territory may cause one's status and entitlement to be contested (Douglas, 2006; O'Neil, Kaufert, & Postl, 1990). Bringing birth home to rural and remote communities has been recommended for the health of Aboriginal women and their communities (Couchie & Sanderson, 2007; Klein, Christilaw, & Johnson, 2002; Kornelson & Grzybowski, 2005). Babies born at home enhance cultural identity through local beliefs and practices, foster family cohesion through shared experience and life stories, and revitalize community spirit and lived endorsement of the wisdom of Elders through the use of accumulated past childbirth knowledge. Given the previous discussion of the difficulty in providing childbirth in the local communities, support of family and friends during childbirth is essential to identity.

Geography, Isolation, and Access to Care

The geography and isolation of the territory are salient to the health of pregnant women. Many of the small communities are accessed by air only and are hours away from perinatal expertise and resources. Weather can affect travel to a larger centre, and with climate change in the Arctic, fog that prohibits safe travel and causes delays is being experienced more often. Some communities in the southern part of the territory are accessed by gravel roads that involve hours of travel through the bush. Local resources in the communities are limited.

It is apparent that access to quality health care is limited by where you live. In one retrospective cohort study in Quebec from 1991 to 2000,

degree of rural isolation where there is limited or no metropolitan influence has been linked with poorer birth outcomes, including stillbirth,
neonatal death, and postnatal death (Luo & Wilkins, 2008). There is no
similar study in the NWT, but there are some indicators that can be
linked. For example, infant mortality for the small NWT communities
was 13 per 1000 live births while for Yellowknife it was 6 per 1000 live
births (GNWT, 2005a). As well, the leading causes of infant death were
reported as conditions originating in the prenatal period, including
short gestation, low birth weight, and respiratory distress. These conditions accounted for 39% while congenital anomalies accounted for 25%
(GNWT, 2005a).

There is limited choice of health care provider when you are pregnant in the territory (Becker & Paulette, 2003; Healey & Meadows, 2007;
Moffitt & Vollman, 2006). As reported in the MES, approximately 31%
of women reported a nurse or nurse practitioner as their primary prenatal care provider; 46%, a family physician; 10%, an obstetrician; and
13%, a midwife (PHAC, 2009). Although some women might have chosen the same type of health care provider as they reported having had
for their prenatal care, others might have selected a different health care
provider (for their prenatal care) if given options. However, there are
no health care provider options in some locations in the territory. If you
live in the remote communities, choice is limited to nurses or nurse
practitioners for prenatal care. If you live in the larger centres such as
Inuvik, Fort Simpson, Fort Smith, Hay River, and Yellowknife, your
choices broaden to encompass nurses, nurse practitioners, family physicians, and possibly midwives if you live in Fort Smith or Yellowknife.
Midwifery remains a limited option since there are only three midwives
in the entire territory.

Choice in where your baby is born is also limited. Many NWT babies are born far from their community and in some cases their territory. Childbirth in their home community is important to northern
women, as has been reported by the midwifery program in Fort Smith
(Paulette, 2007). Findings from a qualitative study with rural women
in Ontario revealed that women in rural communities want care during their childbirth experience that can be obtained locally, is characterized as personal and relational, with continuity of care throughout
their pregnancies and birthing experiences, and allows for informed
choice (Sutherns, 2004). These same sentiments were voiced by northern women from the Beaufort Delta region, who along with other
Inuit women engaged in a call-in talk show that was aired on APTN

in May 2009 (Carry, 2009). Inuit women want maternity care closer to home, supported by providers from their communities who speak their language. As stated above, mothers and Elders agree that babies born locally will revitalize and strengthen community cohesion and improve cultural identity.

Social Support

Support of families, friends, and community is linked to good health (McNicholas, 2002; Raphael, 2004; Richmond, 2009). The anticipation and preparation for birth, the literal and spiritual presence of family at birth and their role in the birth process, the lived experience of birth, and the integration of the birth experience into the larger life experience are important elements for childbirth (Rawlings, 1998). Family-centred maternity care is not an option for many women from remote communities. Pregnant women are evacuated to the regional centres for birth without their family. Fathers are often absent from the birth of their children; in one study conducted with fourteen pregnant women from a remote community in the territory, only two fathers were present for the birth of their babies (Moffitt, 2008). While in Yellowknife and Inuvik awaiting the births of their babies, pregnant women stay in boarding homes/transient centres. In many cases, the pregnant women support each other. When an expectant mother goes into labour, her friends at the boarding home accompany her to the hospital to provide labour support.

Income and Social Status

Poor people are less healthy than rich people (Lynch et al., 2004). Most of the residents of the remote communities are Aboriginal, and Aboriginal people are members of a low-income group, and their health lags behind that of mainstream Canadians (Adelson, 2005). In the remote communities where income is low, cost of store-bought food is high, and fresh produce is often not available, pregnant women have great difficulty maintaining a healthy diet for themselves and their unborn babies.

Good nutrition is linked to good outcomes for mothers and babies. Traditionally, country food provided a valuable source of many nutrients (Berti et al., 2008; Kuhnlein & Turner, 1996; Lambden et al., 2007). However, in many cases traditional diets have been replaced with store-bought food that is processed, lacking in nutrients, and high in sugar. Some women worry about eating traditional local food since reports have surfaced of contaminants in the local animals, fish, and plants they eat (Kuhnlein & Chan, 2000; Northern Contaminants Program, 2009). The risks of eating traditional food that is reported to have unhealthy levels of mercury and persistent organic pollutants (POPs) must be weighed against the benefits of the local food and the disadvantages of eating processed foods. Dietary intake of store-bought processed foods has been linked to higher rates of obesity, diabetes, and cardiovascular disease. There is a decline in the consumption of traditional foods across the territory.

In an assessment of dietary intake in an Inuvialuit population, researchers found that the mean daily intake of many nutrients, including dietary fiber, calcium, and vitamins A, C, and E and total folate, was much lower than the recommended amount; daily intake of fruit and vegetables was low; sugar was added to tea and coffee; sweetened juices and pop were prevalent choices of energy; and butter and margarine were high contributors of total fat intake (Sharma, De Roose, Cao, Gittelsohn, & Corriveau, 2009). The results of this study are being used in a targeted health intervention program in the territory called the Healthy Foods North project. Vitamin D deficiency in babies has been reported as highest in the three northern territories, with maternal contributing factors reported as skin colour, lack of exposure to the sun, and inadequate vitamin D intake or supplementation (Huotari & Herzig, 2008; Ward, Gaboury, Ladhani, & Zlotkin, 2007). It is recommended that all breast-feeding mothers supplement with 800 IU of Vitamin D.

Education and Literacy

Low literacy is related to poor health (Endres, Sharp, Haney, & Dooley, 2004; Ferguson, 2008; Kendig, 2006; Rootman & Ronson, 2005). Health status improves with level of education by increasing employment opportunities, security, and sense of control over your life (Renkert & Nutbeam, 2001; Shohet, 2002). Overall, education levels are improving in the territory as demonstrated by the decrease (34% in 1991 to 29% in 2001) of residents over the age of twenty-five who have less than high school education, as well as increases in the number of residents with some post-secondary education and the number with degrees (14% in 1991 to 16% in 2001) (GNWT, 2005a). Although these are demonstrated improvements, literacy continues to be an issue for northerners.

Renkert and Nutbeam (2001) have defined maternal health literacy as 'the cognitive and social skills which determine the motivation and ability of women to gain access to, understand, and use information in ways that promote and maintain their health and that of their children' (p. 382). Maternal health literacy is vital since a woman's knowledge and understanding of health information directly affects her personal health, the health of her unborn baby, and child health (Ferguson, 2008). Furthermore, women with low literacy have a more difficult time in accessing health care when they cannot understand complex information on forms, when there is limited time with a health care provider offering verbal explanations, and when the health care provider has not detected a low-literacy problem (Ferguson, 2008). These are all concerns that must be addressed in the territory, where there continues to be a literacy problem and where English is often the second language.

Implications from the Review

This review, based on historical influences on health, health status, and social determinants of health, demonstrates that there is little research about the health of pregnant women in the NWT, and that what has been reported suggests the need for more research and more health promotion approaches and strategies. It is important that northern women and communities be included in the development of such a research agenda so that relevant and culturally appropriate steps are taken[7] to improve their health and well-being during pregnancy and childbirth.

From a historical perspective, colonial practices have created pain and suffering for local peoples; if they are to heal and be healthy, reconciliation between Aboriginal peoples and non-Aboriginal peoples needs to be incorporated within all health and healing initiatives. Decolonizing efforts must be enacted, such as working with the population to build local capacity. Future research should be conducted with the full participation of northern women at all levels of the research process.

From a health status perspective, there is a need to implement improved databases. A perinatal surveillance system, as suggested earlier, will assist in reporting patterns, trends, and predictors of the health of pregnant women in the NWT. The indication is that a more detailed account of the health of all northern women is required. A recent strategy has been the development of the Arctic Health Research Network, recently renamed the Institute for Circumpolar Health Research, which was founded in 2005 to advance the health and well-being of northern people and communities. The mandate of the Institute is to build capacities and capabilities of local communities through participatory action research that emanates from research needs as identified by the communities, with results and interventions community driven and owned (Institute for Circumpolar Health Research, 2009).

From the perspective of social determinants of health, there is no doubt that some pregnant women in the territory experience inequities that gravely affect their health (Moffitt, 2008). This is particularly true of Aboriginal expectant mothers living in the remote communities. In the NWT, there has been little attention to social determinants of health. The focus has been on the physical assessment and treatment of mothers and babies without any actions being directed to the deplorable living conditions (poverty, poor nutrition, lack of access to health care, and isolation) of pregnant women and infants. Little is known about what, if any, pre-conception health teaching occurs in the communities of the NWT, and given the grave consequences of substance use and abuse, research and targeted health programming and innovative policy direction is needed.

There has been little change in the medical evacuation policy that stipulates travel for most pregnant women from the small and remote communities of the territory. Gender role, as discussed in chapter 13 of this volume by Heather, Skillen, Cross, and Vladicka, can be contextualized in the North as a requirement to travel for pregnancy and childbirth. This becomes a stressor and a health barrier for pregnant women. Pregnant northern women, like African Canadian women living in Nova Scotia, are marginalized within a persistently colonialized health service that for decades has made little change to develop family-centred maternity care.

The midwifery legislation and the continuity provided by the midwives currently in Fort Smith demonstrate promise for other communities, but at issue is the decreasing birth rate, geographic location, and the isolation. With fewer pregnancies in the remote communities, it is difficult to recruit midwives or perinatal-certified nurses for such specialized care when primary health in the rural and remote areas seems better served with generalist preparation. As well, maternal child health care providers would have difficulty in maintaining competencies to meet the health care needs of pregnant women when the volume of pregnant women is reduced.

As tele-health and video conferencing are improved and extended to all locations, consultation with southern specialists may keep women in their home communities longer. Also, local women educated to provide maternal health services may better support their family and friends than the often understaffed and transient health care service that is now present. As well, it is most important to hear from the pregnant women of the North and to work in partnership with local women to create programs that meet their health needs during pregnancy and childbirth.

As suggested by the World Health Organization (WHO), it is time that 'closing the gap' on health inequity becomes a priority for all countries (Commission on Social Determinants of Health [CSDH], 2008). Social justice for all Canadians includes a healthy environment to grow and live in. This is particularly important during the prenatal period, when the baby is developing. Some of the risk factors for mortality and morbidity in babies, identified by the WHO, are present in the NWT: malnutrition, inadequate stimulation or learning environments, iron deficiency anemia, intrauterine growth restriction, maternal depression, exposure to violence, and exposure to heavy metals (CSDH, 2008). One of the WHO's recommendations for achieving health equity and overcoming these risk factors is to focus on early childhood development (CSDH, 2008). Ultimately, this requires improving the environment of pregnant women in the North so that their health improves along with that of the newborn.

Conclusion

The health of pregnant women in the NWT has been reviewed from historical, health status, and social determinants perspectives. From this review, I have identified directions for future research and health promotion approaches. Although some available indicators of morbidity and mortality show improvement, perinatal data is nonexistent or very difficult to retrieve, and this requires attention so that health promotion efforts, planning, and policy development can occur from an evidence base that facilitates the best practices to meet their needs. I have described many deficiencies and inequities in terms of the social determinants of health that, when improved, will enable positive health outcomes. Pregnant women in the NWT require healthy environments to grow healthy babies. With a coordinated research agenda driven by the local women of the NWT, health for all may become an achieved goal.

Notes

1 The term 'Aboriginal' is used in this chapter to refer to the indigenous people who were the original inhabitants of the land in the Arctic and sub-Arctic regions now known as the Northwest Territories.
2 According to Statistics Canada (2006), the visible minorities in the NWT include Filipino ($n = 690$), Black ($n = 375$), Southeast Asian ($n = 355$), Chinese ($n = 320$), South Asian ($n = 210$), and Latin American ($n = 85$).
3 The division of the Northwest Territories occurred 1 April 1999. Baffin, Keewatin, and Kitikmeot regions, formerly of the Northwest Territories, became the territory of Nunavut.
4 The Indian residential schools are listed in terms of settlements as Akaitcho Hall (Yellownife Vocational School), Aklavik Roman Catholic (Immaculate Conception), Aklavik Anglican (All Saints), Deh Cho Hall (Lapointe Hall), Federal Hostel at Fort Franklin, Fort McPherson (Flemming Hall), Fort Providence Boarding Home (Sacred Heart), Fort Resolution Residence (St. Joseph's), Fort Simpson Anglican (Bompas Hall), Fort Simpson Roman Catholic (Lapointe Hall), Fort Smith (Breynat Hall), Fort Smith (Grandin College), Hay River (St. Peter's), Inuvik Roman Catholic (Grollier Hall), and Inuvik Anglican Hostel (Stringer Hall).
5 Community health representatives are local Aboriginal residents who are primarily responsible for health promotion within the community.
6 The Medical Travel Policy, which includes evacuation for birth, was created by the federal government in the 1970s and continues today under the local government of the NWT.
7 Reconciliation is a process of renewed relationship between the government and the Aboriginal residential school survivors.

References

Aboriginal Healing Foundation. (n.d.) *A residential school bibliography*. Retrieved from http://www.ahf.ca/publications/residential-schools-resources.
Aboriginal Healing Foundation. (2007). *A directory of residential schools in Canada*. Ottawa: Author. Retrieved from http://www.ahf.ca/publications/residential-schools-resources.
Adelson, N. (2005). The embodiment of inequity: Health disparities in Aboriginal Canada. *Canadian Journal of Public Health, 96,* S45–S61.
Becker, G., & Paulette, L. (2003). Informed choice with a focus on rural and northern midwifery in the Northwest Territories. *Canadian Journal of Midwifery Research and Practice, 2*(3), 22–5.

Berti, P.R., Soueida, R., & Kuhnlein, H.V. (2008). Dietary assessment of in-digenous Canadian Arctic women with a focus on pregnancy and lactation. *International Journal of Circumpolar Health, 67*(4), 349–62.

Brett, H.B. (1969). A synopsis of northern medical history. *Canadian Medical Association Journal, 100*, 521–5.

Carry, C. (2009, 13 July). *NutaraqtaarniqNunalingnirmiunutAlianaippuq - Birth a joyous community event.* A screening of a live-to-tape two-hour call-in program about Inuit maternity care at the 14th International Congress on Circumpolar Health Conference, Yellowknife, NT.

Caulfield, L.E., Harris, S.B., Whalen, E.A., & Sugamori, M.E. (1998). Maternal nutritional status, diabetes, and risk of macrosomia among Native Canadian women. *Early Human Development, 50*, 293–303.

CBC News. (2008, 7 November). NWT sounds the alarm about syphilis come-back. Retrieved from http://www.cbc.ca/health/story/2008/11/07/nwt-syphilis.html.

Cnattinguis, S. (2004). The epidemiology of smoking during pregnancy, smok-ing prevalence, maternal characteristics, and pregnancy outcomes. *Nicotine and Tobacco Research, 6* (Suppl2), S125–S140.

Commission on Social Determinants of Health (CSDH). (2008). *Closing the gap in a generation: Health equity through action on the social determinates of health.* Final Report. Geneva,: World Health Organization.

Couchie, C., & Sanderson, S. (2007). A report on best practices for returning birth to rural and remote Aboriginal communities (SOGC Report). *Journal of Obstetrics and Gynaecology Canada, 188*, 250–54. Retrieved from http://www.sogc.org/guidelines/documents/188E-CPG-March2007.pdf.

Daniel, L. (2009). Fatty foods in pregnancy linked to fatter babies. *British Journal of Midwifery, 17*(5), 322.

Daniels, A., Drybones, R., Lafferty, L., Moore, T., & Naedzo, J. (2009, 16 July). Partnership and process in community-based research in the North. Presentation at the 14th International Congress on Circumpolar Health, Yellowknife, NT.

Daviss, B. (1997). Heeding warnings from the canary, the whale and the Inuit. A framework for analyzing competing types of knowledge about childbirth. In E. Davis-Floyd & C.F. Sargent (Eds.), *Childbirth and authoritative know-ledge: Cross cultural perspectives* (pp. 441–73). Berkeley, CA: University of California Press.

Dell, C.A., & Roberts, G. (2005). *Alcohol use and pregnancy: An important Canadian public health and social issue.* Ottawa: Public Health Agency of Canada. Retrieved from http://www.phac-aspc.gc.ca/publicat/fasd-ru-ectaf-pr-06/index-eng.php.

Douglas, V.K. (2006). Converging epistemologies: Critical issues in Canadian Inuit childbirth and pregnancy. In N. Murphy & S. Krivischekov (Eds.), *Circumpolar health 2006: Gateway to the International Polar Year.* Proceedings of the 13th International Congress on Circumpolar Health (pp. 209–14). Novosibirsk, Russia: International Union of Circumpolar Health.

Endres, L.K., Sharp, L.K., Haney, E., & Dooley, S.L. (2004). Health literacy and pregnancy preparedness in pregestational diabetes. *Diabetes Care, 27,* 331–34.

Ferguson, B. (2008). Health literacy and health disparities: The role they play in maternal and child health. *Nursing for Women's Health, 12*(4), 287–98.

Fumoleau, R. (1984). *Denendeh: A Dene celebration.* Toronto: McClelland & Stewart.

Government of the Northwest Territories (GNWT). (2003). *2002NWT drug and alcohol survey.* Yellowknife: Health & Social Services. Retrieved from http://www.hlthss.gov.nt.ca/english/publications/pubresult.asp?ID=146.

Government of the Northwest Territories (GNWT). (2005a). *NWT health status report 2005.* Yellowknife: Health & Social Services. Retrieved from http://www.hlthss.gov.nt.ca/english/publications/pubresult.asp?ID=153.

Government of the Northwest Territories (GNWT). (2005b). *Sexually transmitted infections – The naked truth: A strategic directions document.* Yellowknife: Health & Social Services. Retrieved from http://www.hlthss.gov.nt.ca/english/publications/pubresult.asp?ID=140.

Government of the Northwest Territories (GNWT). (2006). *Northwest Territories early childhood development report for 2004/05.*Yellowknife: Health & Social Services. Retrieved from http://www.hlthss.gov.nt.ca/english/publications/pubresult.asp?ID=177.

Government of the Northwest Territories (GNWT). (2008a). *The 2006 NWT addictions report.* Yellowknife: Health & Social Services. Retrieved from http://www.hlthss.gov.nt.ca/english/publications/pubresult.asp?ID=23.0

Government of the Northwest Territories (GNWT). (2008b). *Health centre services report 2007.* Yellowknife: Health & Social Services. Retrieved from http://www.hlthss.gov.nt.ca/english/publications/pubresult.asp?ID=229.

Government of the Northwest Territories (GNWT). (2009). *Directions for wellness 2007-2008: A summary of First Nations and Inuit Health Branch programs in the Northwest Territories.* Yellowknife: Health and Social Services. Retrieved from http://www.hlthss.gov.nt.ca/english/publications/pubresult.asp?ID=252.

Healey, G.K., & Meadows, L.M. (2007). Inuit women's health in Nunavut Canada: A review of the literature. *International Journal of Circumpolar Health, 66*(3), 199–214.

Heaman, M.I., & Chalmers, K. (2005). Prevalence and correlates of smoking during pregnancy: A comparison of Aboriginal and non-Aboriginal women in Manitoba. *Birth, 32*(4), 299–305.

Huotari, A., & Herzig, K. (2008). Vitamin D and living in Northern latitudes – An endemic risk area for vitamin D deficiency. *International Journal of Circumpolar Health, 67*(2), 164–78.

Institute for Circumpolar Health Research. (2009). *Vision*. Retrieved from http://ichr.ca/about/vision/.

Kakfwi, S. (2006). In the walls of his mind. On *In the walls of his mind* (CD). Yellowknife: Dancing Sky Studio.

Kandola, K. (2006). Prenatal screening for maternal alcohol consumption. *EpiNorth, 18*(2), 15–17.

Kaufert, P.A., & O'Neil, J.D. (1990). Cooptation and control: The reconstruction of Inuit birth. *Medical Anthropology Quarterly, 4*(4), 427–42.

Kendig, S. (2006). Word power: The effect of literacy on health outcomes. *Lifelines, 10*(4), 327–31.

Klein, M.C., Christilau, J., & Johnson, M.B. (2002). Loss of maternity care: The cascade of unforeseen dangers. *Canadian Journal of Rural Medicine, 7*(2), 120–1.

Kornelson, J., & Grzybowski, S. (2005). The costs of separation: The birth experiences of women in isolated and remote communities in British Columbia. *Canadian Woman Studies, 24*(1), 75–80.

Kuhnlein, H.V., & Chan, H.M. (2000). Environment and contaminants in traditional food systems of Northern indigenous peoples. *Annual Review of Nutrition, 20*, 595–626.

Kuhnlein, H.V., & Turner, N.J. (1996). *Traditional plant foods of Canadian Indigenous peoples: Nutrition, botany and use.* Vol. 8 of *Food and Nutrition History and Anthropology* (series ed. Solomon H. Katz). Netherlands: Gordon and Breach.

Lambden, J., Receveur, O., & Kuhnlein, H.V. (2007). Traditional food attributes must be included in studies of food security in the Canadian Arctic. *International Journal of Circumpolar Health, 66*(4), 308–19.

Legacy of Hope Foundation. (2009). *Where are the children? Healing the legacy of residential schools.* Yellowknife: Prince of Wales Northern Heritage Centre.

Lessard, P. (1990). Prenatal care in the western Arctic. In J.D. O'Neil & P. Gilbert (Eds.), *Childbirth in the Canadian North: Epidemiological, clinical and cultural perspectives.* Winnipeg: Northern Health Research Unit, University of Manitoba.

Luo, Z.C., & Wilkins, R. (2008). Degree of rural isolation and birth outcomes. *Paediatric and Perinatal Epidemiology, 22*, 341–9.

Lynch, J., Smith, G.D., Harper, S., Hillimeier, M., Ross, N., Kaplan, G.A., & Wolfson, M. (2004). Is income inequality a determinant of population health? Part 1: A systematic review. *The Milbank Quarterly, 82*(1). Retrieved from http://www.milbank.org/quarterly/8201feat.html.

Lys, C. (2009, 13 July). *Listening to the youth: Understanding the barriers and facilitators to positive, empowered and safer sexual health among female youth in the NWT.*.Presentation at the 14th International Congress on Circumpolar Health, Yellowknife, NT..

Machalek, K., Chatwood, S., Paulette, L., & Becker, G. (2009). *Development of a perinatal surveillance system for the Northwest Territories Canada.* Presentation at the 14th International Congress on Circumpolar Health, Yellowknife, NT.

Mazan, R. (2007). Women at risk: Alcohol patterns among women aged 15 to 44 years, NWT 1996–2006. *EpiNorth, 19*(3), 10–14.

McNicholas, S.L. (2002). Social support and positive health practices. *Western Journal of Nursing Research, 24*(5), 772–86.

Moffitt, P. (2004). Colonialization: A health determinant for pregnant Dogrib women. *Journal of Transcultural Nursing, 15*(4), 323–30.

Moffitt, P. (2008). *'Keep myself well': Perinatal health beliefs and health promotion practices among Tlicho women.* Doctoral diss., University of Calgary.

Moffitt, P., & Vollman, A.R. (2006). At what cost to health? Tlicho women's medical travel for childbirth. *Contemporary Nurse, 22*(5), 228–39.

Northern Contaminants Program. (2009). *Canadian Arctic contaminants and health assessment report.* Ottawa: Indian and Northern Affairs Canada.

NWT Bureau of Statistics. (2006a). *Census.* Yellowknife: Government of the Northwest Territories. Retrieved from http://www.stats.gov.nt.ca/Statinfo/Census/census%2006/_2006census.html.

NWT Bureau of Statistics. (2006b). *Vital statistics.* Yellowknife: Government of the Northwest Territories. Retrieved from http://www.stats.gov.nt.ca/Statinfo/Demographics/VitalStats/revised_vital.html.

O'Neil, J.D., Kaufert, P.L., & Postl, B.D. (1990). *A study of the impact of obstetric policy on Inuit women and their families in the Keewatin Region, NWT.* Ottawa: National Health Research Development Program.

Outcrop. (1990). Northwest Territories data book. Yellowknife: Author.

Paulette, L. (1989). The changing experience of child-bearing in the NWT. *Northern Perspectives, 17*(3). Retrieved from http://www.carc.org/pubs/v17no3/index.html.

Paulette, L. (2007). Fort Smith Health and Social Services Authority midwifery program. *EpiNorth, 19*(1), 7–9.

Premji, S.S., & Semenic, S. (2009). Do Canadian prenatal record forms integrate evidence-based guidelines for the diagnosis of FASD? *Canadian Journal of Public Health, 100*(4), 274–80.

Public Health Agency of Canada (PHAC). (2000). *Canadian perinatal health report.* Ottawa: Author. Retrieved from http://www.phac-aspc.gc.ca/publicat/cphr-rspc00/pdf/cphr00e.pdf.

Public Health Agency of Canada (PHAC). (2009). *What mothers say: The Canadian maternity experiences survey.* Ottawa: Author. Retrieved from http://www.phac-aspc.gc.ca/rh5ssg/pdf/survey/eng.pdf.

Raphael, D. (2004). *Social determinants of health: Canadian perspectives.* Toronto: Canadian Scholars' Press.

Raves, C. (2006). Children and obesity. *EpiNorth, 18,* 1–5.

Rawlings, L. (1998). Traditional Aboriginal birthing issues. *Birth Gazette, 14*(1). Retrieved from EBSCO Host.

Renkert, S., & Nutbeam, D. (2001). Opportunities to improve maternal health literacy through antenatal education. *Health Promotion International, 16*(4), 381–8.

Richmond, C.A.M. (2009). The social determinants of Inuit health: A focus on social support in the Canadian Arctic. *International Journal of Circumpolar Health, 68*(5), 471–87.

Rootman, I., & Ronson, B. (2005). Literacy and health research in Canada. Where have we been and where should we go? *Canadian Journal of Public Health, 96* (Suppl2), S62–S77.

Royal Commission on Aboriginal Peoples (RCAP). (2006). Residential schools. In *Volume 1: Looking forward looking back* (chap. 10). Ottawa: Author. Retrieved from http://www.collectionscanada.gc.ca/webarchives/20071124130216/http://www.ainc-inac.gc.ca/ch/rcap/sg/sgm10_e.html.

Sharma, S., De Roose, E., Cao, X., Gittelsohn, A., & Corriveau, A. (2009, 14 July). *An assessment of dietary intake in an Inuvialuit population to highlight foods for a nutritional intervention program to improve dietary intake: Results from Health Foods North.* Presentation at the 14th International Congress on Circumpolar Health, Yellowknife, NT.

Shohet, L. (2002). *Health and literacy: Perspectives in 2002.* Montreal: Centre for Literacy of Quebec. Retrieved from http://www.staff.vu.edu.au/alnarc/onlineforum/AL_pap_shohet.htm.

Smith, D., Varcoe, C., & Edwards, N. (2005). Turning around the intergenerational impact of residential schools on Aboriginal people: Implications for health policy and practice. *Canadian Journal of Nursing Research, 37*(4), 39–60.

Smylie, J. (2001). A guide for health professionals working with Aboriginal peoples (SOGC Policy Statement). *Journal of Obstetrics and Gynaecology*

Canada, 100, 1–15. Retrieved from http://www.sogc.org/guidelines/public/100E-PS3-January2001.pdf.

Spady, D.W. (1982). *Between two worlds.* Edmonton: Boreal Institute of Northern Studies.

Sperry, J.R. (2001). *Igloo dwellers were my church: The memoirs of Jack Sperry, Anglican bishop of the Arctic.* Calgary: Bayeaux Arts.

Stanton Territorial Health Authority. (2004). *Stanton Territorial Health Authority 2003-2004 annual report: Restoring health with dignity.* Retrieved from http://www.stha.ca/files/services/100/STHA_2003_2004_Annual_Report.pdf.

Stryker, S., & Burke, P.J. (2000). The past, present and future of an identity theory. *Social Psychology Quarterly, 63,* 284–97.

Sutherns, R. (2004). Adding women's voices to the call for sustainable rural maternity care. *Canadian Journal of Rural Medicine, 9*(4), 239–44.

Thomson, M. (1990). Heavy birth weight of native Indians of British Columbia. *Canadian Journal of Public Health, 81,* 443–6.

Ward, L.M., Gaboury, I., Ladhani, M., & Zlotkin, S. (2007). Vitamin D deficiency rickets among children in Canada. *Canadian Medical Association Journal, 177*(2), 161–6.

Watts, N. (2010). High-risk labour and childbirth. In R.J. Evans, M.K. Evans, Y.M.R. Brown, & S.A. Orshan (Eds.).*Canadian maternity, newborn & women's health nursing* (pp. 623–5). Philadelphia: Lippincott, Williams & Wilkins.

Wenman, W.M., Joffres, M.R., Tataryn, I.V., & Edmonton Prenatal Infections Group. (2004). A prospective cohort study of pregnancy risk factors and birth outcomes in Aboriginal women. *Canadian Medical Association Journal, 171*(6), 585–9.

Wilhelm, A., & Hegeman, L. (2004). Exploring fetal alcohol spectrum disorder surveillance in the NWT. *EpiNorth, 16,* 13–16.

Young, T.K., Reading, J., Elias, B., & O'Neil, J.D. (2000). Type 2 diabetes mellitus in Canada's First Nations: Status of an epidemic in progress. *Canadian Medical Association Journal, 163*(5), 561–6.

18 Leisure, Rural Community Identity, and Women's Health: Historical and Contemporary Connections

Deborah Stiles, Steven Dukeshire, and Kenneth S. Paulsen, with Melanie Goodridge, David Hobson, Jamie MacLaughlin, Katriona MacNeil, and J. Cristian Rangel

This chapter describes research undertaken in an effort to respond to Janzen's (1998) identification of the 'health needs and determinants of rural women' (p. iii) as one of the ten key gaps in research on Canadian women's health. In a rural Nova Scotia community we refer to by the pseudonym 'Hampshire,' we employed an interdisciplinary approach tempered with caution (Giacomini, 2004) and a community-based participation research model (Neuman, 2003; Penzhorn, 2002) in an effort to 'hear' (Gubrium & Holstein, 1998) what the women of Hampshire, a rural, Nova Scotia, inland, post-industrial community, were 'saying' about their health and leisure. The findings suggest that rural community identity itself plays a role in shaping rural women's health and leisure. Both Hampshire's rural community identity, as historically constructed, and gender, as rurally configured in the contemporary context, can be seen to be factors in access to, ideas about, and opportunities for leisure. Gender, rural community identity, and health are integrally connected; consequently, in order to understand the health needs of rural women in Canada, and formulate effective rural health policy, we argue that it is necessary to understand the historical and gendered specificities of the rural context.

Background

This research began with a selective review of the literature on community identity in a rural context, rural women's leisure and health, and rural community health. Our goal was to examine the place of key concepts and understandings of this literature in terms of rural communities and their rural yet also industrial development patterns. Logging, mining, farming, and the fisheries have long histories in the Atlantic region as well as the rest of Canada (Brym & Sacouman, 1979; Forbes & Muise, 1993; Frank, 1993). More recent discussions of 'rural restructuring' (Binkley, 1996; Binkley, 2000; Rural Communities Impacting Policy Project, 2003) are only the more recent symptoms of a longer-term economic and social malady affecting Canadian rural communities that have had, historically and over the long term, limited local control over economic development involving extractive industries in their midst (Brym & Sacouman, 1979, pp. 17–20; Stanley, 1993).

Community Identity in a Rural Context

Historians have defined 'rurality' in terms of low population, inhabitants' access to the natural world, and predominant occupations found in the extraction of raw resources like fish and coal or in primary-production agriculture (Samson, 1994, pp. 22–6; Sandwell, 1994). Although the countryside has, over time, become more 'urbanized,' studies such as those discussed by Weinert and Burman (1994) and others make reference to rurally specific socio-cultural differences (Averill, 2003; Gupta & Ferguson, 1997; Hancock, Labonte, & Edwards, 1999; Stiles, 1997). Rurality, in terms of rural and community identity, is conceptualized here as historical and contemporary social patterns and physical configurations of space and household and other structures that connect to rural settings (such as the predominance of single-family dwellings as opposed to large apartment buildings); opportunities for, access to, and participation in natural-world, 'traditional' leisure activities (such as going fishing, sledding or snowmobiling rather than going to the movies); and perceived norms and cultural values linked either explicitly or implicitly to living in an area identified as rural (such as persistent linkages of gender identity with work as part of a capitalist, resource-extraction, industrial or non-industrial economic activity, including woods working, fishing, entrepreneurial endeavours in the arts, professional services, farming, etc.) (Brym & Sacouman, 1979; Sandwell, 1994, 1998; Stiles, 1997, 1998; Weinert & Burman, 1994). As Sandwell (1998) observes in the introduction to her study of rural British Columbia, *Beyond the City Limits*, 'Subsistence activities, household-based economies, gendered hierarchies, and disparate rural identities have continued to shape those [rural] individuals and communities ... well into the twentieth century' (p. 4). And, we would argue, into the twenty-first century.

Community identity in a rural context can be understood as a function of historically shaped demographic and socio-cultural patterns linked to rural persistence patterns and outmigration strategies employed by rural dwellers (Brookes, 1976; Lewis, 2001; Thornton, 1985), gendered change related to migrations or changes in work processes/patterns, access to and use of the natural world (Samson, 1994, pp. 22–7), and gendered social relations constructed, maintained, and, at times, challenged within communities (Beattie, 2000, p. 176; Stiles, 2003, pp. 130–2). Perceptions of, access to, and participation in leisure activities can be understood as rooted historically as well as socially and culturally in the rural context.

Rural Women's Leisure and Health

Culture, class, race, ethnicity, and gender are all linked to overall health and well-being in rural communities (Chávez, 2005). Rurality and gender are also vital in comprehending how women in rural areas navigate the terrains of health—both in terms of community, and of health system access and participation (Thurston, MacKean, et al., 2005; Thurston, Vollman, Meadows, & Rutherford, 2005). Additionally, even a circumscribed review of the literature on rural women's leisure and health links physical activity, and more generally leisure activity, with good health (Freysinger, 1990; Henderson, 2003; Thomlinson, McDonagh, Crooks, & Lees, 2004; Trenberth, 2005).

In rural areas experiencing economic and other challenges, time constraints related to the transportation time needed for such daily life activities as food shopping, school, volunteering, health care, and the like may result in increased household burdens for women, conflicts (or perceived conflicts) over the use of women's time, and lack of opportunities for women for leisure, including physical activity (Henderson, 1996, p. 337). These sets of circumstances may set into motion patterns of inactivity enforced and reinforced by other structural factors (Stiles, Rangel, MacLaughlin, Sanderson, & MacNeil, 2007); however, as Etowa et al. observe in this volume, even with populations that grapple with the 'quadruple jeopardy' effects of geographic distance, racism, poverty, and sexism (p. 300), exercising is an area of rural women's lives where they attempt to effect some positive measure of control over their health (p. 293). The types and experience of leisure (Henderson, 1996, p. 337) as available to and engaged in by women in rural settings, and the ways in which such activities are viewed within the norms, constraints, and contexts of rural community life – including the leisure-health relationship – may also, as suggested by this research project's findings, be influenced by the ways in which a particular rural community or region has experienced leisure historically, and, more specifically, how gender roles and norms have been expressed over time within the rural community context.

Rural Community Health

Rural women and men conceptualize their health in different ways than their suburban or urban counterparts. Rural women may perceive the dimensions that constitute good health differently from perceived norms (Averill, 2003; Thomlinson et al., 2004). Rural women's access to and opportunity for leisure, health care, or health-enhancing services are also a function of historically shaped gender roles. Rural residents in one Canadian study viewed being healthy as a balance of the social, mental, physical, and spiritual parts of life; freedom and autonomy; eating healthily; and being active (Thomlinson et al., 2004). Being rural was part and parcel of individual *and* community identity, and family, friends, and neighbours were considered by the rural residents in this community to be *health* resources (Thomlinson et al., 2004). A recurring theme in rural health appears to be the strong connection between individual well-being and household and community well-being. Arai and Pedlar (1997) noted the importance of understanding the ties between individual health and community health. The link between individual and community well-being may be of even greater significance for women.

Rural communities have experienced and continue to experience adversity in the arenas of underemployment and unemployment, more limited access to health care and health services, the negative effects of rural depopulation, lack of public transportation, higher fuel and food costs, economic downturns external to the community that nonetheless translate into limited work opportunities closer to home, and isolation (Bushy, 1993; Stiles and Cameron, 2009). Yet, the picture for rural dwellers is not all gloom and doom. As Thomlinson and colleagues (2004) showed, and as the responses from focus group participants in the present study suggest, despite all these challenges, rural women in certain respects find a measure of health and well-being in their rural communities.

Living in a rural community in Canada, for example, provides a type of freedom and autonomy that urban areas cannot offer. In Canada much of the rural areas are spaces that all can enjoy (a kind of commons) even if one does not own the land (use of Crown lands in Nova Scotia being but one illustration of this). Rural women, historically, have experienced both freedom from some of the gendered constraints of middle-class, urban women, and more constraints because of their gender (Jensen, 1991). Today, the social context of rurality provides many women with a lifestyle they value. Weinert and Burman (1994) discussed this strength of rural dwellers in terms of their *social* health; even though urbanites had higher ratings in aspects of physical health, rural dwellers appeared to benefit from family interaction, organizational involvement, and social integration (Weinert & Burman, 1994). If these social aspects of health are more robust in rural communities, and social support is more important for women, then the dynamics of rural community health and well-being as well as leisure may be explicitly connected to the overall health of rural women and how rural women view themselves within their rural community.

Following this review of literature, research team members Stiles and Paulsen conducted historical research (Statistics Canada, 1871, 1881, 1891) and consulted a history of the community written by a long-time resident ('Matthews').[1] Peer-reviewed historical scholarship (secondary sources) on Hampshire and other early sites of mid- to late-nineteenth-century rural industrialization then provided context for the qualitative study (Acheson, 1972; Brym & Sacouman, 1979; Forbes & Muise, 1993; McCann, 1993; Stanley, 1993; 'Stevens').

The community-based participatory research (CBPR) model commenced through the hiring of community coordinators from within the community to shape the initial research questions and protocol, and to assist in facilitation of the three focus group interviews (Morgan 1998) held in the community. The sample frame for the focus groups included the approximately 125 women in the community between the ages of nineteen and forty-five years (Statistics Canada, 2001).

The focus group findings were discussed, summarized, and validated by the community coordinators immediately following the last focus group, and a preliminary analysis of the historical research and the focus group data was presented at a 'report-back' meeting and leisure workshop held in the community. There, the women attending provided input into the design and implementation of the mail-out survey, the final phase of the study, whose key components were a twelve-item Sense of Community Index (Perkins, Florin, Rich, Wandersman, & Chavis, 1990) and a twelve-item Sense of Place Scale (Jorgensen &

Stedman, 2001), examining perceived levels of physical, emotional, and social well-being; what types of leisure activities participants engaged in, and how often; and barriers to leisure activities. Participants were also asked to provide demographic information. Due to the small population of women aged nineteen to forty-five years in the community, the sampling frame for the survey was expanded to all women aged nineteen or older, and the survey was mailed out to all 217 households in Hampshire, with an invitation cover letter directed exclusively to the female members of households. Sixty-nine surveys were returned. Characteristics of the sample can be seen in Table 18.1.

Rural Community Identity: Historically Configured

The community of Hampshire has become neither a service hub nor a community focused on creating and maintaining a specific image vis-à-vis tourism (McKay, 1994). Neither is it a community caught up in a specific and current crisis of rural restructuring, as was the case with coastal communities in Nova Scotia and elsewhere in the Atlantic region during the fisheries crisis of the middle to late twentieth century (Binkley, 1996, 2000). Rather, like many rural, inland (in provinces with coastal areas), post-industrial Canadian communities, Hampshire's challenges are rooted in much older historical circumstances. The community was part of some of Canada's earliest industrial developments in the mid-nineteenth century ('Stevens'). It reached its peak population of just under three thousand in 1891, when preliminary tests revealed the possibility of a rich vein of ore that both local but especially internationally placed investors hoped to exploit. Hampshire became the largest community in the immediate area ('Stevens'); its bustling town of original Irish, English, and other settlers was joined by Welsh and other immigrant miners and miners' families. While the majority of the population was this working-class or the older, agriculturally based one, a small contingent of merchants and managers of various ethnicities and religions were also in evidence (Statistics Canada 1871, 1881, 1891).

Hampshire, like many rural communities in this period, was 'vulnerable to external conditions,' as historical geographer Larry McCann has observed (McCann, 1993, p. 126). These externalities, coupled with rural remoteness, led to Hampshire's population beginning to falter even as the regional conditions for industrial development, affected by Canada's National Policy and other factors, took hold and Maritime industry on the whole began to fade (Acheson, 1972; McCann, 1993).

Table 18.1 Characteristics of Survey Respondents (*n* = 69)

Age (years)	19–29	17.6%
	30–39	11.8%
	40–49	11.8%
	50–59	29.4%
	60–69	20.6%
	70+	8.8%
Marital Status	Married/common law	81.2%
	Single	1.4%
	Widowed	10.1%
	Divorced/separated	7.2%
Education Level	Primary to grade 8	7.4%
	Some high school	25.0%
	Completed high school/GED	29.4%
	Some college/university	8.8%
	Completed community coll	14.7%
	Completed coll./univ. degree	10.3%
	Other	4.4%
Annual Household Income	Less than $20,000	14.3%
	$20,000–$29,999	30.4%
	$30,000–$39,999	21.4%
	More than $40,000	33.9%
Work for Pay	No	51.6%
	Yes	48.4%
Household Has Vehicle	No	5.9%
	Yes	94.1%

These vagaries of early industrialization are pivotal to understanding the way in which Hampshire, and other communities like it, changed over time. Chief is lack of, or loss of, local economic control, a lasting feature in rural industrial development/underdevelopment (Brym & Sacouman, 1979, pp. 9–14; 'Stevens'). As David Frank (1993) has noted, even as early as the 1920s in the Atlantic region (including the seeming 'boomtown' of Hampshire), the region was 'marked [by] the culmination of developments that had been in the making for at least a generation … both political and economic power had become concentrated in fewer hands and more distant places' (p. 234).

Today, Hampshire fits the du Plessis definition of 'rural and small town' in being a community of between four to six hundred with a population density of three to five persons per square kilometre (du Plessis, Beshiri, & Bollman, 2001). It is located in a strong Metro

Influence Zone (MIZ), because of its proximity to a town with a population of over ten thousand (Statistics Canada, 2001). It is, but also is not, a 'bedroom community'; that is, it is far enough away from that large town that transportation is difficult for many residents, and thus so is access to certain services, but it is close enough that, over the course of the latter twentieth century, health, social, leisure, and other related services have not been sustained or even considered in Hampshire, as it was assumed that those who wanted them would use (then-) cheap fuel and a car and go to the closest town to obtain them.

Hampshire provides but one example of a Canadian rural community affected not by more recent rural restructuring, but by older historical patterns involving the 'boom' and 'bust' of rural industrialization. In Hampshire's case, it was a boomtown situated in the midst of a rural, hilly landscape ('Stevens'), one that had retained its earlier settlers but had added considerably to its population through the workers and families brought in to supply the skilled labour required by these nineteenth-century industrial developments. Elites and upper management were in the minority; consequently, the community's identity, one it has retained to this day, appears to have maintained well-defined social and economic boundaries shaped by industrially engendered working-class values (Palmer, 1992). The census data and the local history reveal a vibrant mix of cultures, churches, businesses, and associational life throughout the turn of the century, despite industrial decline, a community whose working-class culture significantly shaped community life ('Matthews'; Palmer, 1992).

Given the working-class culture that predominated in Hampshire, the community's embrace of what were working-class and gendered male leisure practices is not surprising. By 1886 there was a cricket team, and following the cricket team, there was a baseball league – both class-based and specifically male-gendered associational life (Howell, 1995, p. 285; 'Matthews'). By the late twentieth century, rural associational life in Hampshire did include women's and co-ed softball teams, but these were secondary to the long-established men's baseball league. Rural and gendered patterns of leisure established so long ago appear to have persisted in Hampshire ('Matthews', pp. 176–80; Stiles et al., 2007), and suggest a rural community identity that continues to privilege male leisure practices (Stiles et al., 2007). This type of male privileging of leisure, noted in a study of women's leisure, health, and well-being in a former gold-mining community of rural Australia, suggests that local and communal options remain limited in some rural communities of 'developed' nations, and the health effects this reality has on women demonstrates the degree to which specific realities of the past continue to influence the present (Warner-Smith & Brown, 2002, pp. 43, 50).

This historical perspective on rural community identity allows more adequate address of the three key themes that emerged from qualitative data analysis of the focus group interviews, themes that were subsequently supported by the survey findings. These three themes, interestingly enough, were less about the *experience* of leisure as perceived by the women, and more about how the community's women viewed the community's identity, what chief health issues they saw as affecting their community, and the gendered dimensions of access to leisure. These three themes can be shorthanded as follows: community identity; rural health is individual *and* communal; and gender shapes our lives – and leisure (Stiles et al., 2007).

Theme 1: Community Identity

Hampshire's past, rich in industrial and associational life, featured fairly prominently, though not exclusively, in the pictures participants were asked to draw of their community in the focus group interviews ('for someone who's never been there before'). The participants' drawings were of ice rinks and ball fields, now fallen into disuse, and features of the natural world, as well as the human-made remnants of the community's rural yet industrial past (most notably, an industrial waste heap that lies near the centre of the community). Nostalgic sites mentioned, such as the 'old school,' the former museum, the former rink, the hall, and churches no longer standing meant that many of the participants – whose grandparents would not even be old enough to be able to recall some of these sites, given that they disappeared so early in the twentieth century – were relying on oral tradition as the basis for their assertions that their community was once a more vital community, one filled with shops, banks, taverns, local jobs, and opportunities for social leisure (churches and social halls, organizations, organized sports), as well as physical leisure (sports for some, but also the rink for skating and the river for swimming).

Knowledge of the natural world and of the community's industrial past also figured prominently in the women's configurations of the community's identity. Their responses suggest that it is an awareness of nature, coupled with a functionality related to the human-made circumstances at hand, which help to define the leisure experiences of rural women. The most prominent feature situating the community landscape was one created as a result of the community's industrial past – an industrial waste heap. It is a hill, where the locals go sledding and engage in partying. The present-day surroundings, as shaped by a rural industrial history, play a role in configuring leisure activities – the industrial waste heap is used as a slope, for sledding – but their prominence in the community also speaks to the prominence of historical memory. 'Can we go to [Mount Haliburton] and sled?' one participant gave as an example, when asked to discuss her picture. Other phrases described the community as 'built on rocks' – the mining legacy – and having 'one main road' – signifying that the 'boomtown' phase never developed beyond providing entrance and exit to the resource extraction industry contained within the town limits.

Theme 2: Rural Health Is Individual and Communal

The question 'How do you define healthy living?' prompted initial, individual, and almost autonomic responses of 'eating right' and 'exercising' from all three groups of focus group participants, much as was expressed by the participants in the study by Etowa et al. in this volume. Yet, one focus group also responded with the revealing "enough money for a healthy lifestyle." Health concerns were also articulated. These included whether individual well water supplies are safe owing to the town's industrial past (and proximity to the industrial waste heap), stress levels, the time it takes for emergency response crews to get to the community, mental wellness and depression, and wait times for medical and health services (available only outside the community).

Leisure activity was evaluated in community and health contexts in our research, and the survey results in particular revealed interesting connections between health, leisure, and community identity. A sense of connection to rural physical space – not necessarily a sense of connection to the people found in that space – was found to be linked to satisfaction with life and the social aspects of health. Community identity was measured using two scales: the Sense of Community Index (SCI) and Sense of Place Scale (SOPS). The SCI assesses overall feelings of belonging/connection to a community (McMillan & Chavis, 1986), and SOPS assesses people's relationship to a spatial setting (Jorgensen & Stedman, 2001). Results from the two scales are presented in Table 18.2.

Table 18.2 Community Identity

Sense of Community Index (/60)	44.34
Reinforcement of needs (/15)	10.93
Membership (/15)	11.38
Influence (/15)	9.86
Shared emotional connection (/15)	11.70
Sense of Place Scale (/60)	40.78
Identity (/20)	12.39
Dependence (/20)	13.19
Attachment (/20)	15.15

Theme 3: Gender Shapes Our Lives – and Leisure

Access to and participation in leisure and women's perceptions of their own leisure as well as of their leisure in comparison to that of men in their community were captured in various responses of the focus groups as well as the survey. The focus group participants, responding to the question, 'What do people in Hampshire do when not working (at job or home)?,' perceived leisure as 'free time.' Activities named by all three focus groups were walking and four-wheeling (ATV riding). Other activities mentioned in two of the three focus groups were fishing, reading, gardening, knitting, watching TV, and casual drinking/partying. Drinking and partying were perceived to be synonymous and were participated in as a regular Friday night activity. Home parties for product sales (e.g., Fantasia™, Tupperware®, or candles) also were mentioned.

After being asked to list all the different activities their community participated in, the women were asked if the list of activities would be 'different for [Hampshire] women versus [Hampshire] men.' The response was as follows. Activities in which both women and men participated – leisure activities perceived by the women as shared activities involving both sexes and a group setting – included four-wheeling, snowmobiling, TV-watching, camping, swimming, board games, using the computer, coasting (sledding), and drinking/partying. Activities gendered exclusively female, according to the women, or participated in by women as 'women's activities,' were the product sales home parties, gardening, family visits, reading, and walking.

Findings from both the focus groups and survey suggest that women and men tend to participate in about the same set of leisure activities,

with the exceptions, noted above, that were gendered exclusively female. On the survey, when asked what leisure activities they and their
partner/spouse engaged in, the women produced lists that were fairly
similar in terms of the amount of time spent in different leisure activities.
However, when comparing the actual amount of time spent on leisure
activities, *according to the women*, men were perceived to be significantly
more likely to engage in drinking/partying, four-wheeling, snowmobiling, fishing, and watching television.

There are two important characteristics to note about these activities.
First, according to the women in the focus groups, three of these five
activities were the leisure activities women most wanted to participate
in: that is, drinking/partying, four-wheeling, and snowmobiling. Yet in
terms of access and participation, women expressed the view that men
were more likely to shed responsibility in order to be able to participate
in these activities. This scenario echoes the situations identified by authors of other chapters. The second important characteristic is that three
of these key activities – four-wheeling, snowmobiling, and fishing – are
directly connected to the rural landscape. In this context, drinking/par-
tying is also an activity that takes place outdoors or in close proximity to
the outdoors (i.e., it takes place in an individual's house, perhaps, but
most likely in the woods or elsewhere, outside, in the community envi-
rons, as there are no pubs or bars in the community). These activities are
an integral part of living in a rural or remote area and are to some degree
dependent on the spatial setting. It is significant that women perceived
that the activities they were more likely to engage in, those that were *not*
shared activities (i.e., participated in with men), were ones that had
essentially no connection to a rural setting. In other words, gendered-
female leisure activities were not connected to the rurality of their environment. From the women's perspective, the leisure activities men were
more likely to engage in, and the ones perceived as shared leisure activities, were the most desirable activities and also most connected to the
spatial environment. Women who lack the opportunity to engage in activities that allow them to relate to the rural geography are thus potentially less likely to develop a strong sense of place, a sense of place and
identity, which is related to social and emotional health and well-being
as well as overall life satisfaction.

Focus group participants with children were also emphatic about the
fact that their leisure was contingent upon the women securing childcare. While both men and women participated in shared activities, the
women contended that men participated more often in these five most

desirable leisure activities, and that some elements of control over leisure participation rested with the men. Examples from the focus groups illustrate this:

> Because the women stay home and look after the kids and do everything. I think the men tend to feel that they have the right and privilege to come and go out the door no matter what's going on and if we can look after the house and get the children looked after, then sure, you can come along, but that's your job to do that.

> So if we can't all, as women, all coordinate to have our kids all gone so we can all get together on the weekend, then we don't get together. They [the men] all still get together ...

Findings from the survey, particularly of the forty-years-and-under group, reflect the statements made in the focus groups, where participants complained about men shedding responsibility at the women's expense to be able to engage in leisure activities that they enjoyed. Indeed, one of the greatest complaints by the young women in the focus groups was that they (not the men in their households) always shouldered the responsibility of finding childcare. It appears that perceived inequality in leisure time is largely dependent on whether or not women have (younger) children.

Similar findings emerged from examination of the impact of barriers on perceived leisure time. Younger women perceived that the barriers had a greater effect on their leisure time; differences in perceived effect decreased as women got older. However, both the differences due to age and differences between women and men are relatively small. The two greatest barriers overall were not enough money and not enough nearby things to do. This certainly reflects the loss of leisure opportunities in Hampshire through the cycle of depopulation (leading to loss of communal leisure activities, such as ball leagues) and loss of services and amenities (such as places to ice skate), as well as economic downturns experienced here as in many rural communities. The importance of life course is captured in the perception of women with children that childcare has a fairly large effect on their leisure activity. That the women perceived this effect as a greater challenge for themselves than for their significant others (who were, it can be understood in the majority of instances, male partners) again echoes the perceptions expressed in the focus groups: men tended to more easily disregard the childcare provisioning required in order to engage in leisure.

Conclusion

The tendencies of rural societies towards more conservative interpretations of gender roles, coupled with the multiple roles that women have to play, may lead to compromised health for women in rural areas (Bushy, 1993). More recent changes in rural gender roles (Halpern, 2001), which have placed the strain of new, multiple responsibilities on women, may be a factor in rural women's not getting the kinds of leisure, including physical forms of leisure activity, that they want or need (Bushy, 1993; Stiles et al., 2007). In order to understand what factors and variables are affecting young rural women's health, it is necessary to understand the role played by community structures and of rurality and rurally configured identity as well as how women view their community and their gender roles as rural women (Neal & Walters, 2006).

It is also informative to note that sense of place rather than sense of community was more strongly related to emotional well-being and satisfaction with life. The finding that men (at least from the women's perspective) have a greater opportunity to engage in the most desired leisure activities and that these activities (such as four-wheeling, snowmobiling, and fishing) rely on place, that is, the rural environment, highlights the intersection of gender and rurality in the perceived differential opportunities to take advantage of the 'rurality' that is their place. The perceived opportunities to engage in leisure activity were also largely affected by women's stage in the life cycle. All in all, the results of our research suggest that gender and rurality interact to produce differential opportunities for leisure. In Hampshire, the connections of the past continue to shape the present to a degree. That they do suggests that the past as well as any present reality related to resource extraction needs to be factored into rural health policy, if it aims to address adequately the social determinants of health. Rural and community identity, as a feature of historically configured social patterns, affects rural women both positively and negatively.

Notes

1 This study was part of Canadian Institutes of Health Research–funded research on the social determinants of health of young rural Nova Scotia women. To maintain the anonymity of the community (as per the Nova Scotia Agricultural College Research Ethics Board–approved protocol) two historical sources that could potentially identify the community to readers

have been identified by pseudonyms. These two sources are cited within the text as 'Matthews' and 'Stevens,' and only these one-word pseudonyms and an explanation are provided in the References list. For more information, contact the lead author at dstiles@nsac.ca.

References

Acheson, T.W. (1972). The national policy and the industrialization of the Maritimes, 1880–1910. *Acadiensis, 1*(2), 3–29.

Arai, S.M., & Pedlar, A.M. (1997). Building communities through leisure: Citizen participation as a leisure pursuit. *Journal of Leisure Research, 29*(2), 167–82.

Averill, J. (2003). Keys to the puzzle: Recognizing strengths in a rural community. *Public Health Nursing, 20*(60), 449–55.

Beattie, M.E. (2000). *Obligation and opportunity: Single, Maritime women in Boston, 1870-1930.* Montreal: McGill-Queen's University Press.

Binkley, M. (1996). Nova Scotian fishing families coping with the fisheries crisis. *Anthropologica, 38*(2), 197–220.

Binkley, M. (2000). 'Getting by' in tough times: Coping with the fisheries crisis. *Women's Studies International Forum, 23*(3), 323–32.

Brookes, A.A. (1976). Out-migration from the Maritime Provinces, 1860–1900: Some preliminary considerations. *Acadiensis, 5*(2), 26–55.

Brym, R.J., & Sacouman, R.J. (Eds.). (1979). *Underdevelopment and social movements in Atlantic Canada.* Toronto: New Hogtown Press.

Bushy, A. (1993). Rural women: Lifestyle and health status. *The Nursing Clinics of North America, 28*(1), 187–97.

Chávez, S. (2005). Community, ethnicity, and class in a changing rural California town. *Rural Sociology, 70*(3), 314–35.

du Plessis, V., Beshiri, R., & Bollman, R.D. (2001). Definitions of rural. *Rural and Small Town Canada Analysis Bulletin, 3*(3), 1–16.

Forbes, E.R., & Muise, D.A. (Eds.). (1993). *The Atlantic Provinces in Confederation.* Toronto/Fredericton: University of Toronto Press/Acadiensis Press.

Frank, D. (1993). The 1920s: Class and region, resistance and accommodation. In E.R. Forbes & D.A. Muise (Eds.), *The Atlantic Provinces in Confederation* (pp. 233–71). Toronto/Fredericton: University of Toronto/Acadiensis Press.

Freysinger, V.J. (1990). A lifespan perspective on women and physical recreation. *Journal of Physical Education, Recreation & Dance, 61*(1), 48–51.

Giacomini, M. (2004). Interdisciplinarity in health services research: Dreams and nightmares, maladies and remedies. *Journal of Health Services Research & Policy, 9*(3), 177–83.

Gubrium, J.F., & Holstein, J.A. (1998). Narrative practice and the coherence of personal stories. *Sociological Quarterly*, 39(1), 163–87.

Gupta, A., & Ferguson, J. (1997). Culture, power, place: Ethnography at the end of an era. In A. Gupta & J. Ferguson (Eds.), *Culture, power, place: Explorations in critical anthropology* (pp. 1–29). Durham: Duke University Press.

Halpern, M.M. (2001). *And on that farm he had a wife: Ontario farm women and feminism, 1900-1970*. Montreal: McGill-Queen's University Press.

Hancock, T., Labonte, R., & Edwards, R. (1999). Indicators that count!: Measuring population health at the community level. *Canadian Journal of Public Health, 90* (Suppl 1), S22–S26.

Henderson, K.A. (1996). *Both gains and gaps: Feminist perspectives on women's leisure*. State College, PA: Venture.

Henderson, K.A. (2003). Women, physical activity, and leisure: Jeopardy or Wheel of Fortune? *Women in Sport & Physical Activity Journal*, 12(1), 113–25.

Howell, C.D. (1995). *Northern sandlots: A social history of Maritime baseball*. Toronto: University of Toronto Press.

Janzen, B.L. (1998). *Women, gender and health: A Review of the recent literature*. Winnipeg: Prairie Women's Health Centre of Excellence.

Jensen, J.M. (1991). *Promise to the land: Essays on rural women*. Albuquerque, NM: University of New Mexico Press.

Jorgensen, B.S., & Stedman, R.C. (2001). Sense of place as an attitude: Lakeshore owners' attitudes toward their properties. *Journal of Environmental Psychology, 21*, 233–48.

Lewis, T.D. (2001, Autumn). Rooted in the soil: Farm family persistence in Burton Parish, Sunbury County, New Brunswick, 1851–1901. *Acadiensis, 31*(1), 35–54.

'Matthews,' Historical source used. Citation details not given here in order to maintain anonymity of community.

McCann, L. (1993). The 1890s: Fragmentation and the new social order. In E.R. Forbes & D.A. Muise (Eds.), *The Atlantic Provinces in Confederation* (pp. 119–54). Toronto/Fredericton: University of Toronto/Acadiensis Press.

McKay, I. (1994). *The quest of the folk: Antimodernism and cultural selection in twentieth-century Nova Scotia*. Montreal: McGill-Queen's University Press.

McMillan, D.W., & Chavis, D.M. (1986). Sense of community: A definition and theory. *Journal of Community Psychology, 14*, 6–23.

Morgan, D.L. (1998). The focus group guidebook. Thousand Oaks, CA: Sage.

Neal, S., & Walters, S. (2006). Strangers asking strange questions?: A methodological narrative of researching belonging and identity in English rural communities. *Journal of Rural Studies, 22*(2), 177–89.

Neuman, W.L. (2003). Social research methods: Qualitative and quantitative approaches. Boston: Allyn and Bacon.

Palmer, B.D. (1992). *Working-class experience: Rethinking the history of Canadian labour, 1800-1991* (2nd ed.). Toronto: McClelland & Stewart.

Penzhorn, C. (2002). The use of participatory research as an alternative approach for information needs research. *Aslib Proceedings, 54*(5), 240– 50.

Perkins, D., Florin, P., Rich, R.C., Wandersman, A., & Chavis, D.M. (1990). Participation and the social and physical environment of residential blocks: Crime and community context. *American Journal of Community Psychology, 18*, 83–113.

Rural Communities Impacting Policy Project. (2003). *Painting the landscape of rural Nova Scotia*. Halifax/Pictou, NS: Atlantic Health Promotion Research Centre/Coastal Communities Network.

Samson, D. (Ed.). (1994). *Contested countryside: Rural workers and modern society in Atlantic Canada, 1800-1950*. Fredericton: Acadiensis.

Sandwell, R.W. (1994). Rural reconstruction: Towards a new synthesis in Canadian history. *Histoire Sociale/Social History, 27*, 1–32.

Sandwell, R.W. (1998). *Beyond the city limits: Rural history in British Columbia*. Vancouver: University of British Columbia Press.

Stanley, D. (1993). The 1960s: The illusions and realities of progress. In E.R. Forbes & D.A. Muise (Eds.), *The Atlantic Provinces in Confederation* (p. 421). Toronto/Fredericton: University of Toronto/Acadiensis Press.

Statistics Canada. (1871). *Census of 1871*. Statistics Canada fonds (RG31-C-1, microfilm reels C9888 – C10570). Ottawa: Library and Archives Canada.

Statistics Canada. (1881). *Census of Canada, 1881*. Statistics Canada fonds (RG31-C-1, microfilm reels C13162 – C13286). Ottawa: Library and Archives Canada.

Statistics Canada. (1891). *Census of Canada, 1891*. Statistics Canada fonds (RG31-C-1, microfilm reels T6290 – T6427). Ottawa: Library and Archives Canada.

Statistics Canada. (2001). *Census of Canada: Census of population, census of agriculture*. Ottawa: Statistics Canada. Retrieved from http://www12.statcan.ca/english/census01/home/Index.cfm.

'Stevens,' Historical source used. Citation details not given here in order to maintain anonymity of community.

Stiles, D., Rangel, C., MacLaughlin, J., Sanderson, L., & MacNeil, K. (2007). Rurality, gender, and leisure: Experiences of young rural women in a Nova Scotia community. *Journal of Rural Community Psychology, E10*(2). Retrieved from http://www.marshall.edu/jrcp/V10%20N2/stiles.pdf.

Stiles, D.K. (1997). *Contexts and identities: Martin Butler, masculinity, class, and rural identity, the Maine–New Brunswick borderlands, 1857-1915.* Doctoral diss, University of Maine.

Stiles, D.K. (1998). Martin Butler, masculinity, and the North American sole leather tanning industry: 1871–1889. *Labour/Le Travail, 42*(Fall), 85–114.

Stiles, D.K. (2003). Rural women, underdevelopment, health knowledge, and modernity: Women and family farms as part of a broader context of change. In A.S.I. Persuric (Ed.), *Perspektive žena u obiteljskoj poljoprivredi i ruralnom razvoju / Women perspectives in family farming* (pp. 130–5). Porec, Croatia: Institute for Agriculture and Tourism.

Stiles, D.K. & Cameron, G. (2009). Changing paradigms? Rural communities, agriculture, and corporate and civic models of development in Atlantic Canada. *Journal of Enterprising Communities: People and Places in the Global Economy, 3*(4), 341–54.

Thomlinson, E., McDonagh, M.K., Crooks, K.B., & Lees, M. (2004). Health beliefs of rural Canadians: Implications for practice. *Australian Journal of Rural Health, 12*(6), 258–63.

Thornton, P. (1985). The problem of outmigration from Atlantic Canada, 1871–1921: A new look. *Acadiensis, 15*(1), 3–34.

Thurston, W.E., MacKean, G., Vollman, A., Casebeer, A., Weber, M., Maloff, B., & Bader, J. (2005). Public participation in regional health policy: A theoretical framework. *Health Policy, 73*(3), 237–52.

Thurston, W.E., Vollman, A.R., Meadows, L.M., & Rutherford, E. (2005). Public participation for women's health: Strange bedfellows or partners in a cause? *Health Care for Women International, 26*(5), 398–421.

Trenberth, L. (2005). The role, nature, and purpose of leisure and its contribution to individual development and well-being. *British Journal of Guidance and Counselling, 33*(1), 1–6.

Warner-Smith, P., & Brown, P. (2002). 'The town dictates what I do': The leisure, health and well-being of women in a small Australian country town. *Leisure Studies, 21*, 39–56.

Weinert, C., & Burman, M.E. (1994). Rural health and health-seeking behaviors. *Annual Review of Nursing Research, 12*, 65–92.

PART FIVE

Theorizing Rurality and Gender

Belinda Leach

In this section the contributors explore innovative theoretical directions for understanding relationships among health, space, and gender. The chapters thus provide a way of thinking about where research into gender, rurality, and health may go in the future, providing some new theoretical foundations for future research. The first two chapters of this section introduce a comparative dimension as well as employing new theoretical framings. Jo Little examines the trend towards locating alternative therapeutic services in rural settings, raising new questions about the relationships among health needs, service provision, and constructions of particular kinds of space. She argues that new therapeutic landscapes – in her study, rural spas – construct understandings of rurality that connect it with both nature and nurturing. However, as she shows, this also tends to incorporate fairly rigid ideas about the healthy and fit gendered rural body that serve to discipline those seeking services, while at the same time running the risk of misrepresenting the actual health status of actual rural bodies. Barbara Pini and Karen Soldatic investigate how differently valued identities – healthy or chronically ill, rural or urban – mark people as belonging in particular spaces. They argue that at the same time that health-related identities, such as 'disabled,' are performed in certain contexts in order to facilitate eligibility for benefits, in other contexts, such as the home, they may be rejected by the same person. While exploring new ways of thinking about rural women's health theoretically, Pini and Soldatic insist on reminding us that no matter how we frame our research theoretically, what is happening to women and men and to their health in rural communities continues to be affected by neoliberal ideas and practices that have profound consequences for funding of health care delivery and for addressing the problems associated with neoliberal economic restructuring – in rural and in urban spaces.

Jo-Anne Fiske and her colleagues advocate for a feminist notion of citizenship that, in contrast to liberal conceptions, highlights practices of social connectivity. In this construction, emotion, interdependence, association, and shared responsibilities are foregrounded, and citizenship then derives from collective engagements, making care a social and political issue and care giving an arena for the performance of citizenship. These authors argue that care giving is ultimately 'the essential democratic act' because it fosters and facilitates interdependency and collective action across public and private spheres. In the final chapter Deborah Thien proposes that rural health research needs to take seriously the significance of emotions to understandings of gender, health, and rurality. She asks, for example, how emotional geographies shape ideas and practices of health in rural settings, what kinds of emotional labour are involved in addressing rural health issues, and how further attention to these issues might contribute to innovative methods for research as well as to recommendations for practice and service delivery.

19 Healthy Rural Bodies?
Embodied Approaches to the Study
of Rural Women's Health

Jo Little

Research on rural women's health in developed countries has to date tended to focus either on the prevalence of particular medical conditions or on the availability and quality of health-related services (Brown, Young, & Byles, 1999; Leipert & Reutter, 2005). Such work has helped to make explicit the spatialization of health and well-being in terms of both illness and treatment and at the same time highlighted the challenges facing service providers and policy makers in meeting the needs of those living in remote areas. For example, it has been important in establishing the vulnerability of rural women to particular medical conditions and showing that certain kinds of illnesses, such as those relating to stress and anxiety, may take a different form in rural than in urban areas. It has also outlined the different experiences of rural women in terms of the kinds of treatment preferred and selected. Investigations of the intersections between health needs and service provision have also started to look beyond conventional approaches to health care in the examination of alternative therapies and community-based action.

Increasingly, research on rural women's health has recognized the broader social and cultural contexts within which health needs, provision, and policy are situated. It has noted the influence of rural social and community relations on the responses to (and sometimes even the causes of) health problems – in particular the limited access to health services available to marginalized groups living in rural areas (see Panelli, Gallagher, & Kearns, 2006). Studies have also shown how cultural constructions of rurality and identity can shape the experience and recognition of illness and the wider sense of well-being amongst rural people. For example studies of mental illness and stress have shown how the construction of 'country folk' as stoical and able to 'soldier on' has influenced both patients' and health providers' willingness to recognize mental conditions among rural residents (see Leipert & George, 2008).

This chapter, in common with others in this volume (specifically chapter 20 by Pini and chapter 22 by Thein), argues that these links with rural cultures and identities are critical to the wider study of rural women's health. Specifically we need to know more about how aspects of rurality, including rural nature, relate to notions of health and about how the relationship between rurality and health is embodied. In developing this understanding, the chapter draws on the idea of therapeutic landscapes and their role in practices of therapy and healing. It argues that therapeutic landscapes incorporate particular constructions of rurality as natural and nurturing that are important in the creation of feelings of health and well-being. In so doing, however, they also serve to discipline the body and the mind into complying with culturally accepted expectations around fitness and appearance. Like Thein, I see emotions as central to the experience of well-being and health. Using the example of the contemporary spa, the chapter examines rurality and nature in the context of embodied therapeutic practices and illustrates how place is intimately tied to ideas about the fit and healthy body. By focusing on the spa, the chapter also shows the importance of everyday spaces and routine leisure activities to the notion of therapeutic landscapes and to disciplining the unruly body in becoming healthy.

The chapter begins by considering directions from the literature that have informed the current study. These directions centre on therapeutic landscapes, well-being, and the body and are drawn mainly from work in geography that has sought to foreground the relationship between health and place. While the ideas and debates discussed here identify a range of theoretical concerns that have underpinned writing on landscape, health, and the body, they are not intended to be comprehensive, but rather are used simply to highlight ideas that have started to influence thinking in this area and hence are useful in developing and extending work on rural women's health. After discussing this background material, the chapter will move on to explore the spa as an example of a therapeutic landscape in which the relationship between rurality, nature, and women's health is played out. The original empirical material on which I draw here is from research undertaken in the UK. The details of the spa experiences I discuss may be far removed geographically from rural Canada. However, the theoretical issues that the research raises and the contribution the study makes to the understanding of wellness and the wider gendered experience of health in rural areas are central to the concerns of this book as a whole and to many of the individual chapters.

Therapeutic Landscapes, Well-Being, and the Rural Body

The study of therapeutic landscapes is now established in the geographical literature, and the concept has been widely researched by those interested in the ways in which space and place become implicated in ideas of health, healing, and well-being. According to Gesler (1996), a therapeutic landscape is defined as one where the 'physical and built environments, social conditions and human perceptions combine to produce an atmosphere that is conducive to healing' (p. 96). Thus particular landscapes and environments are believed to promote health and well-being through a combination of certain valued characteristics (Wakefield & McMullan, 2005). A range of studies has now explored the therapeutic qualities offered by sites and landscapes associated with nature, including water, forests, mountains, and wilderness (see Eyles & Williams, 2008). Recently within this literature the study of certain landscapes as intrinsically healthy has given way to attempts to understand the relational dimension of the self–landscape encounter in which there is a more holistic consideration of health and well-being in people's association with place (Conradson, 2005). Such ideas have extended work on therapeutic landscapes to incorporate greater emphasis on the relationship between health care spaces and identity and on the social construction of illness in the context of different sites and spaces (Kearns & Gesler, 1998).

While initial studies of therapeutic landscapes tended to focus on 'exceptional places,' that is, well-known and iconographic places of pilgrimage, spirituality, and therapy (holy places, spa resorts, and hospitals), there has been a growing tendency to consider the more mundane spaces of well-being (see Wakefield & McMullan, 2005) and to explore the more everyday practices and routines associated with health, therapy, and relaxation (Milligan, 2007; Smith, 2003). This development in the study of therapeutic spaces provides a very useful context for research on contemporary spas as spaces of well-being. In addition, while recent research on therapeutic landscapes has focused on the idea of retreat and on more lengthy periods of escape (see Lea's [2008] work on yoga and massage retreats in southern Spain), this chapter is interested in the recuperative value attached to short spa visits, taken not as a holiday but as 'time out' during the normal working week and everyday life, and in the ways in which this form of recuperation is reflected in the feelings of spa visitors.

The study of the spa as a therapeutic landscape has tended to take a historical approach and to focus on the medicalized properties of the spa waters and on the links between purity and healing (Cayleff, 1988; Gesler, 1998). There has also been some work documenting the social relations that developed in spas (particularly those that developed into 'spa towns'), including an examination of gender relations surrounding spa visits and the use of bathing waters. This chapter is also concerned with the spa as a gendered space but seeks to examine in much more detail how the embodied practices taking place incorporate a notion of health that disciplines the body to conform to dominant notions of masculinity and femininity. In so doing, this work extends ideas on health and the healthy body to thinking about how wellness depends on particular constructions of the fit gendered body. It also draws on ideas of social exclusion in showing how the practices within spas create spaces from which certain bodies that do not conform to the dominant ideas of health and fitness may feel excluded.

There is now a substantial literature exploring the relationship between the more traditional cultural and social constructions of masculinity and femininity existing in rural occupations and communities and the representation and performance of the rural body. Brandth (1995) and Liepins (2000) have shown, for example, the representations of traditional and hegemonic masculinity common in agriculture, while Little (2003) has looked at the ways in which expectations amongst heterosexual couples living in rural communities about the 'suitability' of particular partners as wives or husbands rest on conventional constructions of the male and female body. In this work and in other research on the body in relation to rural leisure and recreation (see Little and Leyshon, 2003), it has been argued that certain bodies are seen as acceptable or 'in place' in the countryside. In the case of agriculture, for example, the 'right' body of the farmer is masculine, fit, and strong and that of the farmer's wife is practical and down to earth. Moreover, physical appearance is shown in such work to embody social/personal characteristics and aspects of identity – the fit healthy farmer's body denoting reliability and strength of will and the less fashionable and 'homely' body of the farmer's wife suggesting tolerance and stability (Little, 2007).

Some rural studies have made specific links between the rural body, health, and fitness, also drawing on the idea of the suitable or appropriate rural body. Edensor (2000), for example, has looked at the early development of the Ramblers Association in the UK and of the rise in walking and hiking as forms of exercise and leisure. He identifies the strong links between health, the body, and the countryside in the emergence of countryside rambling but also notes the ways in which the social and cultural construction of the appropriate rambler's body as one that is fit, healthy, and competent within nature serves to exclude some people from the sport. Bodies that could not cope with either the physical exercise or the demands of remote rural terrain were considered 'out of place' in rural areas. He also notes the presence of a set of moral assumptions concerning exercise and the outdoors that influence the way the rural body is understood and valued.

The growth of work on performance and the body has been increasingly apparent in research on people's experience of and interaction with the landscape. Studies by geographers (see Wylie, 2002) have started to explore the body's affective relationship with the landscape through the performance of walking and moving through the countryside. Such work has begun to consider the more spiritual association between bodies and the landscape and, in so doing, recognized the emotional connections with rurality that are seen as important to the body's well-being. Studies of pilgrimage, for example, have made important links between the embodied performance of walking and being in the landscape, emotion, and well-being, and in so doing reconnected with the literature on therapeutic landscapes (Rose, 2006). In exploring these connections studies have also engaged, both theoretically and empirically, with notions of discipline and regulation. Drawing on ideas by Foucault in particular, researchers have looked at social practices around the control of the unruly body. These, it is suggested, are 'part and parcel of a more general process of surveillance and control in modernity' (Holliday & Thompson, 2001, p. 117) that operates in different ways in different places. These ideas are highly relevant to the examination of the spa in terms both of broad understandings of the body, identity, and control and of the conceptualization of the micro-geographies of the spa as spaces of regulation and discipline.

Finally, it is important to recognize here the potential of work on nature for studies of the rural body. Nature has been alluded to above in discussions of the concept of the therapeutic landscape and has also been shown as relevant to the relationship between representations of the body and the rural landscape. This chapter engages with work on nature in two ways: first, in terms of the qualities of the rural environment and the natural healing properties of the countryside and the therapies that are used in the spa; and second, in relation to the body and the notion of the healthy and fit body as a natural body. Again, the chapter can do no more than acknowledge the rich theoretical debates that have recently explored what is meant by 'nature' – debates that have challenged the dialectical thinking that saw nature as some sort of undisputed, simple reality and shown it rather as complex, socially constructed, and relational (Hinchliffe, 2007). Debates about the meaning of 'nature' have considered not only environments, ecologies, landscapes, and animals, but have also increasingly discussed the concept in relation to the human body as developments in medical science, particularly cosmetic surgery, make questions about the boundaries between the natural and the technological body more and more relevant (Haraway, 1997). The ability to intervene in the appearance and shape of the body clearly has huge implications for emotional as well as physical health. Such ideas are important here in framing the links between well-being and the embodied practices of the spa, particularly those that appear to take a somewhat contradictory line between celebrating the natural body through recourse to technology.

The next section turns to a discussion of the spa and its use and, in so doing, starts to position the study of the spa more centrally in these discussions of the therapeutic landscapes, gender, the body, and nature. It provides the framework for the subsequent discussion of the practices of the spa, showing how an understanding of rural women's health needs to be situated within a broader investigation of a range of embodied practices that sit on the boundaries of leisure and wellness.

The Spa as a Therapeutic Landscape

Recent years have seen a phenomenal expansion in the provision and use of spas in the UK and other Western economies (Mak, Wong, & Chang, 2009). While the enjoyment of spas for therapeutic purposes has a relatively long history, as discussed by some of the earlier therapeutic landscape literature noted above (for example, Gesler, 1993, 1998; Williams, 1999), that use has shifted significantly over time. As the purpose of the spa has changed, so too has its clientele. In the early nineteenth century there was a shift away from the spa as a highly medicalized space to one associated with relaxation and leisure and with a much broader notion of well-being. With this shift came a change in the spa clientele from a wealthy elite to more general appeal. Practices also changed to become much more inclusive and focused on social interaction rather than on individual treatment. With this shift to embrace a wider range of visitors, however, came a decline in general popularity. Later, spas emerged again as spaces of recovery and rejuvenation. They became associated with a more specialist recovery from accidental or self-inflicted abuses of the body in which the 'patient' was hidden from society as part of the healing process. Again, the clientele tended to be the wealthy and elite, celebrities retreating from the stresses of media attention.

The contemporary spa is, however, different again. While some 'old style,' stand-alone spas still exist (famously, the Roman Baths at Bath), many are now part of a bigger leisure complex, attached as an extra facility to hotels, holiday cottages, or fitness centres, and incorporate places to stay and eat. Indeed, the provision of a spa facility is becoming almost a required attribute for larger, upmarket hotels. Evidence of the more widespread provision of spas appears regularly in the pages of magazines and holiday advertizing and leisure guides. Spas may still retain the image of health, recovery, and wellness but are clearly now spaces for a wider type of use and consumption. A major element of the 'spa concept' is the provision of health and, importantly, beauty. The particular emphasis of each spa will vary – some remaining largely hideaways associated with ill health and recuperation, while others emphasize fitness and activity, and still others focus on beauty treatments, relaxation, and pampering. This holistic sense of feeling good involves, as discussed below, the combination of therapies that relax, pamper, but also discipline the gendered body. Spas do this in different ways but all emphasize the holistic and emotional relationship between a fit body and a relaxed mind.

The data used in the second part of the chapter are drawn from research on spas and spa clients in the UK.[1] This research incorporates material from in-depth interviews conducted in two spas in southern England, together with questionnaire data. Both spas were part of bigger leisure or holiday complexes. The larger, the Gloucestershire spa, was part of a business involving a hotel, restaurants, and a bar/pub, while the Devon spa was simply an addition to a small group of holiday cottages. Both spas were expanding businesses, and both were clearly (although slightly unexpectedly) taking advantage of an expansion and diversification in demand.

The interviews were with the spa manager in the case of the Gloucestershire spa and the spa owners/managers (a husband and wife) in the case of the Devon spa. These were semi-structured interviews lasting one and a half to two hours. The interviews provided rich, qualitative data on the spas, probing their particular characteristics and allowing discussion of the views and opinions of the managers/owners, which was particularly important in understanding the ways clients responded to spas as spaces of well-being and as spaces of bodily regulation and discipline.

More basic quantitative data on spa use and the kinds of treatments and therapeutic experiences they offered were gained from the questionnaire. The self-completed questionnaire was distributed to all guests at one spa on two days and was returned by the guests by prepaid envelope. In all just over 50% of distributed questionnaires were returned completed ($n = 50$). The spa where the questionnaire was distributed vetted and approved the questions but played no part in its design or the subsequent analysis of the data. The questionnaire was useful in building up a picture of the nature of the spa's clientele and how the spa was used.

In terms of the relationship between gender and health, one of the most obvious things the spa reveals is the growing importance of relaxation as part of the regular leisure and health routines of women. The two spas visited as part of this research both reported high and growing demand. The Gloucestershire spa operated a membership system and at the time of the research was full, with a membership of 500 and a waiting list of 570 people. The Devon spa had no formal membership but claimed to have many repeat clients and a healthy booking schedule.[2] It was also clear that, of those spa visitors responding to the survey, there was considerable unexploited demand, with 78% of respondents saying they would like to come to the spa more frequently than they currently did. In addition, when asked how important the spa was to them, nearly 40% said it was a high priority and a further 41% said it was a medium priority. Thus less than 20% of spa users saw their visits as representing a low priority in the context of their daily lives and other responsibilities.

While advertising promotes the spa as a space for both men and women (and for families in the case of a minority of spas), the vast proportion of visitors are women – visiting alone or in groups. Ninety-two per cent of completed questionnaires were from women. This is very much a pattern repeated elsewhere; for example, a survey of spas in the United States concluded that 71% of all spa goers in 2003 were women

(McNeil & Ragins, 2005). Visits to the spa by men are generally in support of partners or with a group of friends. The spa itself reflects this gendered usage with a strong bias towards women clients in both the treatments and the spaces of the spa. In addition, women were encouraged to 'hang out' in the spas, frequently spending several hours at the spa in any one visit. Spaces of the spas were promoted as softer feminine spaces through decor, soft furnishings, and touches such as the kinds of magazines and other literature available to guests. Observation in both spas confirmed lounges and bars to be populated by women relaxing in towelling robes while gyms had men in sports gear using exercise machines and weights, thus conforming to rather traditional assumptions regarding gender identity.

Although, as noted above, spas are no longer seen as exclusive, they retain a sense of luxury; indeed their role rests very much on this idea of a treat, even despite the centrality they have gained in the leisure practices of some. While spa visits and membership are expensive, the visitors questioned were not all in high paying jobs (although over 70% were in employment). Amongst the occupations listed by visitors were professional jobs such as IT management consultants, teachers, doctors , and business managers, but there were also non-professional jobs such as hairdressers and cleaners listed. The spa owners in Devon were very conscious of the broad appeal of the spa and noted the diverse range of visitors they received as follows:

> We are not for the mega rich – we have just ordinary people most of the time who want a treat. We have been very surprised by the obvious income level of people who are coming. You're getting people who are earning £6.00, £6.50 an hour and they'll be coming and spending £100, possibly £150 for a day.

Clearly, the price of spa membership puts this out of reach of some people in rural areas. However, what was apparent from the research was the priority attached to spa visits by even those on modest incomes and the sense in which the idea of indulgence was a well-being practice that needed to be protected, as the following section discusses.

Health and the Embodied Practices of the Spa

Clearly, key to the growing importance of the spa as a therapeutic landscape are the health and leisure practices that it supports and advocates. In particular, the spa emphasizes the value of relaxation and 'pampering' as a part of fitness and leisure routines. The notion of fitness as holistic recognizes mental and physical relaxation as contributing to broader feelings of well-being and suggests that exercise needs to be accompanied by rest and 'time out' from busy lives and routines. For women especially, the value of relaxation is seen to be enhanced by the idea that it is a treat or luxury that allows them to focus on their own needs and legitimizes rest as part of a broader fitness regime. As explained by the Devon spa owner:

> There is no question, it [the spa] does relax. From simple things like taking people out of their everyday lives and putting them in an environment where we don't have mobile phones – cups of tea and coffee are brought to you and somebody is running around looking after you. Just that alone is a lovely thing to have … We call it guilt-free relaxation.

The spa, then, was seen as allowing legitimate indulgence in the self, away from daily responsibilities. Crucially, this was believed to have important health and therapeutic implications. According to the spa managers, the emotional release gained from relaxation at the spa was important not only in its own right but as part of overall well-being and physical fitness. As one Devon spa manager said:

> I'd love to get the doctors round here to start to realize the value of what it is we can provide for people … we have, quite regularly, people who are grieving brought along by friends and it's a very nurturing environment. We have examples of women who go through holistic relaxation therapy and they will be in floods of tears through the physical process that is taking place – releasing tension – better than a sedative any day.

The questionnaire revealed that the priorities of the spa clients, especially the women, centred on the relaxation and pampering practices of the spa, rather than on the fitness training and exercise classes provided. Eighty per cent of those questioned listed 'relaxation' as a reason they visited the spa, and more respondents cited 'pampering' than 'fitness' as a motivation for their visit.

The notion of pampering is important here in bringing together therapy, fitness, and relaxation. It suggests that the fit and healthy body is the relaxed body but that, in addition, relaxation is achieved through indulgence and spoiling. Thus pampering legitimates not only relaxation as a part of women's health regime but also luxury. Pampering stresses escape as essential to the maintenance of a 'balanced' life and suggests that luxury can help women to manage the mundane and stressful aspects of life. Such escape was seen as vital to women's emotional state, both in the immediate sense of the feelings associated with the treatments themselves (the luxurious oils, bath robes, and supplies of drinks on demand created, according to those interviewed, calmness, enjoyment, and pleasure) and in the longer term feelings of well-being and happiness that the treatment generated (such a mix of emotional responses has been noted in holistic therapies such as meditation and yoga [see Smith, 2007]). Also central to the idea of pampering was the sense of reward that it incorporated. For many women a 'pamper day' was something that had been earned; frequently it was a gift given by a grateful partner or friend or in celebration of achievement. Indeed, 40% of women responding to the questionnaire had received a pamper day as a gift.

While pampering is based on indulgence, it does not imply an unruly body and is still very much shaped by conventional gendered expectations surrounding body shape and size. This is elaborated upon in the following discussion of the disciplining of the body in the spa. First, however, the chapter looks more directly at the issue of rurality in the relationship between the spa and nature.

Nature and the Spa

This section examines two key aspects of the importance of nature, both as a setting and as a part of spa treatments and therapies, in relation to the spa as a therapeutic landscape. Links are made between nature and the healthy body, but attention is also drawn to the sometimes contradictory use of 'the natural' in the therapies used to encourage a particular form of fit body.

Although the term 'spa' is applied to a range of different fitness and relaxation venues (some attached to conventional hotels or health clubs), stand-alone spas tend to be located either in towns historically associated with spas (for example, Bath or Harrogate) or in rural settings. For such spas, the natural environment is incorporated into the experience, adding to the sense of escape and providing a therapeutic and relaxing environment, and even, at times, a space for particular kinds of treatment. As noted above, nature has for centuries held a central role in the relationship between place, health, and the body not only in terms of the physical benefits of exercise but also in attending to moral, spiritual, and personal development. For example, when discussing the emerging practice of naturism in the early twentieth century, Morris (2009) notes how time in conjunction with nature was believed to encourage individuals to become attuned to their 'instinctive bodily rhythms' and, in doing so, become better equipped to contribute to society (p. 288).

The perceived benefits of close contact with nature were evident both in the interviews with spa managers and in their wider advertising. The setting of the Devon spa was particularly spectacular, and this was drawn on as underpinning the spa's philosophy and explaining its success:

> The setting is fabulous, especially for the pamper breaks. They are invariably inland people coming to the coast. We wish to provide an environment that is relaxing, re-energizing. It's a nurturing environment and it allows you to escape.

Guests staying overnight at the spa accommodation were encouraged to take walks along the cliff top and to enjoy the environment as part of the overall experience. At the Gloucestershire spa, set in farmland, the environment had been incorporated more formally into spa activities with tracks and paths laid out for guests to walk and run and with yoga classes held in the spa garden.

The sense in which nature contributes to the nurturing capacities of the spa is clear in discussions of the actual treatments that take place. In some spas this use of nature is explicit and underpins the holistic philosophy of the spa practices. For example:

> The whole thing about holistic therapy is it's very primitive, very basic. You're dealing with an animal (a human being). The body responds to certain things. It responds to heat, it responds to cold … it responds to the application of pressure, it responds to touch. All our therapies do is utilize those very basic physical responses to produce a sense of well-being, a sense of relaxation. (Devon spa)

As well as encouraging the 'natural' reactions of the body, treatments make use of so-called natural products, and attempts are made to distance the spa practices from the more invasive treatments available at, for example, beauty salons. However, despite the championing of natural therapies, the spas do present something of a contradiction in the bodies that they seek to encourage and facilitate. Desirable natural bodies were seen as those that conform to conventional expectations about size and shape, and, as stressed above in discussion of pampering and relaxation, the healthy body was not a body out of control or undisciplined. Thus, the spa may emphasize holistic natural therapies but in neither the Gloucestershire nor the Devon spas were such therapies seen as out of place alongside conventional beauty treatments. Indeed, both spas offered a range of what would be seen as regular cosmetic treatments, including leg waxing, facials, manicures, and the like. While neither spa offered cosmetic surgery, both were committed to the idea that feeling good also involved looking good and that natural therapy was not necessarily a replacement for other beauty treatments and even surgery, as this might be an important part of clients' sense of well-being.

The next section develops some of these ideas concerning the disciplined spa body, showing how the spa's focus on health emphasizes a particular kind of body both in the way the spa is used and also in the treatments it provides to promote well-being.

The Disciplined Body and the Spa

While the spa is constructed and represented as a place where people can relax and where they are not required to take part in highly prescribed exercise regimes, it is nevertheless a place where the body is regulated and required to conform to certain expectations. This was clear in the way the visited spas were managed. Although the atmosphere in both was relaxed and informal, the micro-geographies of the spas were firmly controlled. Behaviour and clothing in the different areas of the spas were prescribed by explicit and implicit rules. The manager of the Gloucestershire spa saw one of her greatest challenges as balancing the needs of the different spa users and, in particular, protecting the spa as a calm, relaxed, and peaceful environment at times of high demand. The increasing popularity of the spa, especially for women's and birthday parties, presented a particular problem since typically such events encourage bodies to become unruly and threaten the well-being of other spa guests. She summed up by saying:

When my ladies are sitting round in towelling robes they don't want a bloke to walk in and start exercising. You need to separate the spa facilities from the drop-in facilities, otherwise you change the ambience ... I have evicted one member who behaved inappropriately. I told a further two that if they step over the line one more time they'll be gone.

As noted above, there were expectations about the appearance of the fit and healthy body, particularly in relation to women's bodies. There was a clear understanding that the spa body was on display (despite the provision of towelling robes for the clients). Advice on using the spa even suggested that women undertake certain cosmetic treatments (such as leg waxing) *before* going to a spa so that they felt more at ease. Thus the spa was seen as a place where the body could be pampered and treated but not at the expense of appearance. Amongst those responding to the questionnaire, only 10% had *not* used the beauty treatments available at the spa. Moreover, the Gloucestershire spa claimed that the beauty treatments (especially facials and manicures) they provided contributed the highest part of the spa's turnover and were constantly in demand – no longer, it appeared, the preserve of young, fashionable, urban women. Such treatments were seen very much as a regular part of *all* women's routine well-being provision. The Devon spa had recently expanded its range of treatments to respond to the needs of those clients, 'typically career women getting away on holiday,' who 'normally had them elsewhere but had not had time' before coming away.

At both spas the managers were at pains to distance their particular beauty therapies from the 'average' cosmetic treatments, claiming their natural healing philosophies ensured higher quality and efficacy. While the methods of acquiring a particular body may have been seen as more holistic, the body that they sought to achieve was nevertheless conventional. The Gloucestershire spa had recently introduced a treatment, CACI, which seems at odds with the 'natural' philosophy claimed. According to their literature, the CACI is a 'computer aided cosmetology instrument' that uses a micro-current that tones, lifts, and re-educates the muscles. CACI body treatments supposedly 'deal with stubborn areas that exercise has not reached' in an attempt to regulate the unruly body.

The combination of indulgence and discipline was also evident in the provision of food and drink in the spa and the advice given about nutrition. Emphasis was placed on the use of local, organic, and 'healthy' food at the spas and on high-quality presentation. Again, the contradiction between spoiling and health seemed to pervade the provision of food, with, however, the healthy, nutritious meals being supplemented with champagne and cream teas for those on a pamper day. As with the broader pampering philosophy discussed above, such luxury was central to the sense of well-being associated with spa visits.

Conclusion

This chapter has argued that the therapeutic landscape concept offers important insights into ways of thinking about rural women's health. It challenges us to look beyond the issues of illness and service provision that have been central to traditional medical geographies of rural areas in exploring the broader relationships between place, health, and the body. It also extends the study of health to incorporate wider notions of well-being and fitness and the embodied practices through which they are pursued. The therapeutic landscape idea helps us to think about health and place as relational and as shaped by the construction and performance of gender and the body.

The chapter has developed the idea of therapeutic landscapes through a study of the spa. In so doing, it has focused on the growing importance of a holistic sense of well-being to women's health in particular. Relaxation and pampering are now central to women's broader health and fitness regimes and have become, for many, a regular part of their leisure time. They also serve to increase women's emotional well-being and to privilege emotions as crucial to women's health. As this chapter has demonstrated, however, the therapeutic practices used to relax and pamper the body are also a form of regulation. The spa encourages women's well-being but requires that their bodies continue to conform to expected (and highly gendered) norms of size and appearance (see Petersen, 2007). The body is made docile through notions of reward and luxury, and only the disciplined body can access the well-being that the spa provides.

The chapter has argued that the spa has a growing popular appeal, especially amongst women. While pampering practices have in the past been more associated with the wealthy and with an urban construction of femininity, the broadening of appeal to include a wider range of women on lower incomes has been an important part of the recent growth of the spa. Such women may not be able to afford regular spa visits, and so the notion of the spa as a treat holds even more appeal. Moreover, the spa is no longer the preserve offashionable youth but has extended its appeal to older women, and while disciplinary practices still valorize a slim and attractive body, the centrality of indulgence and pampering to contemporary notions of wellness has again ensured the spa's wider appeal.

Finally the chapter has shown the importance of nature in the development of the spa therapies. While not exclusively rural, the spa draws on the rural environment and on nature in situating therapeutic and disciplinary practices. The natural environment is celebrated as enhancing fitness and well-being and, in particular, aiding relaxation and escape. Natural therapies are valorized, similarly, as helping to promote well-being in the holistic treatment of the body and the emotions. The use of nature in this way, however, is not without contradiction since the body that is produced through such natural therapies must still conform to conventional expectations. The boundaries of nature are disrupted and challenged through cosmetic treatments that prescribe the shape and appearance of the healthy spa body.

Notes

1 The research was subject to the ethical guidelines of the School of Geography at the University of Exeter, UK.
2 The research took place shortly before the 'credit crunch' and recession hit the UK economy. This may have made a difference to the popularity of the spas, although both businesses still exist at the time of writing.

References

Brandth, B. (1995). Rural masculinity in transition: Gender images in tractor advertisements. *Journal of Rural Studies, 11*, 123–33.

Brown, W., Young, A., & Byles, J. (1999). Tyranny of distance? The health of mid-age women living in five geographical areas of Australia. *Australian Journal of Rural Health, 7*, 148–54.

Cayleff, S. (1988). Gender, ideology and the water-cure movement. In N. Gevitz, (Ed.), *Other healers: Unorthodox medicine in America* (pp. 82–98). Baltimore: Johns Hopkins University Press.

Conradson, D. (2005). Landscape, care and the relational self: Therapeutic encounters in rural England. *Health and Place, 11*, 337–48.

Edensor, T. (2000). Walking in the British countryside: Reflexivity, embodied practices and ways to escape. *Body and Society, 6*(3–4), 81–106.

Eyles, J., & Williams, A. (Eds.). (2008). *Sense of health, place and quality of life.* Burlington, VT: Ashgate.

Gesler, W. (1993). Therapeutic landscapes: Theory and a case study of Epidauros. *Environment and Planning D: Society and Space, 11,* 171–89.

Gesler, W. (1996). Lourdes: Healing in a place of pilgrimage. *Health and Place, 2,* 95–101.

Gesler, W. (1998). Bath's reputation as a healing place. In R. Kearnes & W. Gesler, (Eds.), *Putting health into place: Landscape, identity and well being* (pp. 17–35). Syracuse, NY: Syracuse University Press.

Haraway, D. (1997). *Modest_Witness@Second_Millennium. FemaleMan_Meets_ OncoMouse: Feminism and technoscience.* New York: Routledge.

Hinchliffe, S. (2007). *Geographies of nature: Societies, environments, ecologies.* London: Sage.

Holliday, R., & Thompson, G. (2001). A body of work. In R. Holliday & J. Hassard (Eds.), *Contested bodies* (pp. 117–34). London: Routledge.

Kearns, R., & Gelser, W. (1998). *Putting health into place: Landscape, identity and well-being.* Syracuse, NY: Syracuse University Press.

Lea, J. (2008). Retreating to nature: Rethinking 'therapeutic landscapes.' *AREA, 40*(1), 90–98.

Leipert, B., & George, J. (2008). Determinants of rural women's health: A qualitative study in southwest Ontario. *Journal of Rural Health, 24*(2), 210–18.

Leipert, B., & Reutter, L. (2005). Developing resilience: How women maintain their health in northern geographically isolated settings. *Qualitative Health Research, 15*(1), 49–65.

Liepins, R. (2000). Making men: The construction and representation of agriculture-based masculinities in Australia and New Zealand. *Rural Sociology, 65*(4), 605–20.

Little, J. (2003). 'Riding the rural love train': Heterosexuality and the rural community. *Sociologia Ruralis, 43,* 401–17.

Little, J. (2007). Constructing nature in the performance of heterosexuality. *Environment and Planning D: Society and Space, 7*(5), 851–66.

Little, J., & Leyshon, M. (2003). Embodied rural geographies: Developing research agendas. *Progress in Human Geography, 27*(3), 257–72.

Mak, A., Wong, K., and Chang, R. (2009). Health or self indulgence? The motivations and characteristics of spa-goers. *International Journal of Tourism Research, 11,* 185–99.

McNeil, K., & Ragins, E. (2005). Staying in the spa marketing game: Trends, challenges, strategies and techniques. *Journal of Vacation Marketing, 11,* 31–9.

Milligan, C. (2007). Exploring the place of the Common Place. In A. Williams (Ed.), *Therapeutic landscapes: Geographies of health* (pp. 255–72). Guildford, UK: Ashgate.

Morris, N. (2009). Naked in nature: Naturism, nature and the senses in early 20th century Britain. *Cultural Geographies, 16,* 283–308.

Panelli, R., Gallagher, L., & Kearns, R. (2006). Access to rural health services. *Social Science and Medicine, 62,* 1103–14.

Petersen, A. (2007). *The body in question: A socio-cultural approach.* London: Routledge.

Rose, M. (2006). Gathering dreams of presence: A project for the cultural landscape. *Environment and Planning D: Society and Space, 24*(4), 537–54.

Smith, M. (2003). Holistic holidays: Tourism and the reconciliation of body, mind, spirit. *Tourism Recreation Research, 28,* 103–8.

Smith, P. (2007). Body, mind and spirit? Towards an analysis of the practice of yoga. *Body and Society, 13*(2), 25–46.

Wakefield, S., & McMullan, C. (2005). Healing in places of decline: (Re) Imagining everyday landscapes in Hamilton, Ontario. *Health and Place, 11*(4), 299–312.

Williams, A. (Ed) (1999). *Therapeutic landscapes: The dynamic between place and wellness.* Lantham, MD: University Press of America.

Wylie, J. (2002). An essay on ascending Glastonbury Tor. *Geoforum, 33,* 441–54.

20 Women, Chronic Illness, and Rural Australia: Exploring the Intersections between Space, Identity, and the Body

Barbara Pini and Karen Soldatic

This chapter brings a rural dimension to the literature on women and chronic illness by drawing on the story of an Australian rural woman who has chronic fatigue syndrome, or myalgic encephalomyelitis (ME). Integral to this literature is Moss and Dyck's (2002) book-length exploration of the lives of forty-nine women who had been diagnosed with either ME or rheumatoid arthritis (RA), along with their other writings on the topic (e.g., Dyck, 1995a, 1995b; Moss 1997; Moss & Dyck, 1996, 1999a, 1999b, 2001). In framing the chapter around this collective scholarship we focus on three interrelated themes it has emphasized and examine these through the lens of rurality. These are the themes of space, identity, and the body.

Given that Moss and Dyck (2002) are geographers, it is not surprising to find that one of the most significant of the ideas that they have brought to the study of women and chronic illness is the concept of space, and the way in which spatial use and experience shift in relation to changes in health. They have found, for example, that chronic illness may lead women to relocate from their home or modify the home, while external spaces such as that of the neighbourhood become restricted to them. Also highlighted is the high likelihood that chronic illness leads to a shift in employment status, which then negatively affects one's engagement in social spaces. More recently, Crooks (2004) has added to this scholarship, detailing the way in which neoliberal policy reforms of recent years have significantly curtailed the capacity of chronically ill people to engage meaningfully in a range of public spaces such as leisure, work, and recreation. Further, as Joanne Fiske and colleagues demonstrate in chapter 21 of this book, the negative consequences of such reforms are potentially aggravated in a rural context.

In nominating spatiality as a critical dimension in the study of women and chronic illness, Moss and Dyck (2002) simultaneously emphasize the importance of identity and the complexity, multiplicity, and dynamism of identity. It is a point Moss (1999, p. 158) makes in an autobiographical piece about her own experience of ME. She obviously shares a great deal with her research participants who also have ME, but realizes that as she finds herself 'listing pages of adjectives' to describe herself there are also many other aspects of herself that render her different from those she interviews. These various identities mark people as belonging or not belonging in particular spaces. For example, the identity of the *healthy person* is highly valued in contemporary society and would be seen as legitimate in workspaces, whereas this is not the case for the identity labelled *chronically ill* (Crooks & Chouinard, 2006). In this sense, identities do not occur in the absence of power relations; they are policed by ourselves and by others. This is clear from Crooks, Chouinard, and Wilton's (2008) description of chronically ill women's negotiation of the identity *disabled*. The women explain that they perform such an identity for the state and medical authorities in order to access welfare, but also they resist such an identity with strategies such as redefining disability in extreme terms or claiming disability in some spaces and not others (e.g., the workplace but not the home).

For Moss and Dyck (1999a) the notions of space and identity are taken up as part of what they label a 'radical body politics' (p. 162). In this respect, the body, as materially and discursively constituted, is a third intersecting if not overarching element of their analytical edifice. The engagement of the terms 'radical' and 'politics' gestures towards their concern with interrogating the normative and the operation of power as they relate to embodiment. In affording such centrality to the body in their work, these feminist geographers distinguish themselves from those who in advocating a social model of disability assert that 'disability is wholly and exclusively social,...,disablement [that] has nothing to do with the body' (Oliver 1996, pp. 41–2). The conceptual distinction between the body and disability that is central to the social model thesis has been viewed as critical in challenging the traditionally dominant medical model and its conflation of disability with impairment. However, within the disability studies literature, feminist scholars have mounted a strong argument that the social model has been diminished by a refusal to recognize and theorize disability as embodied (e.g., Crow, 1996; Thomas, 1999). Such a case is evident, not only in the work of Moss and Dyck (2002), but also in a broad range of geographical writing on disability and gender that has focused on the 'retrieval of the body in disability studies' (Hansen & Philo, 2007, p. 495) and highlighted the interconnectedness of spatial locations, identity, and the body.

As Moss and Dyck (2002) explore the stories of chronically ill women through the framework of space, identity, and the body, their analysis remains embedded in the materiality of broader social, political, and economic relations. Dyck (1995a) explains, for example, that the capacity of women with ME to restructure space in light of their illness is circumscribed by their financial situation and/or level of support from family and friends. Similarly, Moss (1997) notes that the poverty experienced by an older woman with arthritis whom she interviews 'compounds her invisibility' (p. 30), for she lacks the resources to go out or entertain friends at home. In the following section, as we detail the story of a chronically ill woman living in rural Western Australia, examining aspects of space, identity, and the body, we retain a similar focus on the material. This means contextualizing her narrative by reference to an extended period of dramatic rural restructuring that has seen a significant withdrawal of government services, decreased employment opportunities, population decline, increased poverty, and heightened social problems in many rural areas of the country (Cheers, 2001; Gray & Lawrence, 2001; Hall & Scheltens, 2005; Tonts, 2005).

We first met Sharon[1] at a public forum convened by People with Disabilities Western Australia and Physical Disability Australia, two disability advocacy organizations, to discuss the public inquiry into the national restructuring of disability services (PWDWA, 2010). The public forum drew together a diverse range of participants, many of whom lived with disability and chronic illness. As Sharon detailed her situation to the forum, it became clear that her narrative provides key insight into the way in which chronic illness is shaped not just by gender but also by rurality. Interested in understanding Sharon's story further and in bringing it to a broader audience, we sought an interview and subsequently travelled to her home to talk further with her. The relatively unstructured narrative approach we utilized in conducting the interview sought to draw to the fore the subjective and lived experience of disability and chronic illness (Malacrida, 2009; Sakalys, 2000), and it is therefore this emphasis we privilege in the following recounting of Sharon's story.

Sharon's Story

Sharon is a forty-six-year-old woman living on acreage an hour north of Perth. The area has changed significantly in recent years as a result of urban encroachment along with the influx of those seeking a rural life-style close to the city centre. The land on which Sharon lives is part of what had been her family's working farm going back five generations. A relative continues to graze cattle on the land today, and it is also leased to a horticulture business. Sharon's mother lives on the property in a house beside Sharon and her four children, two of whom are in their late teens and the other two in primary school. Her husband works as a tradesman in a nearby community. While Sharon and her husband had lived in the city in the early years of their marriage, they returned to Sharon's family land to build a home as a result of the high cost of property and because of her attachment to the place.

Sharon recalls first noticing she was sick at eighteen, when she was diagnosed with glandular fever. This original illness meant she was un-able to work for three months in her job as a laboratory assistant. The illness lingered but Sharon returned to work after a doctor told her, 'It is all in your head. You just need to pull your socks up.' Her work role allowed her some autonomy, which she used to manage her sickness and maintain a pretence of 'good health.' For example, she remembers 'bad days' where she had to lie on a sick-bay bed or 'okay days' where she would still have to sit down but could continue with her work, and then some 'good days' where she busily attempted to catch up on tasks. Seeking to further banish the illness, Sharon not only continued em-ployment, but joined a gym and took up scuba diving in an effort, she said, to 'get physically back to where I was.' Over the next few years the rhetoric of self-admonishment was heightened considerably as Sharon became involved in a fundamentalist sect that preached that sickness was a result of weakness, and ultimately represented evil.

While Sharon's strategies to manage her illness may appear to be in-tense, as Johnson and Johnson (2006) suggest, women who have an am-biguous chronic illness are required to 'learn how to manage them [the illnesses] within a context of a health care system and social culture that are hostile to the legitimacy of their illness experience' (p. 159). From Sharon's narrative we learn that her early experience of her illness and the struggle to seek an official medical diagnosis were, in many in-stances, undermined by the medical professionals with whom she came into contact. Even though Sharon could clearly identify changes within her body, the first medical doctor suggested a probable medical diagno-sis but did not seek further investigation. With support from family members, Sharon sought a second opinion. However, this did not lead to an official acknowledgement of an enduring illness. Instead, the sec-ond medical professional Sharon consulted told her:

You have definitely had something in the past, but now I think it is all in your head. You just need to pull your socks up and make yourself go to work.

What Sharon experienced in this clinical encounter has been well documented in the feminist literature on chronically ill women, that is, doctors trivializing and de-legitimizing her own experience of her body as well as seeking to regulate and control her body by suggesting the illness is not 'real' (Moss and Dyck, 1999b, p. 378). In this respect Sharon's situation would have been magnified because of the rural context, as there are few alternatives in relation to health care. Her options for seeking out a medical professional who might have afforded her an opportunity to be heard were very limited because of her geographic isolation.

In 1984 and then in 1991 Sharon faced further periods of extended ill health and was unable to work. She was told by medical professionals that she had a post-viral illness. Eventually, when Sharon's youngest child was three years of age she became, as she tells us, 'acutely ill.' She had left the sect and was now under immense stress due to a traumatic family situation. When her health deteriorated she sought more medical help. This was seven years ago, however, and since this time Sharon has not been well enough to be in full-time employment. Indeed, she has had extended periods of up to two years where she has been 'severely ill.' During such a stage she says, 'I can't support myself or hold myself up. I can't formulate words. I'm really foggy. I can't make decisions or read letters.' She added:

Like I said for two years I spent a lot of time just lying under that tree, cause I was getting it ... most days as bad days. For that two years I couldn't read and I couldn't think but I could watch leaves move and just enjoy the artistic part of the leaves. That's about all. That's how bad my brain was.

Despite experiencing seven years of acute ill health, Sharon has only recently begun receiving any government support: two hours of cleaning every week. When we commented that this was very, little Sharon observed, 'It's a lot when I didn't have anything. It's made a big difference in our lifestyle. A big improvement.' The fact that two hours of assistance can be viewed so positively is indicative of the enormity of the desperation Sharon and her family have experienced over the years.

Sharon sadly reflects on the negative impact the illness has had on all of her children as well as her own relationship with the children, recalling, in particular, how her eldest daughter has had to 'be mum,' preparing meals, organizing her siblings for school and bedtime, and assuming responsibility for a myriad of household chores. Sharon informs us that one of the children had a developmental delay in his early years while another has more recently developed severe migraines. She suggests that some of her children's health concerns have been related to her illness, and to the broader issue, of a lack of appropriate services. Without an official medical diagnosis, Sharon and her family were deemed ineligible for a range of disability supports and home care services, which has resulted in an inordinate burden on family members. She was therefore left to deal with the stress of her own undiagnosed illness, which was magnified by the stress that an unexplained illness creates in negotiating familial relationships (Thorne, 1993, p. 25).

Her situation is reflective of the precarious notion of well-being afforded to women with a chronic illness whose condition refuses to be identified by a standard medical assessment process (Moss and Dyck, 2002). As Thorne, McCormick, and Carty (1997, p. 8) argue, this continues 'to create programs that ignore the social and family context in which illness is lived.' For women such as Sharon, it also results in lack of access to services, compounding her own illness by medical neglect and by increasing ill health among family members, and in a high level of social isolation since her social space is restricted, a situation compounded by her rural location.

Given Sharon's rural location, transportation has been particularly problematic. In this respect she has relied a great deal on her own mother to drive her to doctors' appointments, to buy groceries, and to ferry the children. Each morning the children need to be driven to the bus stop along the long dirt road that leads to the family home, and despite Sharon's efforts to do this 'no matter how unwell I was,' some days the children have not been able to attend school. This is not only about the children having to walk in poor conditions and for a long period, but also about Sharon's concern for their safety as they stand alone on what is a remote country road. When inquiring about the children's absence, school administrators counselled Sharon to ask one of the other mothers to assist, but she explained that she was reluctant to do so on a number of counts. First is her ongoing and broader concern that the nature of her illness is such that her capacity can fluctuate dramatically. She claimed, 'It is very hard to ask for help because one day

I'd be well and the next day I'd be sick. It's hard to justify.' Second is the fact that the house is so isolated, and until very recently the dirt road had large, deep puddles of water that were a major obstacle for vehicles not built to deal with extreme off-road conditions. A third factor underlying her reluctance to seek assistance from other mothers is her concern that she would not be able to offer any reciprocity. A final reason for that reluctance is that she has largely tried to hide her illness, or at least its extent, in an effort to avoid being misunderstood, judged, or dismissed. Undoubtedly Sharon's illness has also isolated her from the types of social networks that might have been able to provide her with support and assistance.

Sharon's social isolation and her experience of her body as a woman with a chronic illness residing within a rural landscape are also mediated by her identity as a mother. In their review of the literature on gender and rurality, Little and Panelli (2003) elucidate the centrality of motherhood in the rural. They note that rural women are generally 'seen first as mothers' (p. 284). For women with disabilities, this positioning is highly problematic as idealized notions of motherhood frequently leave many disabled women feeling inadequate in their performance of the 'good mother' (Malacrida, 2003). For Sharon, however, the experience of motherhood with a chronic illness is far more complex. In fact, she reveals the ways in which her isolated rural location simultaneously provided a safe place for her and her children and also facilitated her ability to avoid the levels of surveillance that many mothers with disability and chronic illness experience (see Malacrida, 2009). Reflecting upon the relationship between her chronic illness, her role as mother, and her rural location, she comments:

> In some ways better, in some ways worse. The better would be that I have had a beautiful outlook. That I, hmm ... I haven't got neighbours with an expectation on me for having a nice clean house or a clean car like it can be in suburbia. My kids have had a lot of freedom and they have been safe in lots of ways. So if they had been in suburbia it would have been really hard to have ... I wouldn't have had as much control, all those kinds of things. So they have been free even though I have been unwell.

Even though the rural setting provided Sharon with a level of reprieve, she later reflects upon the ways in which her chronic illness has affected her ability to be the all-encompassing caring and reliable mother. Sharon recollects her experience of all four children having head lice at the same time. Able-bodied mothers may regard this as one of the and mundane tasks of mothering; however, Sharon's narrative reveals how these activities are both emotionally and physically exhausting when you are chronically ill.

> Lice was a really big issue for me. I think it was one of the hardest things I have had to deal with. Hmm ... because I knew how to get rid of lice, that wasn't the issue. It was that I wasn't well enough to do it. I was able to control it to the point where it wasn't affecting other kids in the classroom but I couldn't actually get rid of it. The only way I knew to get rid of it was with the conditioner method, plus I didn't want to be using the insecticide ones because that wasn't good for my health. I was actually told by one of the doctors not to use the pyrethrin-based ones. But it is so physical ... that was the one movement that would really do me in, plus you have to wash all of the towels and my daughter's hair, she had such thick hair it used to take me a whole day just to do her hair. I was just in this rut of trying to get rid of it. I would get so exhausted. It would take me about two weeks to try to get over de-licing the kids hair. It was so so hard.

Managing the expectations of everyday life as a good wife, a good mother, and a good rural woman has, on different occasions, subjected Sharon to a heightened level of stress within her relationship with her partner. She emphasizes this point when she reflects upon her relationship during the period of her children's head lice:

> I mean you think why I couldn't ask my husband to do it, but he was so tired bringing in income to look after us all. He is coming home to mess and no meal half the time and then come home and I would ask him could you help me ... he would just lose the plot. It was better not to ask him.

Sharon raised the issue of the 'messiness' of the house and her husband's attitude towards this a number of times throughout the interview. At one point she stated, 'My husband as well, he is so worn out as he just had to work, you know, really hard. And he was coming home to absolute chaos.' She added that the situation was magnified because of the lack of an official medical diagnosis, observing that 'I had a partner who didn't believe I was sick.'

It is not surprising that Sharon has become quite tenacious at not only identifying her bodily changes, but also searching for a possible diagnosis that could rationally explain her bodily state. The ongoing negotiation of her unexplained bodily differences as a woman with an ambiguous chronic illness has had a profound effect on her sense of self. When we sat down at the kitchen table to begin the interview, she produced numerous letters along with a vast array of information received from various local medical professionals and specialist doctors. Moreover, she had compiled a large volume of information about her condition, even completing an essay on the subject of chronic fatigue for a short course she had recently undertaken. Sharon's intent to demonstrate the authenticity of her condition illustrates the deep level of emotional upheaval that comes with the uncertainty of not being believed.

As discussed in the above sections, Sharon's access to what is a very limited level of support has been facilitated by the fact that she has only recently been afforded an official medical diagnosis, 'chronic fatigue syndrome.' Asked about the diagnosis, Sharon provides insight not only into the power of the medical establishment, but also into the marked asymmetries of power between doctors and women with a disability. She recalls her appointment with a clinical immunologist in June 2007 and her anxiety that she would leave his office without the important documentation validating her illness. At the time she remembers thinking:

> I so desperately needed some help that I said, 'I need to walk out of here with something. Don't send me away with nothing … Please write something down on this letter.' Now, having the letter has made all the difference and doors have opened up.

At this appointment, as with many others she has had with doctors over the period of her illness, Sharon was feeling reasonably well. As she explained, that she had to sit in a waiting room meant that by the time she saw a doctor she appeared to be well, as many of her symptoms would subside. This necessarily exacerbated fears about credibility and the authenticity of her illness, fears she has had to endure for more than twenty-eight years. In relating this, she expresses the deep relief that results from finally experiencing a medical encounter that not only legitimized her understanding of her body but provided the vital documentation to gain access to appropriate supports. Most significantly, however, she now feels that

> I have come out of this mentally and emotionally very strong, because I felt it was the only way to get through it. It gave me the opportunity, as I had lots of time on my hands, to self-reflect. I mean if you can't read and you can't …

Despite having obtained the critically important medical endorsement of her illness, Sharon has continued to have to negotiate the potentially punitive gaze of the medical fraternity. She recounted seeing a locum GP from whom she simply required a referral to see a specialist about lesions that had erupted on her skin.

> I had a doctor who made me cry. He wasn't my normal doctor. I had to see him as I had to get a referral for the lesions on the day … He seemed pretty common-sense and I had seen him with my daughter for her migraines. And I thought I'd go with what he says as I like that common-sense approach. He kind of rolled his eyes about getting help from silver chain. He gave me a really hard time.

For a number of years Sharon had been treated by a medical doctor who employed natural therapies and was recommended in 2003 by her GP as someone who treated patients experiencing fatigue. As she recollects the initial consultation with this doctor, she reveals that much of the previous treatment she had received from mainstream medical people was marked by marginalization and/or indifference, noting:

> At least he was listening to me and he was very thorough. I had to fill out pages on my symptoms. He was a very intelligent man, I felt very happy seeing him.

Ultimately the vitamin supplements recommended by this doctor did not greatly alleviate Sharon's illness; they were also expensive and therefore placed a significant burden on family finances. Further, Sharon's engagement with natural remedies meant that she had no *official* medical diagnosis that could be used to garner government support and services.[2]

As she had done as an eighteen-year-old, Sharon worked to hide, contain, and manage her illness at an individual level. In this respect she felt her rurality allowed her to conceal the extent of her illness. She commented, 'You are a bit hidden. If I lived in suburbia people might have noticed.' Such a comment contradicts the extensive literature detailing the gendered dynamics of rural community life and rural volunteer work (Dempsey, 1992; Little, 1997a; Little & Austin, 1996; Poiner, 1990). This literature has highlighted that there is a high level of expectation that rural women will be extensively involved in specific activities and practices and considerable surveillance to ensure that this expectation is met. Sharon noted that when she was growing up her mother had been very active in the community and that 'people would have noticed.' However, it appears that the dramatic changes that have taken place in the area – a shift away from a population focused on farming to one focused on tourism/lifestyle – have seen the disbanding of many of the more traditional rural groups (e.g., Country Women's Association) once active. Today there is a transitory and more mobile population in the area, and this population is not necessarily connected to each other by background, values or practices, or perhaps they are connected to each other in ways that are alien to people such as Sharon.

What is most obvious from the newly built prestigious houses in Sharon's vicinity is the presence of a very wealthy cohort seeking to embrace the rural idyll and living on acreages with orchards or hobby farms. Sharon indicated that there was a great deal of socializing amongst women who constituted this group, and she had been invited to participate in their activities when she first returned to the district. However, she explained that the leisure practices pursued by these new entrants to the rural arena are very expensive (e.g., crafts, lunches) and consequently preclude her involvement.

While Sharon experienced some aspects of her invisibility as positive, the classed dimensions of her position should not be overlooked. That is, it is likely that she is more easily rendered invisible by her class status. Traditionally, and increasingly in Sharon's case, the middle class is normalized and the working class has become an unseen or at best shadowy presence (Bryant & Pini, 2008). This is also the case of Sharon's illness. It is certainly clear that the district is changing, but Sharon's invisibility to the local population of 'rural women' is likely also to be a result of the fact that she has suffered ill health for an extended period. This was most evident in our conversation when Sharon talked about her earlier role in a volunteer service group. She gained a great deal of satisfaction from her participation in the organization and had taken on a leadership position before she became so seriously ill she had to curtail her involvement. Recalling the decision, she stated, 'I started getting crook [ill] and I was letting them down all the time. It was really hard because I was part of the group.' Thus, Sharon became a 'floater' for the organization, filling in when and if required to undertake particular tasks, but in this capacity, she said, 'You're not really part of it anymore.' Sharon eventually resigned fully from the group because of ill health and recalled a comment from one of the organizational leaders:

She said, 'It's been a bit hard with you Sharon but you've really come good.' So I felt like really, she hadn't understood why I kept letting her down.

Sharon has intermittent contact with other people with chronic fatigue syndrome, and during our interview compared her own situation positively with one such person who lives in a unit in the city. The expansive outlook of green trees and rolling paddocks along with the quiet of the rural landscape, she said, were important to her when she was very ill in that they had a restorative impact. This is not to suggest, however, that Sharon experiences the rural uniformly as a 'therapeutic landscape' (see Little, chapter 19 of this volume). She explains how she has needed to deal with no running water in the house due to either loss of power or the collapse of a liner in the water tank. Moreover, the distances involved in attending to daily household tasks in her rural location are physically demanding. Sharon provides insight into the demanding physicality of rural life, and how this affects her body, when she describes rudimentary tasks such as emptying the garbage bin:

> The bin is not collected near the house but needs to be taken up the road to the boundary of the property. When I have been too ill to do this I have had to deal with the overflow of rubbish.

The relationship between the physicality of the rural landscape and the embodied physicality of rural women has been elaborated upon by Grace and Lennie (1998) in an Australian study focusing on questions of identity and farming women. They have argued that the physicality of the rural environment means that 'many Australian rural women develop impressive levels of practical and managerial competency, physical strength, self-reliance and robust determination' (p. 363). Clearly, the capacity for Sharon to embody and perform such traits – and with them the archetypal identity of 'rural woman' – is severely curtailed by her illness. Indeed, Sharon herself noted that there was a significant disjuncture between her embodied self and the rural landscape, which she described as 'such a physical place to be.'

As Sharon has experienced better health she has begun to reconnect with the world of work. In 2009 she participated in a vocational education and training program focused on assisting women with re-entry to the workforce. Following this, in 2009 she completed a preparatory course for entry to first-year university. She spoke enthusiastically about these educational opportunities and the studies she might pursue in areas such as environmental science or community development. At the same time, she recognized that the chances of further education, and indeed, a career of her choice, were limited by a range of intersecting factors including discrimination and lack of workplace flexibility. She wondered aloud, for example, 'At the end of it [university] would someone employ me with my health background?'

Also influencing Sharon's decisions about her future are shifting government policy. In a set of moves that will resonate with Canadian readers, Australia has significantly reformed access to entitlements for people with a disability under welfare-to-work legislation (Soldatic & Pini, 2009). Under the terms of changes introduced by the former conservative Howard government in 2005, Sharon has been assessed as having the capacity for between sixteen and twenty-two hours a week of employment, and as a consequence is not entitled to any disability welfare payments that are prescribed to less than 15 hours of work per week. Such limited support would not have been the case prior to 2005. Aside from the fact that Sharon says it would be impossible for her to commit to this amount of ongoing work, there is the reality that the labour market is highly circumscribed for Sharon because of her rurality, the long period of time she has been out of the workforce, and her ongoing illness.

Conclusion

In introducing this chapter we focused on the work of Moss and Dyck (2002) and their claims that notions of space, identity, and embodiment are central to understanding the experience of chronic illness for women. Sharon's story provides empirical support for such a thesis, particularly as it demonstrates the way identity and embodiment are shaped by the very dynamic and multiple discursive and material dimensions of rurality. As Deborah Thein argues in chapter 22 below, dominant social and cultural assumptions about rurality prescribe and privilege particular emotional behaviours and competencies many of which are gendered (and racialized). The harshness of the Australian landscape is connected if not conflated with the bodies of the rural inhabitants of this landscape, so they are viewed as hardy, physically active, resilient, capable, competent, and strong. In a similar respect, Parr, Philo, and Burns (2005) reveal how the Scottish Highlands area is seen to embody a particular profile or character as sturdy and tough. For those with mental health problems, studied by Parr et al. (2005), this version of rural embodiment is almost impossible for them to perform, as is seen in Sharon's case. Hers is a body of fatigue and fragility. It is also an unreliable body that needs assistance and support. Sharon's body thus violates deeply entrenched imaginaries of the rural. Her failure to conform to the bodily norms of rurality has seen her rebuked and chastised both overtly and covertly by medical practitioners, community members, and family. It has also resulted in her minimizing or denying the extent of her illness.

There is, of course, a specifically gendered dynamic to Sharon's transgressively rural body and rural identity, for she is judged not only against hegemonic ideals of rurality, but also according to hegemonic ideals of rurality and gender. This latter notion is an ideal of femininity that gives emphasis to the traditional and familial with strong social and moral codes attached to enacting the roles of wife and mother. Such is the pervasive power of conventional discourses of rural femininity mobilizing around beliefs about the *good mother* and the *good wife* that these may affect rural women's employment aspirations or use of child-care (Little, 1997b; Halliday & Little, 2001). When chronic illness renders fulfilling the definitions of motherhood and wifehood espoused in the rural problematic, sanctions and recriminations are likely from the self as well as others. For Sharon this has been experienced in her interactions with her children and husband, so that even within the home-space she has had to discipline her body to prepare an evening meal or drive the children to the bus stop and extracurricular activities. At a broader community level Sharon has also felt the regulative impact of rural and gendered constructions of motherhood and wifehood, as is so potently illustrated in her efforts to de-lice the children's hair despite the debilitating implications this had for her. So cognizant is Sharon of the potential for judgment and censure that she finds some solace in her rural isolation because her house (and its state of cleanliness) is not on constant view for the community.

As Sharon has struggled with the way discursively constituted notions of rurality have positioned her as inadequate and lacking, she has also been affected by the material aspects of her rural location. This includes the fact that there is little choice of available medical professionals, limited public transport, restricted employment opportunities, and few support service options. Such themes find resonance in the Canadian experience as evidenced by the contributors to this book. In Australia and in Canada this material disadvantage has been greatly aggravated by the dramatic reconfiguration of the welfare system over the past decade, which has seen decreased government support for people with a disability. The financial strain and physical, social, and emotional distress Sharon experiences in rural Australia are thus likely to be indicative of what Chouinard and Crooks (2008, pp. 173–88) describe as 'the growing peril' of people with a disability and their service and advocacy organizations in the 'increasingly harsh neoliberal environment' that characterizes the contemporary Canadian state.

In seeking to extrapolate from Sharon's story, we are greatly hindered by the lack of data on women with disabilities and/or chronic illness living not just in rural Australia but also in rural Canada. This is an invisible group, particularly in terms of official data gathering. There is even less information available on specific groups of people with a disability, such as women with disability and chronic illness. This, of course, has significant ramifications for understanding the social determinants of health for the specific population group 'rural women with a chronic illness.' In the absence of such information, Sharon's narrative provides an important impetus for a more comprehensive focus on the lives of chronically ill rural women.

Acknowledgements

We would like to thank Sharon for agreeing to be interviewed for this study.

Notes

1 'Sharon' is a pseudonym, the use of which was an agreed condition of the interview.
2 In Australia natural therapies, even when prescribed by registered medical practitioners, are not covered under the broader public health system, Medicare, nor can the costs of natural supplements be recovered through the publicly funded pharmaceutical benefit scheme, a system that subsidizes registered prescription medications.

References

Bryant, L., & Pini, B. (2008). Gender, class and rurality: Australian case studies. *Journal of Rural Studies, 25*(1), 48–57.

Cheers, B. (2001). Globalisation and rural communities. *Rural Social Work,* 6(3), 28–40.

Chouinard, V., & Crooks, V.A. (2008). Negotiating neoliberal environments in British Columbia and Ontario, Canada: Restructuring of state-voluntary sector relations and disability organizations' struggles to survive. *Environment and Planning D: Government and Policy, 26,* 173–90.

Crooks, V.A. (2004). Income assistance (the ODSP) and disabled women in Ontario, Canada: Limited program information, restrictive incomes and the impacts upon socio-spatial life. *Disability Studies Quarterly, 24*(3), np.

Crooks, V.A., & Chouinard, V. (2006). An embodied geography of disablement: Chronically ill women's struggles for enabling places in spaces of health care and daily life. *Health and Place, 12*(3), 345–52.

Crooks, V.A., Chouinard, V., & Wilton, R.D. (2008). Understanding, embracing, rejecting: Women's negotiations of disability constructions and cateogrizations after becoming chronically ill. *Social Science and Medicine, 67*(11), 1837–46.

Crow, L. (1996). Including all our lives: Renewing the social model of disability. In J. Morris (Ed.), *Encounters with strangers: Feminism and disability* (pp. 206–26). London: Women's Press.

Dempsey, K. (1992). *A man's town: Inequality between men and women in rural Australia.* Melbourne: Oxford University Press.

Dyck, I. (1995a). Hidden geographies: The changing life-worlds of women with multiple sclerosis. *Social Science and Medicine, 40*(3), 307–20.

Dyck, I. (1995b). Putting chronic illness 'in place': Women immigrants' accounts of their health care. *Geoforum, 26*(3), 247–60.

Grace, M., & Lennie, J. (1998). Reconstructing rural women in Australia: The politics of change, diversity and identity. *Sociologia Ruralis, 38*(3), 351–70.

Gray, I., & Lawrence, G. (2001). A future for regional Australia: Escaping global misfortune. London: Cambridge University Press.

Hall, G., & Scheltens, M. (2005). Beyond the drought: Towards a broader understanding of rural disadvantage. *Rural Society, 15*(3), 348–58.

Halliday, J., & Little, J. (2001). Amongst women: Exploring the reality of rural childcare. *Sociologia Ruralis, 41*(4), 423–37.

Hansen, N., & Philo, C. (2007). The normality of doing things differently: Bodies, spaces and disability geography. *Tidjschrift voor Economische en Sociale Geografie,98,* 493–506.

Johnson, J., & Johnson, K. (2006). Ambiguous chronic illness in women: Community health nursing concern. *Journal of Community Heath Nursing,* 23(3), 159–67.

Little, J. (1997a). Employment, marginality and women's self-identiy. In P. Cloke & J. Little, (Eds.), *Contested countryside cultures: Otherness, marginalisation and rurality* (pp.138–57). London: Routledge.

Little, J. (1997b). Constructions of rural women's voluntary work. *Gender, Place and Culture*, 4(2), 197–209.

Little, J., & Austin, P. (1996). Women and the rural idyll. *Journal of Rural Studies*, 12(2), 101–11.

Little, J., & Panelli, R. (2003). Gender research in rural geography. *Gender, Place and Culture, 10*(3), 281–9.

Malacrida, C. (2003). *Cold comfort: Mothers, professionals and ADD.* Toronto: University of Toronto Press.

Malacrida, C. (2009). Gendered ironies in home care: Surveillance, gender struggles and infantilisation. *International Journal of Inclusive Education,* 13(7), 741–52.

Morris, J. (1999). *Pride against prejudice.* London: Women's Press.

Moss, P. (1997). Negotiating spaces in home environments: Older women living with arthritis. *Social Science and Medicine, 45*(1), 23–33.

Moss, P. (1999). Autobiographical notes on chronic illness. In R. Butler & H. Parr (Eds.), *Mind and Body Spaces* (pp. 155–66). London: Routledge.

Moss, P., & Dyck, I. (1996). Inquiry into environment and body: Women, work and chronic illness. *Environment and Planning D: Society and Space, 14,* 737–53.

Moss, P., & Dyck, I. (1999a). Journeying through ME: Identity, the body and women with chronic illness. In E.K. Teather (Ed.), *Embodied geographies: Spaces, bodies and rites of passage* (pp. 157–92). London: Routledge.

Moss, P., & Dyck, I. (1999b). Body, corporeal space, and legitimating chronic illness: Women diagnosed with M.E. *Antipode, 31*(4), 372–97.

Moss, P., & Dyck, I. (2001). Material bodies precariously positioned: Women embodying chronic illness in the workplace. In I. Dyck, N. Lewis, & S. McLafferty (Eds.), *Geographies of women's health* (pp. 231–47). London: Routledge.

Moss, P., & Dyck, I. (2002). *Women, body, illness: Space and identity in the everyday lives of women with chronic Illness.* Lanham, MD: Rowman and Littlefield.

Oliver, M. (1996). Defining impairment and disability: Issues at stake. In C. Barnes & G. Mercer (Eds.), *Exploring the divide: Illness and disability* (pp. 39–54). Leeds: Disability Press.

Parr, H., Philo, C., & Burns, N. (2005). 'Not a display of emotions': Emotional geographies in the Scottish Highlands. In J. Davidson, L. Bondi, & M. Smith (Eds.), *In emotional geographies* (pp. 87–101). Aldershot, UK: Ashgate.

Poiner, G. (1990). *The good old rule: Gender and other power relations in a rural community*. Sydney: Sydney University Press/Oxford University Press.

PWDWA. (2010). Productivity Commission inquiry into disability support and care. *The Advocate* (Winter), 1.

Sakalys, J. (2000). The political role of illness narratives. *Journal of Advanced Nursing, 31*(6), 1469–75.

Soldatic, K., & Pini, B. (2009). The three Ds of welfare reform: Disability, disgust and deservingness. *Australian Journal of Human Rights, 15*(1), 77–96.

Thomas, C. (1999). *Female forms*. Buckingham: Open University Press.

Thorne, S. (1993). *Negotiating healthcare: The social context of chronic illness*. Newbury Park, CA: Sage.

Thorne, S., McCormick, J., & Carty, E. (1997). Deconstructing the gender neutrality of chronic illness and disability. *Health Care for Women International, 18*(1), 1–16.

Tonts, M. (2005). Government policy and rural sustainability. In C. Cocklin & J. Dibden (Eds.), *Sustainability and change in rural Australia* (pp. 194–212). Sydney: UNSW Press.

21 Health Policy and the Politics of Citizenship: Northern Women's Care Giving in Rural British Columbia

Jo-Anne Fiske, Dawn Hemingway, Anita Vaillancourt, Heather Peters, Christina McLennan, Barbara Keith, and Anne Burrill

While Canadians perceive universal health care as constitutive of national identity, economic globalization and the decline of the welfare state bring into question if, and how, the right to health care should continue. Governments employ a neoliberal ideology to rationalize service cuts and for-profit care through deploying market principles of economic efficiency; they represent the intrusion of profit regimes as offering 'choice' for all Canadians and reconstitute patients as customers and consumers. Through framing social policy in neoliberal discourses, care giving is depoliticized and citizens' right to health care is marginalized (Rylko-Bauer & Farmer, 2002; Pini & Soldatic, chapter 2 of this volume). In consequence, neoliberal repositioning of health care into the private realm strikes at the heart of Canadian identity and calls for an interrogation of citizenship (Crites, 2005).

Feminist political economists contest neoliberal constructs of citizenship that deny health care as a basic right. They call for studies of care giving that take into account the 'context of the context' and the 'setting of the setting' (Armstrong, 2001, p. 123). Moving beyond neoliberal assumptions of the autonomous individual, whose relationship with the state is constituted as a contract undertaken to maximize self-interest, feminists advance arguments that incorporate the interdependent citizen whose community membership is constituted through participation and a consciousness of belonging. In this construct of the citizen-subject, family settings and care practices, not the state, are granted priority in conceptualizing citizenship (Hankivsky, 2004). Relationships and connectivity are understood to be ways in which citizenship is enacted and a sense of identity and extrafamilial relations in the local community are sustained (Tronto, 2005). In contrast to neoliberal understanding of citizenship in terms of individual rights, boundaries, and exclusion, feminists argue citizenship is best construed as a practice of social connectivity (Armstrong, 2001). Within a feminist perspective, public/private boundaries that constitute liberal conceptions of citizenship are problematized: rationality, independence, separation, and self-interest are eschewed in favour of emotion, interdependence, association, and shared responsibilities (see Thien, chapter 22, this volume). Citizenship thus emerges from contributions to social well-being, and is understood as relational or social citizenship (Ben-Ishai, 2007; Kingwell, 2000; Sevenhuijsen, 1998). This model of citizenship positions care giving as an arena in which citizenship is performed and sees care giving as the 'essential democratic act' because care facilitates interdependent relations, forges collective social actions and public participation, and 'cuts across the public and private spheres' (Hankivsky, 2004, p. 7).

Reliance on volunteer care, the unpaid, freely given work individuals do to provide for others in need, is a central strategy of neoliberal states seeking to reduce spending and cut taxes through deinstitutionalization (Hankivsky, 2004). However, despite its importance, informal volunteer care in rural regions has not been well studied. As Little (chapter 19, this volume) states, rural women's health research increasingly focuses on cultural and social contexts and community responses to policy and service provision. The goal of this chapter is therefore twofold: to show how volunteer care-giving practices in four rural resource communities of northern British Columbia constitute essential democratic action, and to interrogate the capacity of feminist discourses to meaningfully capture women's commitment to caring. We ask: How do volunteer care givers represent their personal care-giving experiences? Do their representations reflect the polemical debates that mark public discourse, and if not, can feminist discourse fairly represent volunteer care givers' experiences and community engagement?

Background

This chapter arises from a larger research project exploring practices and social relations of paid and unpaid care givers within rural and remote resource communities during an economic cycle of rapid decline following a period of economic expansion. We interviewed fifty-eight women ranging in age from twenty-seven to seventy-three regarding their paid and unpaid care-giving relations. Thirty-five of the fifty-eight participants carried multiple care responsibilities; paid workers were active volunteers and often care givers to family members. Overwhelmingly, participants were Caucasian women, although in three of the communities a small number of First Nations women participated. The interviews focused on individuals' typical care routines and duties.

For this chapter we selected narratives of volunteer care giving and analysed them by means of thematic coding; passages of the narratives were organized by related ideas, or themes, and then in a reiterative process examined and compared with one another. Themes that conceptualized how the women explained and felt about their care giving were compared to themes that identified what they did and for whom. This method was guided by the axial coding practices described by Strauss and Corbin (1998).

The Community Context

The economy of northern British Columbia is founded on resource extraction, which is subject to boom/bust cycles and vulnerable to the global economy. At the time of our research, Prince George, Prince Rupert, Quesnel, and Fraser Lake were coming out of a period of economic decline – a brief respite, as by 2008 economic crises had taken hold once again. Historically each of the communities relied heavily on forestry and mining, while Prince Rupert enjoyed a rich fishing industry as well. By 2002, fishing and forestry in particular were in crisis. Fish stocks were seriously depleted and huge tracts of forests in northern British Columbia were devastated by the mountain pine beetle (a devastation continuing to the present), and forestry suffered further from two decades of soft lumber trade disputes with the United States; in consequence the region lost jobs and infrastructure (Ewart & Hemingway, 2008). The three smaller communities are far from ideal for accessing essential care. Distances to the main service centre, Prince George, a city of 74,000, are considerable; Prince Rupert (population 13,000) lies 715 kilometres to the west, Fraser Lake (population 1400) 150 kilometres to the west, and Quesnel (population 10,000) 119 kilometres to the south. Travel can be hazardous, particularly in winter. All four communities serve outlying villages, hamlets, and First Nations reserves; in the winter, several villages and hamlets are accessible only by plane from Prince Rupert. Public bus service is limited; flying is costly and major airlines connect the communities through Vancouver, adding to cost and travel time. The Northern Health Authority, which serves the entire region under study, connects communities with designated buses for patients and companions, although not always on an ideal schedule. Medical services are also limited. All communities rely on a combination of itinerant specialists from southern areas and sending patients to large urban centres in the south. Local services vary dramatically. For example, Fraser Lake has no emergency care, and the diagnostic medical centre served by four family physicians is open Monday to Friday only. Emergency hospitals lie an hour's journey to the east and west of Fraser Lake, and most acute patients are transferred to the regional hospital in Prince George, two hours by road to the east.

Each community is marked by social transience; professionals often remain only for short periods, and with economic uncertainty the labour force is by necessity highly mobile. Resource industries organize work in rotating shifts and often require workers to be away from home during the work week or longer. When the economy fails, households are disrupted as family members migrate to opportunities elsewhere. Younger adults often leave behind elderly kin who are reluctant to leave their homes or who cannot afford to move to more expensive locales. Each community also grapples with the consequences of provincial deinstitutionalization policies that have closed residential institutions for special needs adults for whom independent living is impossible. As institutions close elsewhere, communities experience an influx of individuals whom the government chooses to return to their community of origin, often without consideration for personal circumstances such as alienation from family or the complete absence of family members remaining in the area.

The smallest two communities, Fraser Lake and Quesnel, have sought to redefine themselves as ideal retirement communities: they are located in spectacular scenery, have low living costs, and are known for their strong community spirit. Housing prices are low relative to metropolitan areas in the southern part of the province; however, basic amenities are restricted to food stores, local doctors, sparse recreation facilities, and a number of service groups. Despite their newly created identity as retirement communities, Fraser Lake and Quesnel have little to offer seniors who are advanced in age or have care needs due to chronic illness, dementia, or poor mobility. Fraser

Lake has no designated assisted living services, and Quesnel's services cannot meet demand. Like Fraser Lake, Quesnel relies on the centralized services in Prince George an hour and more away by highway.

Health provision in the three smaller communities is hampered by centralization of administration and specialists in Prince George, a practice that conforms to the management model that seeks cost efficiencies. Government offices have closed or been relocated to larger regional communities, and many agencies once providing face-to-face service are now only available by telephone or Internet. Home care work is similarly centralized; administrative offices in the larger communities assign and monitor care workers in outlying villages. As employees of the Health Authority, care workers can be assigned clients at considerable distance from their homes.

'Care deficiencies,' as Hochschild (1995, p. 332) has labelled the weaknesses in social policy, are a growing concern in rural communities isolated from urban services. During periods of economic decline, rural resource-based communities feel the loss of services most acutely. As governments cut back, women take up the slack through care provision for family and friends, volunteer services, and paid caring labour that brings with it increased workloads and stress (Hanlon, Halseth, Clasby, & Pow, 2007; Leipert & Reutter, 2005; Pini & Soldatic, chapter 20). Studies have shown that within this northern health region, home support (care provided in a client's home to allow the client continued residence there) lies well below provincial averages in terms of hours of care and range of services provided (Cohen, Murphy, Nutland, & Ostry, 2005). In the context of diminishing public services, the four communities have come to rely heavily on volunteer labour. As is often the case, networks of women form a central core of volunteers; they belong to a range of associations and networks, share social activities, and engage in local political action as advocates for particular interests and general community well-being. Volunteer work is divided by age; in each community women providing care directly to seniors tend to be middle aged and 'young' seniors, while children's education and recreation attract younger parents as volunteers. Service groups with a long-standing presence in the communities, such as the Women's Institute and Rotary, are in rapid decline, as they hold limited appeal to younger community members. Volunteer work, moreover, is beyond the capacity of some families, where shift work and long periods of out-of-town employment prevent any regular participation in the community; this also makes home care for family and community members exceedingly challenging.

Women's Volunteer Experiences

In the four communities women's care-giving activities encompassed a broad range of activities that connected them to their communities. Their volunteer activities ranged from informal relationships with neighbours and friends, to membership in voluntary associations, to assisting health and other services in a range of supportive activities. In Fraser Lake, the smallest of the four communities, women's volunteer activities included running charity events and working for the Canadian Legion, which among other services provides meals on wheels, organizes fundraisers to assist families travelling outside the region for critical care, and holds memorial services and funeral dinners. Other volunteer activities included assisting and advocating for the mentally ill, driving community members to medical appointments, driving as much as 100 kilometres to shop for others, routinely cooking for neighbours, tending farm animals, and assisting with home building and maintenance. In Quesnel, in addition to a similar range of community engagements found at Fraser Lake, women were volunteer palliative care aides, comfort companions to chemotherapy patients, leaders of networks working with the disabled, and active helpers in the local transition home. In the larger city of Prince George, volunteers worked with organized service groups and agencies, joined the governing boards of non-profit groups, held memberships in regional and provincial associations, and associated with one another through ad hoc groups and informal networks. They supported a broad range of individuals who were socially and economically excluded from the mainstream community: the homeless, seniors in long-term care, sex trade workers and youth at risk on the street, and special needs adults and children.

Across the communities women undertook responsibilities from opening their homes to temporary residents to aiding family and friends with babysitting and offering respite to families stressed by home care responsibilities. They also offered respite to women who contracted with the health authority to operate care facilities in their homes. The women's lives revolved around working for others with whom they had strong family and extra-family ties. A woman described the link between her paid caring work and volunteer work in this way:

I've always been raised with that kind of social conscience ... I also just see in this kind of weird way that I, I find making money off somebody's pain, you know, the work I do, cause that's what's happening. Then I absolutely feel um, a moral obligation to be giving back.

Uncomfortable with being paid to care for someone suffering pain, she undertook volunteer care giving as a way to give back to the community.

Not only did care giving absorb a substantial amount of time, other activities were subordinated to care-giving schedules. A number of retired volunteers committed twenty hours or more weekly to their community service, and some described routines that engaged them for a full work week. Women in the labour force spoke of care duties they assumed either early in the morning before going to work or immediately after work. One woman spent entire nights with a palliative patient, while others spent evenings at meetings, visiting, or preparing meals for others. Volunteers juggled work schedules to offer respite to primary care givers, often to help offset costs of hiring care aides or temporary nurses. Others, who were not in the paid labour force, scheduled volunteer work around their husbands' work shifts when they could, and when they could not the men either assisted them in their tasks or 'got used to' their wives' routines.

Although few explicitly described their care giving in terms of citizenship, the emphasis they placed on commitment to community resonates with feminist concepts of relational citizenship. Care giving prompted some women to become more active at all levels of governance from local community associations to federal election campaigns; one woman translated her paid and unpaid experience of caring into policy development work 'at a national level or provincial level ... looking at early child development.' At the heart of their narratives of their typical care routines lay a strong sense of belonging to their communities. They were aware that their efforts to provide for others and to establish and sustain reciprocal care relationships contributed to healthy and safe communities. In one community, women worried about the impact of illegal drugs. Families with members selling drugs became isolated from the care they needed, while elderly neighbours to drug dealers did not feel safe leaving their homes in the evenings. Not surprisingly, committed volunteers found time to assist seniors who felt unsafe and made frequent visits to allay the seniors' fears.

Significantly, when asked to define care giving, women found it difficult to draw boundaries around their multiple volunteer roles, family needs, and interdependence with friends and relatives. A younger woman with small children told us:

Time off, when you're trying to reprieve from, you know, your um, workplace, you're in conflict as to whether you just go and escape and be, or
whether you spend that time going to connect with people ... you know,
the, the time and energy that um, that my mom requires, there's lots
of pressure.

Volunteering to assist others was experienced in holistic relationships.
Strong connections with others were viewed as developing reciprocal
relationships; giving services to others meant getting support in return:
'it's hard to explain because it's really supposedly a thankless job, but
it's not ... you get so much in return.' Repeatedly, volunteers focused
on the broad social contributions that linked their multiple engagements and the value of their work to the community as a whole. And
while they spoke positively, even defensively, of the emotional returns
they enjoyed as a consequence of their busy lives, they also reflected on
the context in which their commitments were made. As much as they
were attached to their communities, they were aware of the economic
and political shortcomings that shaped volunteer care-giving experiences. One woman explained it this way:

There was always cutbacks to, you know, government supports under an
NDP government as well, but, um, since 2001 with the BC Liberals it's
even worse, you know. So there's even fewer supports for women to, to
strike out on their own. And I think that that's also hugely emotionally
taxing on women. So it really undermines, you know, their strength and
their ability to be organized and to have the opportunities and to, you
know, to, to do what they have to do every day.

Care-Giving Discourses

Community Connections

Women who provided volunteer care in private homes or through community service located themselves within discourses of nurturing
women whose caring relationships are grounded in compassion and
emotional well-being. Women framed their narratives of care for family
and friends in terms of the quality of personal relationships and emotional rewards: 'the work feels really important. Relationship feels really important.' They spoke of living with or near to family members
whom they 'helped' and 'supported.' Maintaining good relationships
and being good to others, whether family, close friends, or neighbours,

motivated the women to provide assistance: 'I feel like a million bucks when I walk out of there usually, you know ... I probably get way more out of it than the people I sit with [in palliative care].' Engaging in social activities, a walk or drive in the park, or taking tea and baked goods to loved ones and friends are examples of the informal assistance women described. Sharing experiences emerged in narratives as the signifier of the meaning of caring: it was not the tasks the women engaged in on behalf of others but the quality of the time spent with others. The women constituted caring relationships as ones that brought them 'appreciation' and 'satisfaction.' Whether 'looking in on' neighbours or volunteering, they found the connections they made with others 're-warding' and 'worth it.'

Commitment to community was given as a reason to be involved in volunteer activities. It was a way 'to give something back.' Caring, they stated, is not an option but a personal responsibility, 'something that is just part of life.' Women reflected on their caring roles within the community context; volunteering and 'looking in on' others created connections, provided a sense of belonging, and contributed to community safety. Through visiting, talking, and sharing common experiences in looking after others, they avoided loneliness and were able to engage in formal associations and informal networks.

Neoliberal Discourse

Neoliberal discourse, as Harvey (2005) has argued, carries a broad appeal. Neoliberalism foregrounds a rhetoric of human dignity and individual freedom and argues these are under threat from all forms of government intervention and reliance on collective responsibility. Framed within a rhetoric of choice and the creative power of the individual, neoliberalism 'proposes that human well-being can best be advanced by liberating individual entrepreneurial freedom and skills within an institutional framework characterized by strong private property rights, free markets and free trade' (Harvey, 2005, p. 2). Women frequently drew on concepts found in neoliberal ideology. They spoke of elders' desires to be independent and to exercise personal choices in their care. Some seniors sought independence from family as well as from paid health care providers. One woman said: 'Their health starts going, their family steps in and says, "You're gonna do this or you're gonna do that."' Volunteers also valued individual autonomy from both public and private paid care giving. One volunteer expressed this as being 'able to be free to give him [her neighbour] care when he wanted it not when she was told to.' Women also defended the gendered constructs of their caring activities. Drawing on traditional notions of woman as nurturer, they spoke of having 'natural' qualities that men lacked. Intimate care in particular was seen as their domain; those who had raised children described providing toileting assistance to seniors and the disabled as a natural progression from infant care. 'I really do think the ladies do a good job. That's our job ... That's maternal touch' were the words of one woman.

The women did not, however, accept the political constructs of neoliberal ideology. They did not take up the market discourses the state uses to rationalize its health reform; they rejected the construct of health care patients as 'consumers' and 'customers.' Many of the women, in particular those simultaneously volunteering and employed in caregiving positions, were deeply suspicious of for-profit models of senior care. They resisted government claims that private firms could, and would, provide quality, affordable services. A woman described her experience with a for-profit agency in this way:

> [The for-profit agency] has some really excellent workers, but they don't get paid very much. They get paid eighty fifty an hour. [The agency] collects double that plus more. So ... the agency makes more money than the actual care giver who's doing the lifting and the cleaning.

Several women also spoke of the invisibility of their community contributions. Voluntary palliative care is one example of an invisible service. One palliative volunteer spoke of her work as 'fl[ying] under the community radar.' The privacy of the service, lack of support networks for the patient, and night-time volunteer schedules all contribute to the hidden nature of this service. A 'taken for granted' stance of community leaders in regard to volunteer labour, some suggested, meant that community leaders had come to rely on volunteers as 'business as usual,' as the norm. They felt community leaders perceived this as routine women's work or as an accepted way to rationalize and not pay for expensive services. Another woman told us: 'personal care giving that we were giving I ... don't begrudge. But I am still very, very angry about the lack of help, the lack of response from public health, the lack of help from the medical world.'

While women specifically gendered their assistance to others, they also recognized the support men gave to them. To some extent women embedded their appreciation of men's care giving within neoliberal gender frames. Men appeared in their stories as critical to successful care giving but not as central actors. Women described husbands and brothers as supports for primary care giving. Although her partner worked away much of the time, a woman told us that 'when my husband's around, he's a great help. He's terrific.' They listed tasks commonly construed as masculine as examples of the support they received: men repaired and maintained homes of the elderly and ill, worked on vehicles, cut fire wood, maintained yards, and the like. Men also took on tasks that in the past were construed as feminine but now are approached by many in the community as gender neutral. Cooking, hunting, fishing, and berry picking by men all contributed to support for women providing care and for those receiving care. Men drove paid care givers to their work, particularly in winter when roads are dangerous; babysat grandchildren, nieces, and nephews; and arranged work shifts to meet wives' volunteer commitments.

Despite the strong support some volunteers received from men, women's care giving in these communities reflects a national pattern. Studies over the past two decades consistently demonstrate that women of all ages are far more likely to be care givers than men. National studies have found that women account for three-quarters of health care volunteers (Armstrong & Armstrong 2003; Romanow, 2002). However, men's care work has not been fully explored; the roles that men play, as described by the participants, are often seen as ancillary tasks rather than direct aspects of care. More research is needed to understand men's participation in care through such work as home and equipment maintenance, cooking, and transportation.

Feminist Discourse

Inter Pares (2004) summarizes feminist discourse as one that 'reveals and clarifies how gender determines or influences the social and political relationships and structures of power and the differential economic effects that flow from these relationships and structures' (p. 4). Feminist political economic discourse frames women's unpaid labour as a burden with heavy social and economic consequences for female care givers, particularly rural care givers (Hankivsky, 2004). Feminist discourse used by researchers to describe volunteer care giving as a burden and exploitation was rejected, for the most part, by the participants in this study. They disputed the notion of caring as 'unpaid labour'; such language, they implied, failed to capture the emotional attachment that

bonded givers and recipients of care. While acknowledging and up-
holding a gendered nature of care giving, they rejected conceptual
frameworks that implied they were subordinated as a consequence of
caring and refused to accept their care giving as primarily a burden.
They deployed a range of expressions to suggest that looking after others was 'just something you did' as a family member and good neighbour, and as 'just part ... of life, you know.' They did not describe their
volunteer labour as exploitive nor as secondary to other forms of commitment. Neither did they experience the gendered nature of their
work as secondary to that of men; rather, they incorporated their husbands and brothers into their care-giving activities in terms of equitable
partners sharing social responsibilities. This was particularly marked
in the shared labour of women and men in fundraising and other community activities.

Failure to explicitly articulate feminist (a term they resisted frequently) conceptualizations of care giving as a burden, labour, or exploitation is at odds with the volume and depth of the commitments
and the experiences women described. This was made clear as active
volunteers spoke about the intensity of their service and the state's reliance on their community contributions. They recognized that their efforts compensated for diminishing services and lack of community
infrastructure, which one woman described in this way: 'there's lots of
care givers and that changes with the way the government system cov-
ers [services].' Active volunteers were repeatedly called upon to fulfil
multiple roles, many of which took women from their home communities to attend meetings elsewhere. They listed drawbacks of volunteering in well-known discourses of burn out, juggling multiple
expectations, taking time from family and social events, and above all
losing time for themselves. Repeatedly we heard comments similar to
this: 'you get really, really tired ... You need a break ... But then it's, it's,
when you think about it now, you think how did I survive? But you
always seem to.' They worried that a lack of young volunteers left their
communities vulnerable. They identified the transient nature of community populations as increasing the challenges they faced. The frequent entry and departure of local residents left gaps in their social
networks, and they felt keenly the emotional loss when friends to
whom they were deeply attached moved away.

Women constructed their identities within the context of relational
citizenship in phrases consistent with feminist discourse. The majority
of the women described caring as a meaningful activity that shaped

who they saw themselves to be as individuals, community members, and neighbours. This was particularly important to women who defined care giving very broadly. In a perspective of caring that included a wide range of activities – meals on wheels, fundraising, memberships in non-profit governing boards, anti-poverty groups – women achieved identities as valued community members and leaders. They presented themselves as community citizens deeply connected to one another and proud of their achievements. Volunteer work broadened social bonding and the individuals cared for became 'just like family.' In this context the community as a whole took on particular meaning and became a place to protect.

Rural Care Deficits

Although the women appeared to espouse some values propounded in neoliberal discourse with respect to their care-giving roles, they explicitly rejected neoliberal policies when speaking of rural community needs. The explanations they offered for problems within rural health care delivery and social services are more aligned with feminist political economy. 'Health care,' Armstrong (2001) states, 'is not only about what happens in the formal system, nor can the formal system be understood without reference to household and communities, to informal care' (p. 125). Just as feminist political economists turn to the state to explain the current context of health care, so did the women in this study. They identified three forces that account for rural care deficits: a lack of infrastructure that leaves individuals, families, and communities vulnerable to economic boom/bust cycles; rationalization of health budgets that has shifted care from publicly funded institutions to family and community; and centralization of government services in distant urban centres. Notably, they did not turn to neoliberal values to explain family and individual needs in terms of personal, moral, or financial failure, nor did they hold individuals, communities, or women accountable for their own care.

Diminishing Infrastructure

As supported in a study by Leipert and Reutter (2005), and similar to the case in Australia discussed by Pini and Soldatic in chapter 20 of this volume, the women identified six elements of diminishing infrastructure: reduced hospital care and shortages of alternative services, rising inequities as a result of deinstitutionalization, poor wages for care givers as care shifted from professional nurses to care aides, increased reliance on informal care, lack of public transit, and centralization of local services.

Reduced Services

Several women spoke of hospital wards being shut down for cost savings, which resulted in longer waits for hospital care. At the same time they experienced a shortage in other care facilities and services (e.g., extended care homes), which the government promoted as viable alternatives to hospitalization. They identified inequities between what hospitals offered and the personal costs borne at home. Families who provided unpaid care at home had to purchase prescribed medications and personal supplies, bandages, and diapers, for example, all of which are normally provided without cost to patients in hospitals.

As other studies have clearly demonstrated, volunteer unpaid labour compensates for diminishing infrastructure and deinstitutionalization (Hankivsky, 2004). To reduce budgets, home care workers employed by the health authority were restricted in their duties. Paid care workers were no longer able to offer holistic services to their clients and their families. Once able to provide light housekeeping duties, which allowed them to support or enhance safe personal environments, and to prepare simple meals, they were now constrained to providing only 'essential' personal care, bathing, intimate needs, and help with medications. The low wages paid home care workers resulted in frequent staff turnover in rural areas, creating disruptions in personal care for the patient.

Deinstitutionalization

Not only did rationalization of health budgets shift care from publicly funded institutions to paid home care workers, it also meant a significant shift from institutional care to informal family and volunteer care, as evidenced in the four communities of our study. As is often the case in rural communities, rural regions in British Columbia offer considerably fewer hours of paid care per week than do urban areas, a deficit taken up by unpaid workers (Cohen et al., 2005). When volunteers, who are not necessarily well trained, replace trained home care workers, the capacity to regulate home care and provide protection for vulnerable individuals and families is diminished. Volunteer workers spoke of offering respite for families who could not afford paid care givers. They spoke of the relatively low wages home care workers received and how even these wages lay beyond the reach of households who required more than the services provided by the health authority. Volunteers identified serious lack of infrastructure as contributing to the stress on communities, on families, and on their own personal well-being. Redress for stretched volunteers, the women said, lies in financial support for home care. More paid workers were required and regulations against a holistic approach to care giving need to be reconsidered. The lack of nutritious meals is but one example of a problem that needs to be addressed. Volunteers with programs such as meals on wheels advocated for a return to earlier practices that would have trained, paid workers available more frequently, for longer periods of time, and enabled to provide holistic care.

Public Transportation

As others have also learned, the most serious deficit for many was lack of effective public transportation (Michalos et al., 2007). The health authority in northern British Columbia had recently introduced a network of buses to carry patients and their companions to medical appointments; however, this service did not cover the full range of health-related services that community members required. Nor did the service benefit community members forced to travel out of their communities to purchase essential home care items or to visit family in residential facilities located as far as two hours from home. Families unable to provide their own transportation relied on friends and volunteer associations to drive them between communities. Volunteering to compensate for lack of public transportation comes at a personal cost; volunteers assume costs for fuel, vehicle maintenance, and personal expenses while transporting others.

Centralization of Services

Lack of public transport exists simultaneously with shifts to centralization of services. With closure of government offices and diminished services in smaller communities, travel needs increase. Accompanying centralization of services is increased reliance of government offices on telephone and Internet communications. Standard practice in regional offices is to receive phone messages and to return calls in accordance with government office routines. For volunteers this creates added pressure to be available to assist seniors and others in making calls and to be available to receive the return calls. In rural areas this is particularly problematic as care givers often are assisting individuals who do not reside in close proximity. Limited access to and experience with computers, as well as unreliable Internet access, make Internet communications a challenge for many.

Centralization of services disadvantages rural areas beyond the additional costs borne by families and the alienation experienced by patients institutionalized far from home. Centralization has also meant that rural residents are less able to participate in the decision making that shapes health and social policies and ultimately determines the quality and quantity of services and programs. Public consultation on policy initiatives is central to democratic processes. Structured inequities in democratic representation means smaller communities are not represented in the formation of policy and practices; consequently their particular needs are less likely to be met, a problem others have documented (Michalos et al., 2007). Volunteers experience these inequities through the additional toll on their time as they are forced to travel to consultations and through frustrations that follow from inadequate and inappropriate service models.

Compounding the lack of democratic representation and program inadequacies are the challenges of coping with lack of coordination of services. In British Columbia, managing care is not solely the responsibility of the health ministry; ministries addressing child and family development, housing, and social development are also involved in care management. Authorities for the various regimes managed by the ministries are not centralized in the same locations, nor do their service area boundaries coincide. The need to work with administrative offices located in a number of towns and to coordinate volunteer care in different service districts creates additional pressure on volunteers and smaller communities as they juggle travel to several locations and cope with a range of uncoordinated programs.

Poor coordination of services and programs is further exacerbated by government practices of developing short-term programs through annual cycles of grant competitions. Non-profit agencies not only spend considerable time developing project proposals in a context of uncertainty, they frequently find themselves competing against one another. As government priorities are redefined, the agencies reinvent themselves and their programs to meet ever-shifting expectations. Complex regulations and governing practices further complicate the context in which volunteers provide care; health and social service regulations are often at odds with one another, difficult to follow, and presented in terms incomprehensible to many community members. Some regulations are viewed as highly intrusive and unnecessary (e.g., rulings that seek to prohibit community potluck dinners for fear of food contamination) and contrary to community well-being. As a consequence of these government practices, volunteers are once again stretched as they participate in the formulation of proposals and programs while reorganizing their activities to match evolving programs and retraining to meet fluctuating standards (e.g., obtaining food security and first aid certification).

The inequitable power relations that privilege urban areas over rural and south British Columbia over north are readily understood by volunteer care givers and those who receive their support. In this context, volunteers view the state as having failed them in their most essential social contribution: building strong, healthy communities through interdependent relations of care. When asked what they wanted, study participants responded with clear expectations. They wanted infrastructure and not-for-profit services that will enable them to serve others and enjoy the fulfilment that comes through this service. As much as they may appear to espouse values that are rhetorically deployed by neoliberal governance with regard to the right to provide care, they find much in common with a feminist political economy that holds government authorities responsible for enabling them to offer services safely and effectively and without stretching community capacities beyond reasonable limits.

Conclusion

Feminist political economists conceptualize care giving as multidimensional practices: as unpaid domestic and voluntary labour, paid labour, a burden, a sacrifice, and as women's work (Armstrong, 2001; Hankivsky, 2004). As we have demonstrated above, this discourse does not fully resonate with the care givers in our study. Their failure to align with feminist discourse, even as their experiences appear to support it, reminds us that discourses always operate in contested terrains.

Discourses are marked by complexity and tensions; they compete for meaning and as they are taken up acquire new meanings that are often unintended and on the surface appear to be contradictory.

More complicated understandings and nuances are revealed with respect to relations of power and domination in volunteer care giving. Gendered volunteer labour, contrary to feminist political economists' expectations (Armstrong, 2001), is not necessarily experienced as relations of subordination. Women's narratives in this study revealed that a shift is taking place from traditional gendered roles of female reproductive labour versus male productive labour. In the communities in this study, men provide ancillary services and supports for women's voluntary care giving; as men participate in tasks once construed as feminine, reproductive labour shifts towards gender neutrality. Women took up identities as nurturers that are readily framed and explicitly exploited by neoliberal market models, but did so with pride and deep satisfaction. They resisted being subordinated through claims of feminine specificity as care givers by acting on the assumption that their work matters, a claim asserted by feminists since the 1960s, and that leadership extends from the value they place on their social contributions to community well-being.

How women claim space as citizens lies at the centre of understanding state structures and relations of power between the metropolis and the rural, the state and the individual. Feminist political economy conceives of citizenship as arising out of and being practised through connectivity (Armstrong, 2001; Tronto, 2005). Reciprocal relations of interdependence are forged through women's care-giving practices. The shift in governing practices from public services to private care and community responsibilities is understood on similar terms both by women living the shift and by feminist political economists. While women claim that as citizens it is their right to provide care, they also hold the state accountable to them. Just as they seek to create and sustain reciprocal relations within community, through mobilizing via local organizations and informal networks to fight for needed resources, they call upon the state to reciprocate for their civic contributions.

In sum, empirical studies documenting care givers' experiences and perceptions of their community relations reveal care as the 'essential democratic act' (Hankivsky, 2004, p. 7). Rural women of northern British Columbia conduct their caring relations within the frame of relational citizenship and extend personal care giving to democratic actions. Justification for women's leadership and having a voice in decision making arises from demonstrating sustained responsibilities for others. Relational citizenship as practiced by volunteering women in rural resource communities seeks to dissolve social distances through the broad incorporation of care giving in community life. In this case study, women's public action substantiates Hankivsky's (2004) claim that care giving lies at the heart of democratic processes that radiate from family to community to the polity at large. Through care giving, women claim space in the public sphere in a range of structured and informal relationships that give meaning to their lives and create, sustain, and enhance community.

Acknowledgments

The authors acknowledge the Social Sciences and Humanities Research Council for funding this research (grant # 410-2004-1646). Thanks are also due to the women we interviewed, for their time and knowledge that were graciously shared with us, and to the communities, including the many organizations that facilitated the research process.

References

Armstrong, P. (2001). Evidence-based health care reform. In P. Armstrong, H. Armstrong, & D. Coburn (Eds.), *Unhealthy times: Political economy perspectives on health and care in Canada* (pp. 121–45). Toronto: Oxford University Press.

Armstrong, P., & Armstrong, H. (2003). *Wasting away: The undermining of Canadian health care* (2nd ed.). New York: Oxford University Press.

Ben-Ishai, E. (2007). *Towards a revised conception of social citizenship: An autonomy focused model.* University of Michigan. Retrieved from http://www.cpsa-acsp.ca/papers-2007/Benishai.pdf.

Cohen, M., Murphy, J., Nutland, K., & Ostry, A. (2005). *Continuing care: Renewal or retreat: BC residential and home care restructuring, 2001-2004.* Vancouver: Canadian Centre for Policy Alternatives. Retrieved from http://www.policyalternatives.ca/sites/default/files/uploads/publications/BC_Office_Pubs/bc_2005/continuing_care.pdf.

Crites, V. (2005). The Canadian identity and the right to health care: From wait-lists to social citizenship. Unpublished master's thesis, University of Victoria.

Ewart, P., & Hemingway, D. (2008, 12 June). *Devastating mill shutdowns: What can towns like Mackenzie do?* Retrieved from http://www.opinion250.com/

blog/view./9649/7/devastating+mill+shutdowns:+what+can+towns+like +mackenzie+do%3F.

Hanlon, N., Halseth, G., Clasby, R., & Pow, V. (2007). The place embeddedness of social care: Restructuring work and welfare in Mackenzie, BC. *Health & Place, 13*, 466-81.

Hankivsky, G. (2004). *Social policy and the ethic of care.* Vancouver: UBC Press.

Harvey, D. (2005). *A brief history of neo-liberalism.* Oxford: Oxford University Press.

Hochschild, A.R. (1995). The culture of politics: Traditional, post-modern, cold-modern and warm-modern ideals of care. *Social Politics, 2*, 331–46.

Inter Pares. (2004). *Towards a feminist political economy.* Inter Pares Occasional Paper, no. 5. Ottawa: Inter Pares. Retrieved from http://www.interpares. ca/en/publications/pdf/feminist_political_economy.pdf.

Kingwell, M. (2000). *The world we want: Virtue, vice and the good citizen.* Toronto: Viking, Penguin Group.

Leipert, B., & Reutter, L. (2005). Women's health in northern British Columbia: The role of geography and gender. *Canadian Journal of Rural Medicine, 10*(4), 241–53.

Michalos, A., Hatch, P.M., Hemingway, D., Lavallee, L., Hogan, A., & Christensen, B. (2007). Health and quality of life of older people, a replication after six years. *Social Indicators Research, 84*(2), 127–58.

Romanow, R.J. (2002). *Building on values: The future of health care in Canada. Final report.* Ottawa: Commission on the Future of Health Care in Canada. Retrieved from http://publications.gc.ca/pub?id=237274&sl=0.

Rylko-Bauer, B., & Farmer, P. (2002). Managed care or managed inequality? A call for critiques of market-based medicine. *Medical Anthropology Quarterly, 16*(4), 476–502.

Sevenhuijsen, S. (1998). *Citizenship and the ethics of care: Feminist considerations on justice, morality and politics.* London: Rutledge.

Strauss, A., & Corbin, J. (1998). *Basics of qualitative research techniques and procedures for developing grounded theory* (2nd ed.). London: Sage.

Tronto, J. (2005). Care as the work of citizens: A modest proposal. In M. Friedman (Ed.), *Women and citizenship* (pp. 130–45). New York: Oxford University Press.

22 Well Beings:
Placing Emotion in Rural, Gender, and Health Research

Deborah Thien

'What happens when complexity is treated as a resource rather than a problem ...?' (Williams, 2009, p. 262)

Inspired by sociologist Simon Williams' provocative question, this chapter examines how emotion is a productive resource, both as a theoretical lens and as an under-examined material feature of care giving, health, and well-being, when considering rural women's health research. Through a discussion of emotional geographies, the discursive figuring of rural spaces as spaces for feeling, and the ongoing production of feeling subjects, I argue for a closer attention to emotion as 'a complex aspect of social life' (Fullagar, 2008, p. 48). Bringing emotion into the frame highlights a new and meaningful way to generate detailed considerations of rurality, gender, and health, raising questions about a number of implications for rural women's health. For example, how do notions about and practices of health depend upon what might be called 'emotional geographies,' as Davidson, Bondi, and Smith do in their eponymous collection (2005)? How do women negotiate their own and others' presumptions of women's place in 'emotion work' (Hochschild, 2003) specifically, and the gendered aspects of rural life more broadly (Thien, 2005c), when attending to emotional health in a rural landscape? How might such theoretical framings of emotion lead to specific recommendations for methodological practice and development in rural women's health and gender studies? And what then can researchers with an interest in emotion contribute to 'well beings' in rural settings? In exploring these concerns, this chapter seeks to extend the breadth of feminist and health research, develop the field of emotional geographies, and add a new perspective to thinking about rurality, gender, and health.

Background: Locating Emotion in Rural Women's Health Research

A major finding of Janzen's *Women, Gender & Health: A Review of the Recent Literature* was the lack of evidence addressing the 'health needs and determinants of rural women' (Janzen, 1998, p. 34). Nearly ten years later, Beverley Leipert and her colleagues, in their call for attention to pharmacological issues for rural women, offer an excellent overview of the now documented health concerns rural women face: low numbers of rural physicians, gender-related health issues, privacy concerns in small communities, travel considerations, occupational and socio-cultural factors, life-stage (e.g., teens, seniors), prescribing practices and a related lack of counselling services, and high rates of cardiovascular disease, cancer, mental health issues, obesity, spousal violence, alcohol, and substance abuse (Leipert, Matsui, & Rieder, 2006). As this long list demonstrates, the last decade has produced significant strides in evidencing rural women's lives and health needs. Existing research examines women's experiences of rural spaces (e.g., Little & Austin, 1996; see also Little, chapter 19 of this volume), rural women's health (e.g., Leipert & Reutter, 2005), women as health practitioners in rural places (e.g., Leipert, 1999), and geographies of rural mental health (e.g., Milligan, 1999; Parr, 2002; Wilson, 2003). However, while feminist research on spaces and practices of care (e.g., Bondi, 2009a; Dolan & Thien, 2008; Thien & Hanlon, 2009; and see Fiske et al., chapter 21 of this volume) comes closest, the particular dimensions of emotion as it relates to and illuminates gender and health in rural, isolated, or remote geographies have yet to be fully articulated. The few exceptions in health-related fields (e.g., Riddell, Ford-Gilboe, & Leipert, 2009; Wainer & Chesters, 2000) and in geographic research (Bondi, 2009a; Little, Panelli, & Kraack, 2005; Parr, Philo, & Burns, 2005; Thien, 2005b) lead the way to a specific and systematic attention to emotion in relation to rural women's health.

What does it mean to speak of the geographies of emotion? Emotion, by definition, *is* movement:

> A moving out, migration, transference from one place to another; a moving, stirring, agitation, perturbation (in physical sense); a political or social agitation; a tumult, popular disturbance; any agitation or disturbance of mind, feeling, passion; any vehement or excited mental state; a mental 'feeling' or 'affection' (e.g., of pleasure or pain, desire or aversion, surprise, hope or fear, etc.).(Oxford English Dictionary, 1989, s.v. 'emotion')

Emotion can be understood as a continual taking place of always dynamic, felt relations between bodies, places, events, things. Geographers Eric Laurier and Hester Parr (2000) argue: 'Emotions can be understood as complex manifestations of corporeal and psychological aspects of human beings which are simultaneously felt and performed as relations between self and world' (p. 98). These definitions, incorporating body and mind, self and external other, are indicative of important and recent shifts in thinking about emotion. Earlier studies of emotion were strongly influenced by Descartes' seventeenth-century metaphysical positing of a mind-body separation (Descartes, 1986). Within this oppositional binary framework, emotion was defined predominantly by its mutual exclusion with reason, leading to emotion's association with the body, not the mind, and its subsequent positioning as instinctive, not deliberative (Thien, 2011). These ideological divisions have been maintained by 'common-sense' gendered associations: between men, superior mental capacities, and reason, and between women, the disorderliness of embodiment, and emotion (Harding & Pribram, 2002; Lupton, 1998). Alison Jaggar (1989) argues that the circulation of these powerful discursive forces has invited subsequent undermining of both women and emotion, in a lineage of scientific reasoning that includes Descartes, Kant, and others. On the westernized socio-cultural map, emotion is found in the feminized 'realm of the personal' (Probyn, 2005, p. 135), while masculinist knowledges are valorized as central, normative, and authoritative. As a consequence, scholarship on emotion has been sidelined at best, and emotion often deliberately excluded from scholarly investigations in the name of scientific objectivity.

Yet, more and more it is apparent that 'our emotions *matter*,' as Liz Bondi and her colleagues note (Bondi, Davidson, & Smith, 2005, p. 1). Feminist geographers, invigorated by debates about health, caring, and daily life, have sought to offer new understandings of emotion's subjects and spaces (for two representative collections of this work, see Davidson, Bondi, & Smith, 2005; Smith, Davidson, Cameron, & Bondi, 2009a). Under the broad category of emotional geographies, this emerging research has encouraged a more nuanced consideration of the complex ways in which emotions and spaces are relationally constituted, seeking to 'understand how the world is mediated by feeling' (Thien, 2005a, p. 451); that is, to make sense of emotion as a way of being and knowing in the world (Bondi, 2005, 2009b; Davidson & Bondi, 2004).

What do geographies of emotion have to offer to rural women's health? As Leslie Kern (2012) argues: 'Emotions are ways of knowing, understanding and communicating with the world around us. They shape our choices and practices in complex interactions with social, cultural, economic and political factors' (p. 29). In this chapter, I argue that research into the complexities of this socio-spatial dynamic offers two major conceptual contributions invaluable for understanding and assessing the complexities of ge ndered realities, particular rural places, and diverse health circumstances.

The first contribution is to challenge the simplistic dualism of feminized emotion and masculine reason and thus to call into question the resulting, 'natural' division of gendered subjectivities and spaces for 'healing and feeling' (Milligan, Bingley, & Gatrell, 2005, p. 49). This conceptual shift makes space for rural places to be productively complicated instead of too simply drawn. This can be done effectively by contrasting discursive constructions of rural caring and support with empirical examples of localized rural realities (e.g., Parr et al., 2005; Thien, 2005b). That is, as is discussed further below, the very character of rural places as spaces where certain feelings (such as well-being or hardiness) are presumed can be assessed and evaluated through specific examples with demonstrated effects on rural women's health.

The second contribution is to dispel the mirage of a self-producing and self-narrating rational agent who propels (him)self unfettered through neoliberal space to a place of health and well-being. Instead, by foregrounding the emotional subject, I emphasize the co-constitution of identities and spaces, that is, I foreground the 'spatial imperative of subjectivities' (Probyn, 2003, p. 298); this in turn allows reflection on the implications of the 'feeling subject' (Thien, 2009a, p. 207), considered here in the context of gender and health. In other words, as I will describe in more detail below, women's specific and diverse rural health experiences can be more directly acknowledged through addressing the particular and emotional valences of health and well-being. The following two sections respectively explore these possibilities.

Locating Rural Feeling: Rural Spaces and Well Beings

Beginning with 'an imagination that is attuned to, rather than turned from, emotion' (Leathwood & Hey, 2009, p. 438), it is apparent that rurality poses challenges for women's health not least because of the way that rurality itself is ideologically or discursively constructed as a space for feeling. Rural spatial imaginaries range from the cosy corners of a dreamy idyll to the vastness of desolate scenes. The rural is, on one hand, a bucolic landscape potentially encompassing 'all health-enhancing beaches, mountains, mineral spas, forests, gardens and supportive communities' (Wainer & Chesters, 2000, p. 142); on the other hand, rural places may be spaces of 'rural hardship, deprivation, lack of services and physical and psychological dangers' (Wainer & Chesters, 2000, p. 143). Thus, on the side of rural benefits, geographer David Conradson (2005) reports the 'emotional gains' for those who experience the English rural as a therapeutic landscape (p. 37). But Poon and Saewyc (2009) report that British Columbia's rural areas 'are disadvantaged in employment rates, median incomes, and access to health care providers' (p. 122), and this leads to perceptions, if not experiences, of a lack of care in these rural places.

The intractability of *ideas* of rurality that hold sway across the geographies of many Western societies, whether positive or negative, can serve to mask the diverse experiences of rural places, with the results unevenly felt. For example, in rural places, the rigours of geographical distance from neighbours, services, and other amenities are often assumed to be accompanied by the benefits of neighbourliness (Parr, 2002). While the costs of traversing rural spaces may serve indeed to limit or restrict opportunities for health care, the presumed interpersonal proximity assumed to engender close and caring relations may not suffice to ameliorate such disadvantages, depending on where and how one is positioned in a rural emotional geography (Dolan & Thien, 2008, p. 39; Thien, 2005b). In other words, how rural places are constructed as spaces for feeling will differ according to the specificities of place. Drawing inspiration from Edward Casey, Thien and Hanlon (2009) explore how places can be understood as 'the spatial ordering and focusing of human intention, experience and behaviour' (p. 158). Rural communities will differ according to how they have come to be, including their emotional and cultural geographies; ties (past, present, future) with industry; variable economic contexts; and levels of participation. As this suggests, the complexity of factors underpinning a designation of 'rural' underscore the misleading simplicity of rurality as known and measurable place.

As one example, in Canada, an increasingly urbanized country since the Second World War, rural places have changed in dramatic if uneven ways, affected first by wartime industrialization, then the urban development and concentration of post-secondary education, followed by rapid professionalization (Cowen, 2008, p. 15). The resulting material changes to rural places further cemented rural imaginaries, positioning rural places as innocent retreats and simultaneously terrifyingly wild spaces, in contrast to urban scenes of sophistication and control.

Rendered discursively as simple and wild, rural places transmit strongly gendered signals with implications for health and well-being. Part of the notion of the rural 'simple life' is a valuing of 'patriarchal views of the family, including traditional roles about gender relations and gender inequality' (Riddell et al., 2009, p. 135). In a rural Australian study, the authors contend, 'traditional rural masculinity is associated with hardness and a taboo against seeking help with problems, leading to a reliance on women's skills in emotional work' (Wainer & Chesters, 2000, p. 144). In the Shetland Isles of northern Scotland, women describe their strategies for emotional well-being as shaped by a place that is characterized by its masculinist economy and the high premium placed on hard men, hard drinking, and imperviousness to the elements (Thien, 2005b). Other similar, but not identical, reports of gendered relations in rural places include mining communities in Australia (Gibson 1991) and military populations in England (Woodward 1998), where feelings are at least publicly limited and restricted in line with local expectations. In rural places, whether this evokes the simple pastoral or the fearsome wild, the very notion of rurality coupled with the conditions of non-urban life shape an emotional geography that locates emotion in feminized, private places. Unsurprisingly, such gendered characterizations of rural places and their projected capacities or limitations for feeling have differential effects on rural life.

Feeling Subjects: Gender, Care, and Rurality

Research has shown that women endure a 'double disadvantage' due to their gender and their rural situation (Chapman & Lloyd, 1996, p. 2). In the Western Isles of Scotland, research with female health workers indicated how 'the pressures of paid and home work demonstrate the lack of boundaries between the two. Women are expected to care for patients, relatives, friends and neighbours on a continuous basis' (McKie, 1996, p. 32). For those women who do health work professionally, the 'pressures of maintaining their professional and family caring role in remote and rural island communities can result in a range of social and psychological pressures' (McKie, 1996, p. 34; see also Leipert, 1999). For women with ill health who may need care giving, other pressures come to bear. Pini and Soldatic (chapter 20 of this volume) present a narrative of a rural Australian woman with chronic fatigue syndrome.

They argue that her illness disabled her expected performance as a caring/care-giving rural woman and mother. In this way, rurality is not only in and of itself cast as an emotionally charged geography, but also becomes an uneven and gendered arena for the performance of emotional competence, of emotional health or its lack.

Caring, a highly emotionally resonant symbolic and material practice, is most frequently embodied by women. In part, this is due to how people 'do gender,' and how 'we' do it differently through the enactment of multiple possible masculinities and femininities in our everyday practices, in our relations with others, in our use of language, and through our use of space (Dolan & Thien, 2008; Haraway, 1997, p. 28; Thien, 2009b, p. 72). Connell and Messerschmidt (2005) elaborate: 'Gender is always relational ... [for example,] patterns of masculinity are socially defined in contradistinction from some model (whether real or imaginary) of femininity' (p. 848). Such circulating normative models give shape to a collective reality, 'operat[ing] in the cultural domain as on-hand material to be actualized, altered or challenged through practice' (p. 849). As regards emotion, normative practices of gender locate femininity as emotional and masculinity as unfeeling. The material results include the feminization of care and care work with clear consequences for how women feel, especially for how women feel well.

While such gender-polarized scripts are not easily mapped onto individual women's or men's experiences, 'idealized expressions of masculinity and femininity contain strongly prescriptive notions of appropriate emotionality, developed through social, spatial and political means' (Thien, 2009a, p. 216; see also Lupton, 1998). We (differently) learn to read, interpret, and express emotion in relation to these gender-normative contexts; what may seem naturally occurring, 'seemingly instinctual,' can be instead understood as 'cultural achievement' (Sheller, 2004, p. 225). In our daily affairs, including negotiating health and well-being and navigating our particular positions in the world, we are all 'theorists of emotion' (Gobert, 2009, p. 73) making sense of these historical and cultural versions of emotion in embodied and relational ways (see Thien, 2011).

Gendered subjectivities are constituted in and through these sense-making processes: countless moments of differentiation and reification take place (Ng, 2000), such that, for example, women's domestic or caring work, whether paid or unpaid, is perceived as an extension of women's 'natural' feeling capacity. Furthermore, the busywork of these generative processes produces both material (witness low wages for

and long hours of care work) and symbolic devaluing of these feminized skills (read as naturally occurring instead of practiced) in contrast
to the valuing of men's productive labour (Dolan & Thien, 2008, p. 39).
In rural places, these 'care roles extend beyond the domestic and familial realm to include the reiteration of a feminized rural landscape contingent on the reproduction of neighbourliness and intergenerational
stability' (Dolan & Thien, 2008, p. 39; see also Thien, 2005c).

Scholarship on care, particularly feminist attention to the gendered
aspects of caring, has contributed significantly to formulating new on-
tological frameworks that regard care as a fundamental feature of social
relations; recognize care as a set of engaged relational processes; and
acknowledge difference in the (gendered) forms that care takes in particular social and spatial contexts (see Thien & Hanlon, 2009 for a brief
summary of this work). Fiske et al (chapter 21, this volume) argue for
positioning care giving as an act of citizenship. Focusing on volunteer
care giving, they note that carers practice their citizenship by gaining
access to the public sphere (traditionally a masculine sphere) and taking an active part in community decision making and leadership. Their
participants claimed the value of caring was in part the 'emotional attachment that bonded givers and recipients of care'; thus, they rejected
the notion that caring could be dismissed as 'unpaid labour' instead
arguing that such a designation did not adequately convey the depth of
meaning and emotional connection forged in the relational practices of
caring. Payne (2009) offers a counterpoint to this, critiquing an understanding of emotional labour as 'skilled' labour, and instead claiming
that such emotion work is ubiquitous. But, as Bondi (2008) argues,
while emotion work in caring may be widespread, it is both various
and complex in its manifestations: '[There is some emotional contact or
interaction] in many contexts in which people work and receive services, but many forms of care work involve unusually intimate and/or
sustained contact between those involved' (p. 259) Furthermore:

> Expertise in specific caring tasks may be essential, but in many instances
> the capacity to bear witness to suffering and to view the recipients of care
> as experts of their own experience are also of great importance in the pro-
> vision of care. This calls upon care-givers to consider their subjective posi-
> tioning relative to the recipients of their care, including how this positioning
> might be perceived and how it might feel to those involved. (p. 262)

In rural geographies, such understandings of care and of the emotional work involved are part of the daily formation and maintenance,

in conscious and unconscious ways, of strongly gendered emotional expectations, all of which shape the nature of women's experience (Dolan & Thien, 2008). No wonder, then, that rural care 'has the potential to oppress both carers and cared for' (Bondi, 2008, p. 250). In her examination of the development and delivery of rural counselling services in Scotland, Liz Bondi (2009a) notes of rural places: 'Intimate knowledge and close social connectedness is widely assumed to generate 'caring communities,' in which women in particular provide a plentiful supply of informal care and are swift to recognize care needs' (p. 164). Thus, the rural may be experienced as 'a specific space of power and oppression that is co-implicated with processes of gendering identity' (Dolan & Thien, 2008, p. 39).

Emotions have particular import when we consider that it is 'the repetition of gender relations that regulate[s] feminine subjectivity as women are related to, and relate to, themselves through such norms' (Fullagar, 2008, p. 37). The overdetermined 'nature' of woman as emotion(al) has writ women as expert navigators of emotional terrain, making an experientially and conceptually well-worn path for women to take care of others in spaces of health and heart. Men are encouraged, on the other hand, to 'display their masculinity in a form that includes physical prowess and avoidance of emotional expression' – a set of expectations that lead, among other outcomes, to violence against self and others (Benoit & Shumka, 2009, p. 8).

Arlie Hochschild (2003) understands this emotional theorization process as a series of 'feeling rules' in her feminist sociological exploration of 'emotional labour.' Drawing from the symbolic interactionism of Goffman, the psychological work of Freud, and extensive empirical research, she argues that people operationalize such rules, wherein cultural assessments of appropriate feeling are made, in conscious and unconscious ways to ensure we correctly manage feeling (pp. 56–7). In Hochschild's analysis, emotion management has particular gendered significance; she argues that women have developed their emotion management skills in exchange for economic security, performing affective labour in exchange for financial reward (p. 20). In this way, the assumption of emotion as inherently, naturally female is revealed instead as a play of power; 'woman' and 'emotion' are uncoupled and reconfigured.

While Hochschild's framing of emotional labour is undoubtedly important, this work can be further extended to consider the always spatial context of emotion and subjectivity. That is, as Elspeth Probyn (2003) argues, 'we experience our subjectivities, the ways in which we are positioned in regard to ourselves as subjects, in terms of both space and time … our bodies and our sense of ourselves are in constant inter-action with how and where we are placed' (p. 290). Such studies sug-gest the value of emotion as a means of articulating the complexity of identities and their social and spatial relations.

Simone Fullagar (2008), a sociologist who examines women's narra-tives of recovery from depression, argues that emotion serves as a means of 'questioning dominant models of subjectivity that privilege rationality, singularity, and psychological notions of inner truth' (p. 48; see also Thien, 2005b), while also playing a vital part in understanding depression in the context of social relationships. In her analysis of rural and urban Australian women, she concludes that such models of the self invite women to fashion themselves as 'weak,' 'emotional,' and 'de-pendent' in line with gendered discourses governing well-being (p. 38). In this self-governance of feeling, Fullagar's respondents are demon-strating they are emotionally 'civilized' (Lupton, 1998, p. 172). Deborah Lupton (1998) contends that a civilized emotional self is one 'cognizant of when it is appropriate to repress the expression of one's feelings and when it is appropriate to reveal them, and to act accordingly'; that is, such a self has the ability to recognize socially normative emotionality (p. 172).

As this discussion suggests, rural care is conceptualized in highly gendered ways. Yet, despite the 'crucial importance of relationships in all kinds of care,' it remains 'widely recognized but generally under-theorised' (Bondi, 2008, p. 251), not least in its emotional implications for different(ly) feeling subjects. In Wainer and Chesters' (2000) analy-sis of Australian rural places, they are alert to the consequences of shift-ing rural mores for men, who might be 'vulnerable to mental health problems due to changing cultural understandings of masculinity and femininity' (p. 143). In their study of partner support in colorectal can-cer, Emslie and colleagues (2009) analysed in-depth interviews with married or cohabiting respondents with colorectal cancer in the UK in order to compare men's and women's accounts of partner support. They found that gender-normative expectations about the performance of care, and indeed the emotionally laden expectations of care itself, were subject to debate: 'The simplistic notion that male caregiving can be equated to practical or instrumental care while female caregiving is emotional or expressive can be challenged' (p. 1174). In a related analy-sis, Cheryl Lousley (2009) offers an illuminating examination of rural masculinity and emotion vis-à-vis an investigation of Canadian literature. Her arguments suggest that hegemonic understandings of emotion that equate dexterity of emotional expression with women fail to recognize masculine forms of embodied emotionality. She argues: 'Masculinities should no longer be discussed in terms of a retreat from or restraint in emotion, but rather as particular articulations of emotion' (p. 230). In contrast to normative and gendered models of emotionality, she finds that 'emotional embodiment [is] central to constructions of masculine identity' as well as to what she characterizes as the 'imagining [of] moral lives in rural places' (p. 240). Similarly, research with Royal Canadian Legions, veterans' clubs devoted to memorializing wartime losses, in rural areas and small towns suggests that Legions offer counter-normative spaces for male feeling (Thien, 2009a). Clearly, considering gendered dimensions of emotion in rural places is important, in both material and ideological terms, and must be carefully examined through ongoing thoughtful empirical research.

Reframing emotion as both 'individually lived' and 'socially derived through relationships with others within specific structural conditions' such as those of the rural locale (Philipose, 2007, p. 63) and in specific spaces encourages a more nuanced consideration of complex ways in which emotions and spaces are relationally constituted, which in turn offers new purchase on women's health experiences and understandings. From this perspective, the subject is always in motion; the emotional self or feeling subject is ever forming, not in a time-space vacuum but always becoming intelligible synchronously with places and objects encountered. Consequently, constellations of individuals, their feelings, and the places of or for feeling can be assessed as distinctly, if not always collaboratively, or self-consciously constituting the dynamic processes of feeling subjects (Thien, 2009a). This conceptual consideration of the feeling subject has been given empirical grounding through ethnographic and geographic explorations of emotion-laden experience, from agoraphobia (Davidson, 2000, 2001), obsessive-compulsive disorder (Segrott & Doel, 2004), and delusion (Parr, 1999), to emotional well-being (Thien, 2005b). Collectively, this work highlights the ways in which the feeling subject is neither body nor mind, but rather a mobile force blurring bodily and psychic boundaries.

In Joyce Davidson's (2000) work, for example, she posits agoraphobia as fundamentally a 'gender-specific boundary problem' (p. 38) wherein women feel insecurely bounded and require external devices (a hat, a home) to feel self-contained. Davidson suggests that women's agoraphobic experience 'disturbs taken-for-granted understandings of self as securely, straightforwardly bounded' (p. 31). In an examination of emotional well-being in Shetland's North Sea island communities, women's narratives of intimacy also highlighted the permeability of boundaries, between, for example, their senses of public and private selves in socially proximate rural societies (Thien, 2005b). These local accounts of managing interpersonal intimacy (such as dating, friendship, or divorce) demonstrated that overlapping and dynamic personal and community spaces of intimacy have varying effects on people's sense of emotional well-being, often in highly gendered terms. As Elspeth Probyn (2003) has argued, 'thinking about subjectivity in terms of space of necessity reworks any conception that subjectivity is hidden away in private recesses' (p. 290). We are, feeling subjects are, a communal affair. Emotional geographies offer this explicit consideration and thus reworking of the subject of gendered and health discourses as a profoundly *feeling* subject.

Implications

> Emotions are vital (living) aspects of who we are and of our situational engagement within the world; they compose, decompose, and recompose the geographies of our lives. (Smith, Davidson, Cameron, & Bondi, 2009b, p. 10)

In this chapter, I have drawn on emotional geographies and other research to raise conceptual issues about emotion with material and theoretical implications for rural women's health research. I have suggested that a more explicit attention to emotion works to challenge foundational binaries (male/female, emotion/reason) that bedevil the practices, experiences, and analyses of rural women's health and well-being. In deliberately stretching these naturalized divisions, flexible and dynamic gendered subjectivities, or 'feeling subjects' (Thien, 2009a, p. 207), can make new sense of the spatialities of emotion. Additionally, exploring the gendered geographies of rurality allows rural spaces for health to be productively complicated by exposing the gendered and emotionally laden underpinnings of rural discourse, as well as by examining empirically detailed research in rural places.

The emotional geographies framework I put forward, then, extends a series of poststructuralist challenges to the historically configured masculine rationality of science by emphasizing the spatial contexts of persistent and pernicious alliances that have dismissed women as emotional, their caring skills as obligatory nature, and their own health as of only tangential importance. By placing emotion in the foreground of critical thought, emotional geographies and other research on emotion seek to challenge the notion of emotion as naturally feminized, naturally caring, and instead to explore the cultural fabric of daily emotional practice.

An emphasis on emotion gives insight not only into diverse rural experiences, but also into their socio-spatial and socio-political contexts. Feminist scholar Liz Philipose, in her examination of pain in lived experiences of global politics, draws on the work of Frantz Fanon and others to locate emotion in the 'colonial present' (Gregory, 2004, p. xv) and to consider how emotion is not only gendered but also racialized. She argues that emotion offers a key moment of departure for transforming experiences from marginalized to meaning-full: 'Without highlighting the emotions of political actors, the import of political claims is often unrecognizable. Further, the subjectivity of political actors is denied when we make pain and emotion marginal to the work of political transformation' (Philipose, 2007, p. 64). In contrast, then, to the ideologically inferior status of emotion and the subsequently marginalized gendered and racialized feeling subjects, emotion can be seen as having a vital role in highlighting an overarching claim to human well-being. Set in the dynamic relations of the rural, wherein gendered and spatial fortunes are inextricably interwoven, this move also goes someway (somewhere) towards (re)claiming rural places as sites of and for women's health and wellness.

Considering the emotional geographies of rural places offers a means to consider 'other' relational aspects of subjectivity in relation to, not in isolation from, gender. As Keith Halfacree (2007) notes, 'the rural [is] much more heterotopic than is often appreciated' (p. 99), or indeed even acknowledged. Geographer Deborah Cowen (2008) argues of the Canadian landscape: 'Ideologies of the rural have served to deny both urban images of national identity and Aboriginal presence on the land in favour of images of "empty" landscape open for European settlement or solitude' (p. 192). In this context, the paucity of geographical health research in the area of indigenous well-being is unsurprising. Kathleen Wilson (2003) writes into this erasure via her spatial analysis of the health and well-being of an Anishinabek (Ojibway and Odawa) community in northern Ontario, Canada. Findings from her in-depth interview-based research into the cultural beliefs systems of these indigenous peoples (including their identification of emotional healing associated with the land) suggest that further analyses must 'acknowledge diversity, difference and the existence of multiple identities and their role in shaping health' (p. 85). Wainer and Chesters (2000) also emphasize the significance of affective consequences of land and loss of land for indigenous Australians: 'The dispossession and violence done to Aboriginal people since European invasion/settlement has had a strong adverse effect on [their] mental health in rural places' (p. 143). For such marginalized populations, place and the associated complex nuances of diverse feeling subjects are a crucial consideration in striving towards improved emotional health and well-being.

Conclusion

In this chapter, I have argued that not only is emotion a valuable consideration in an assessment of rural health and gender, but also that an emphasis on emotion can function to illuminate anew the intricate interplay of gender, rurality, and health. For people in rural places, distinctions of health and well-being may be unevenly felt by differently feeling subjects in ways that belie the normative discourses of rurality. Considering gender, rurality, and health in the relational framework of emotional geographies offers insights for how researchers can further develop rural women's health and gender studies. Placing emotion in gender, rural, and health research ultimately offers another perspective from which to strive for enhanced rural health and well-being across a diversity of gendered rural experiences. As Fullagar (2008) puts it: 'Understanding what constitutes a more liveable life for different women is a socio-political issue' (p. 35). Rather than being problematic, the resulting complexity invites inclusive, wide-ranging, and creative approaches for assessing, theorizing, and improving rural women's health.

References

Benoit, C., & Shumka, L. (2009). *Gendering the health determinants framework: Why girls' and women's health matters.* Vancouver: Women's Health Research Network.

Bondi, L. (2005). Making connections and thinking through emotions: Between geography and psychotherapy. *Transactions of the Institute of British Geographers, 30*(4), 433–48.

Bondi, L. (2008). On the relational dynamics of caring: A psychotherapeutic approach to emotional and power dimensions of women's care work. *Gender, Place and Culture, 15*(3), 249–65.

Bondi, L. (2009a). Counselling in rural Scotland: Care, proximity and trust. *Gender, Place and Culture, 16*(2), 163–79.

Bondi, L. (Ed.). (2009b). *The international encyclopedia of human geography.* London: Elsevier.

Bondi, L., Davidson, J., & Smith, M. (2005). Introduction: Geography's emotional turn. In J. Davidson, L. Bondi, & M. Smith (Eds.), *Emotional geographies* (pp. 1–16). Aldershot, UK: Ashgate.

Chapman, P., & Lloyd, S. (1996). *Women and access in rural areas: What makes the difference? What difference does it make?* Aldershot, UK: Avebury.

Connell, R.W., & Messerschmidt, J.W. (2005). Hegemonic masculinity: Rethinking the concept. *Gender & Society, 19*(6), 829–59.

Conradson, D. (2005). Landscape, care and the relational self: Therapeutic encounters in rural England. *Health & Place, 11*(4), 337–48.

Cowen, D. 2009. *Military workfare: The soldier and social citizenship in Canada.* Toronto: University of Toronto Press.

Davidson, J. (2000). '… the world was getting smaller': Women, agoraphobia and bodily boundaries. *Area, 32*(1), 31–40.

Davidson, J. (2001). *Agoraphobic geographies: An exploration of subjectivity and socio-spatial anxiety.* Unpublished doctoral diss., University of Edinburgh.

Davidson, J., & Bondi, L. (2004). Spatialising affect; affecting space: An introduction. *Gender, Place and Culture, 11*(3), 373–4.

Davidson, J., Bondi, L., & Smith, M. (Eds.). (2005). *Emotional geographies.* Aldershot, UK: Ashgate.

Descartes, R. (1986). *Meditations on first philosophy: With selections from the Objections and Replies,* trans. & ed. J. Cottingham. Cambridge: Cambridge University Press.

Dolan, H., & Thien, D. (2008). Relations of care: A framework for placing women and health in rural communities. *Canadian Journal of Public Health, 99,* S38–S42.

Emslie, C., Browne, S., MacLeod, U., Rozmovits, L., Mitchell, E., & Ziebland, S. (2009). 'Getting through' not 'going under': A qualitative study of gender and spousal support after diagnosis with colorectal cancer. *Social Science & Medicine, 68*(6), 1169–75.

Fullagar, S. (2008). Leisure practices as counter-depressants: Emotion-work and emotion-play within women's recovery from depression. *Leisure Sciences, 30*(1), 35–52.

Gibson, K. (1991). Company towns and class processes: A study of the coal towns of Central Queensland. *Environment and Planning D: Society and Space, 9*, 285–308.

Gobert, R.D. (2009). Historicizing emotion: The case of Freudian hysteria and Aristotelian 'purgation.' In M. Smith, J. Davidson, L. Cameron, & L. Bondi (Eds.), *Emotion, place and culture* (pp. 59–76). Aldershot, UK: Ashgate.

Gregory, D. (2004). *The colonial present: Afghanistan, Palestine, Iraq.* Malden, MA: Blackwell.

Halfacree, K. (2007). Still surprises in store: Revisiting the ordinary in rural geography. *Documents d'Anàlisi Geogràfica, 50,* 87–103.

Haraway, D.J. (1997). *Modest_ Witness@Second_ Millennium.FemaleMan_ Meets_ OncoMouse: Feminism and technoscience.* New York/London: Routledge.

Harding, J., & Pribram, E.D. (2002). The power of feeling: Locating emotions in culture. *European Journal of Cultural Studies, 5*(4), 407–26.

Hochschild, A.R. (2003). *The managed heart: Commercialization of human feeling.* Berkeley, CA: University of California Press.

Jaggar, A.M. (1989). Love and knowledge: Emotion in feminist epistemology. *Inquiry: An Interdisciplinary Journal of Philosophy, 32*(2), 151–76.

Janzen, B.L. (1998). *Women, gender & health: A review of the recent literature.* Winnipeg: Prairie Women's Health Centre of Excellence.

Kern, L. (2012). Connecting embodiment, emotion and gentrification: An exploration through the practice of yoga in Toronto. *Emotion, Space and Society, 5*(1), 27–35.

Laurier, E., & Parr, H. (2000). Emotions and interviewing in health and disability research. *Ethics, Place and Environment, 3*(1), 98–102.

Leathwood, C., & Hey, V. (2009). Gender/ed discourses and emotional subtexts: Theorising emotion in UK higher education. *Teaching in Higher Education, 14*(4), 429–40.

Leipert, B.D. (1999). Women's health and the practice of public health nurses in northern British Columbia. *Public Health Nursing, 16*(4), 280–9.

Leipert, B.D., Matsui, D., & Rieder, M.J. (2006). Women and pharmacologic therapy in rural and remote Canada. *Canadian Journal of Rural Medicine, 11*(4), 296–300.

Leipert, B.D., & Reutter, L. (2005). Developing resilience: How women maintain their health in northern geographically isolated settings. *Qualitative Health Research, 15*(1), 49–65.

Little, J., & Austin, P. (1996). Women and the rural idyll. *Journal of Rural Studies, 12*(2), 101–12.

Little, J., Panelli, R., & Kraack, A. (2005). Women's fear of crime: A rural perspective. *Journal of Rural Studies, 21*(2), 151–63.

Lousley, C. (2009). 'I love the goddamn river': Masculinity, emotion and ethics of place. In M. Smith, J. Davidson, L. Cameron, & L. Bondi (Eds.), *Emotion, place and culture* (pp. 227–43). Aldershot, UK: Ashgate.

Lupton, D. (1998). *The emotional self: A sociocultural exploration.* London: Sage.

McKie, L. (1996). Women, health and health work in island communities. In P. Chapman & S. Lloyd (Eds.), *Women and access in rural areas: What makes the difference? What difference does it make?* (pp. 32–44). Aldershot, UK: Avebury.

Milligan, C. (1999). Without these walls: A geography of mental ill-health in a rural environment. In R. Butler & H. Parr (Eds.), *Mind and body spaces: Geographies of illness, impairment and disability* (pp. 221–39). London: Routledge.

Milligan, C., Bingley, A., & Gatrell, A. (2005). 'Healing and feeling': The place of emotions in later life. In J. Davidson, L. Bondi, & M. Smith (Eds.), *Emotional geographies* (pp. 49–62). Aldershot, UK: Ashgate.

Ng, R. (2000). Restructuring gender, race, and class relations: The case of garment workers and labour adjustment. In S. Neysmith (Ed.), *Restructuring caring labour: Discourse, state, practice, and everyday life* (pp. 226–45). Toronto: Oxford University Press.

Oxford English Dictionary. (1989). 2nd ed. (online). Retrieved from http://oed.com:80/Entry/61249.

Parr, H. (1999). Delusional geographies: The experiential worlds of people during madness/illness. *Environment and Planning D: Society & Space, 17*(6), 673–90.

Parr, H. (2002, March). *Rural madness: Culture, society and space in rural geographies of mental health.* Paper presented at the annual meeting of the Association of American Geographers, Los Angeles, CA.

Parr, H., Philo, C., & Burns, N. (2005). 'Not a display of emotions': Emotional geographies in the Scottish highlands. In J. Davidson, L. Bondi, & M. Smith (Eds.), *Emotional geographies* (pp. 87–102). Aldershot, UK: Ashgate.

Payne, J. (2009). Emotional labour and skill: A reappraisal. *Gender, Work & Organization, 16*(3), 348–67.

Philipose, L. (2007). The politics of pain and the end of empire. *International Feminist Journal of Politics, 9*(1), 60–81.

Poon, C.S., & Saewyc, E.M. (2009). Out yonder: Sexual-minority adolescents in rural communities in British Columbia. *American Journal of Public Health, 99*(1), 118–24.

Probyn, E. (2003). The spatial imperative of subjectivity. In K. Anderson (Ed.), *Handbook of cultural geography* (pp. 290–9). London: Sage.

Probyn, E. (2005). *Blush: Faces of shame.* Minneapolis, MN: University of Minnesota Press.

Riddell, T., Ford-Gilboe, M., & Leipert, B.D. (2009). Strategies used by rural women to stop, avoid, or escape from intimate partner violence. *Health Care for Women International, 30*(1–2), 134–59.

Segrott, J., & Doel, M.A. (2004). Disturbing geography: Obsessive-compulsive disorder as spatial practice. *Social & Cultural Geography, 5*(4), 597–614.

Sheller, M. (2004). Automotive emotions: Feeling the car. *Theory Culture & Society, 21*(4–5): 221–42.

Smith, M., Davidson, J., Cameron, L., & Bondi, L. (2009a). *Emotion, place and culture.* Aldershot, UK: Ashgate.

Smith, M., Davidson, J., Cameron, L., & Bondi, L. (2009b). Introduction: Geography and emotion – emerging constellations. In M. Smith, J. Davidson, L. Cameron, & L. Bondi (Eds.), *Emotion, place and culture* (pp. 1–18). Aldershot, UK: Ashgate.

Thien, D. (2005a). After or beyond feeling?: A consideration of affect and emotion in geography. *Area, 37*(4), 450–6.

Thien, D. (2005b). Intimate distances: Considering questions of 'us.' In J. Davidson, L. Bondi, & M. Smith (Eds.), *Emotional geographies* (pp. 191–204). Aldershot, UK: Ashgate.

Thien, D. (2005c). Recasting the pattern: Critical relations in gender and rurality. In J. Little & C. Morris (Eds.), *Critical studies in rural gender issues* (pp. 75–89). Aldershot, UK: Ashgate.

Thien, D. (2009a). Death and bingo? The Royal Canadian Legion's unexpected spaces of emotion. In M. Smith, J. Davidson, L. Cameron, & L. Bondi (Eds.), *Emotion, place and culture* (pp. 207–25). Aldershot, UK: Ashgate.

Thien, D. (2009b). Feminist methodologies. In R. Kitchin & N. Thrift (Eds.), *International encyclopedia of human geography* (vol. 4, pp. 71–8). London: Elsevier.

Thien, D. (2011). Emotional life. In V.J. Del Casino, Jr., M. Thomas, R. Panelli, & P. Cloke (Eds.), *A Companion to Social Geography* (309–25). Wiley-Blackwell.

Thien, D., & Hanlon, N. (2009). Unfolding dialogues about gender, care and 'The North': An introduction. *Gender, Place and Culture, 16*(2), 155–62.

Wainer, J., & Chesters, J. (2000). Rural mental health: Neither romanticism nor despair. *Australian Journal of Rural Health, 8*(3), 141–7.

Williams, S.J. (2009). The 'neurosociology' of emotion? Progress, problems and prospects. In D. Hopkins, H. Kuzmics, H. Flam, & J. Kleres (Eds.), *Theorizing emotions: Sociological explorations and applications* (pp. 245–67). Chicago: Campus Verlag, University of Chicago Press.

Wilson, K. (2003). Therapeutic landscapes and First Nations peoples: An exploration of culture, health and place. *Health and Place, 9*(2), 83–93.

Woodward, R. (1998). 'It's a man's life!': Soldiers, masculinity and the countryside. *Gender, Place and Culture, 5*(3), 277–300.

Contributors

Natalie Beausoleil is an associate professor of social sciences and health in the Division of Community Health and Humanities, Faculty of Medicine, Memorial University. She earned her MA and PhD in sociology from the University of California in Los Angeles (UCLA). Informed by feminist and critical perspectives, she has done extensive research in the area of body and health in contemporary Western society, in the fields of health promotion and the prevention of disordered eating and eating disorders. Her research focuses on the experiences and meanings of the body, health, and fitness for women and youth. She has recently written about the dominant discourses of health and beauty conveyed by health professionals, educators, and policy makers. Dr Beausoleil is part of an international network of critical obesity scholars. She is also a visual artist and researcher on arts and health.

Matthias Beck is professor of public sector management at Queen's University Belfast. His main research interests are risk management and risk regulation with a particular focus on the public sector, public-private partnerships, and state-business relationships in transitional and developed economies. He was the principal investigator of a National Institute for Health Research (NHS) Service Delivery and Organization program report entitled *The Role and Effectiveness of Public-Private Partnerships (NHS LIFT) in the Development of Enhanced Primary Care Premises and Services.* He is the editor of the *Journal of Risk and Governance* and is on the editorial boards of the *International Journal of Public Sector Management, Policy and Practice in Health and Safety,* and *Work, Employment and Society.*

Rachel Rapaport Beck is a policy analyst with the College of Midwives of Ontario. She has worked for over fifteen years in women's health with a focus on maternity care. Previously, she was a research and policy associate at Prairie Women's Health Centre of Excellence.

Wanda Thomas Bernard is a professor with the Dalhousie University School of Social Work. Her research with black men and the violence of racism has had significant impact not only on academic work but also on agency and community-based practice. She has made major academic and professional contributions to the field of black masculinity, to the investigation of black women's health and well-being, and to an Africentric understanding of the strengths of black families, including black men's experience of mothering. She has received numerous awards and certificates and much recognition over the years for her trendsetting work, including the Order of Canada Award in 2005.

James Brophy is an adjunct assistant professor with the Department of Sociology, Anthropology and Criminology at the University of Windsor and is affiliated with the University of Stirling and the University of York. He earned his PhD from the University of Stirling. He worked for eighteen years as a director for the Occupational Health Clinics for Ontario Workers. He is currently employed by the National Network on Environments and Women's Health at York University; and his current research focus is occupational and environmental risk factors for breast cancer. He is an international board member for *New Solutions: a Journal of Environmental and Occupational Health Policy* and an editorial board member for the *Journal of Risk and Governance*. He has co-authored, along with Margaret Keith and others, two books: *Workplace Roulette: Gambling with Cancer* and *Barefoot Research: A Worker's Manual for Organizing On Work Security.*

Angeline Bushy holds a BSN degree from the University of Mary in Bismarck, North Dakota; an MSN degree in rural community health nursing from Montana State University in Bozeman; an MEd in adult education from Northern Montana College in Havre; and a PhD in nursing from the University of Texas at Austin. She is a fellow in the American Academy of Nursing and a clinical specialist in public health nursing. She has worked in rural facilities located in the north-central and intermountain states; presented nationally and internationally on various rural nursing and rural health issues; published six textbooks and numerous articles on that topic; and is a lieutenant colonel (ret.) in the US Army Reserve.

Anne Burrill has a graduate degree from the University of Northern BC. She is a social planner with the City of Williams Lake and a sessional instructor with the School of Social Work at the University of Northern BC. Her research interests are in the fields of community development, social policy, women's issues, and women's care giving.

Barbara Clow is executive director of the Atlantic Centre of Excellence for Women's Health, Halifax, and associate professor research in the Faculty of Health Professions at Dalhousie University. She has a PhD in the history of medicine from the University of Toronto and has presented and published on various dimensions of the history of health and healing, including the history of cancer, alternative medicine, and thalidomide. In the past ten years, she has pursued a program of research and publication on diverse aspects of women's health, including the gendered dimensions of health care reform in Canada, the implications of public policy discourse for the health and well-being of women in Canada, the social determinants of African Canadian women's health, the role of gender in the HIV/AIDS pandemic, and the impact of women's unpaid care-giving work.

Jennifer Cross is an instructor in the University of Alberta Collaborative BScN Program at Red Deer College in Alberta, and holds a master's degree in nursing. She has conducted qualitative research about farming women's perceptions of their health in relation to their work and in relation to work restructuring. Areas of teaching and interest include population health, community development, mental health, and the health of vulnerable populations in rural and urban contexts.

Rick Csiernik is professor, School of Social Work, King's University College at the University of Western Ontario. He has written and edited 8 books, authored over 100 peer reviewed articles and book chapters and has been an invited presenter to over 150 national and international conferences and workshops. He has been on the King's University College Honor Role of teaching eleven consecutive times and is past recipient of the McMaster University Instructor Appreciation award.

Ewa Dabrowska is lecturer in the Department of Health Studies and Contemporary Studies at Laurier Brantford, where she teaches courses in human geography. She holds a PhD in geography from Wilfrid Laurier University and an MSc from Jagiellonion University, Krakow. Her research and teaching interests are engaged with the study of social and cultural landscapes of rural communities, social vulnerability, and global environmental change. Using philosophy of inclusion, she explores issues relevant to the health needs and capacities of vulnerable populations. She has published articles on ethnicity, inclusivity, and environmental risk in Ontario Mennonite communities.

Karen Dyck has provided psychological services to rural and northern Manitoba communities for over fifteen years and is the founding chair of the Rural and Northern Psychology Section with the Canadian Psychological Association. She is an associate professor and the director of the Rural and Northern Psychology Program in the Department of Clinical Health Psychology, Faculty of Medicine, at the University of Manitoba. Within this role she provides a range of clinical services and is also involved in program development and evaluation, research, and educational presentations. She is also actively involved in the training and supervision of practicum students, pre- and post-doctoral residents, and new faculty within the Rural and Northern Psychology Programme.

Josephine Etowa is an associate professor and the Loyer Da Silva Research Chair in Public Health Nursing at the University of Ottawa, and a founding member and past president of the Health Association of African Canadians. As a nurse, midwife, lactation consultant, researcher, and educator, she has worked in various capacities within the Canadian health care system and abroad. Her research is grounded in over twenty-four years of clinical practice in the area of maternal-child and public health nursing. Her research is in the area of inequity in health and health care with a particular focus on the health of visible minority women. She has published extensively and is co-author of *Anti-racist Health Care Practice* (2009). Dr Etowa's distinguished contributions have been recognized with a number of awards, including the Atlantic Centre of Excellence for Women's Health (ACEWH) Leadership Award 2006 and the College of Registered Nurses of Nova Scotia (CRNNS) Centennial Award of Distinction (2009).

Jo-Anne Fiske is a professor of women's studies and dean, School of Graduate Studies at the University of Lethbridge. Trained in medical and legal anthropology, she devotes her research to addressing issues of the state, social inequities, and social policy. Her research focuses on feminist political economy and feminist anthropology with special attention to Aboriginal women's health and legal status, rural women and care giving, and structures of marginalization. She has published in numerous journals, including *Feminist Studies, Atlantis, BC Studies,* the *American Indian Research and Culture Journal,* and the *Journal of Legal Pluralism.* She is a member of the National Network of Aboriginal Mental Health Research and serves on the board of the British Columbia Center of Excellence for Women's Health. She is currently working on projects related to homelessness, health and citizenship, and gambling cultures of rural communities.

Amber Fletcher is a Ph.D. candidate at the University of Regina. She holds a BA honours degree in women's studies from the University of Regina and a master of arts in women's studies from York University in Toronto. Her interdisciplinary research combines women's and gender studies with political sociology to understand how Saskatchewan farm women are affected by, and respond to, major changes in agricultural policy and climate. Her doctoral research is supported by a Joseph-Armand Bombardier Canada Graduate Scholarship from the Social Sciences and Humanities Research Council (SSHRC) and a PEO International Scholar Award. In 2011 she received the Governor General's Award in Commemoration of the Persons Case for her work on gender equality issues. She grew up on a farm near Kelvington, Saskatchewan.

Cheryl Forchuk is associate director, Nursing Research, Arthur Labatt Family School of Nursing, and professor, Department of Psychiatry at the University of Western Ontario. She is an assistant director of the Lawson Health Research Institute, the research arm of the London hospitals. She received her bachelor of science in nursing and bachelor of arts in psychology from the University of Windsor; her master of science in nursing from the University of Toronto with a clinical specialty in mental health; and her PhD from the College of Nursing at Wayne State, Detroit, Michigan. Her research explores issues related to mental health and mental illness, including therapeutic relationships, interprofessional education, housing/homelessness issues, poverty, and the transition from hospital to community.

Nikki Gerrard is a community psychologist who recently retired from being coordinator of the Rural Quality of Life Program, Adult Community Mental Health and Addiction Services, Saskatoon Health Region. She is an adjunct professor in the Department of Community Health and Epidemiology, College of Medicine, University of Saskatchewan. She sees individual clients in private practice and, as a community psychologist, is also interested in the psyche of the community and spends a lot of her time developing community strengths, through community development, education, research, and organizing. She worked with rural people doing farm stress work for eleven and a half years. Her research interests include racism and sexism, together, in mental health systems, resiliency in rural people, and women's psychology.

Michael Gilbertson earned his master of science degree in ecology from Queens University in Belfast and his PhD from the University of Stirling. As a biologist, his career included research into the injurious effects of persistent toxic substances on the health of fish, wildlife, and humans, which he has studied in relation to the United States–Canada Great Lakes Water Quality Agreement. He has published widely in scientific journals and government documents.

Carolyne Gorlick is an associate professor of social policy, School of Social Work, King's University College at the University of Western Ontario. Her research has focused on low-income women and their children moving together on a path framed by risk, endurance, hope, and transitions. Specifically, this involved a longitudinal study of low-income single mothers and their children, a national study of Welfare to Work programs in Canada, and a CURA research project on housing and homelessness, all funded primarily by Social Sciences and Humanities Research Council of Canada (SSHRC) or Health and Welfare Canada. Special funding awards received include SSHRC/Therese F. Casgrain Fellowship on Women and Social Policy and SSHRC/Special Postdoctoral Fellowship on Urban Poverty.

Cindy Hardy is an associate professor in the Department of Psychology at the University of Northern British Columbia and a registered clinical psychologist specializing in child, youth, and family mental health. Her current projects are focused on knowledge translation as a strategy for advancing and supporting the work of child and family practitioners in rural and northern British Columbia and on evaluation of demonstration projects designed to support children and families affected by fetal alcohol spectrum disorders. Dr Hardy teaches undergraduate and graduate courses in psychopathology, clinical psychology, and professional ethics.

Joanne Havelock is originally from Winnipeg, Manitoba, and currently resides in Regina, Saskatchewan. She has over two decades' experience as a policy analyst with the provincial government in the areas of health, environment, and the status of women. Her work in policy analysis and communications with Prairie Women's Health Centre of Excellence included conducting gender-based analysis, coordinating the Rural Women's Issues Committee of Saskatchewan and the Regina Photovoice project, and collaborating in research and recommendations concerning the implementation of midwifery. Currently she is engaged as a consultant and planner related to women's issues, health, poverty, community development, and the environment. She is one of the founders of the Women's Information Network of Saskatchewan.

Margaret Haworth-Brockman is executive director of Prairie Women's Health Centre of Excellence, where she leads a program of research, policy advice, and communications. She was co-leader of a national project exploring rural women's health issues in Canada, and has been engaged in community activities and research projects about rural women ever since. Other key areas of research include issues related to Aboriginal women's health, gender in health planning, and women's health indicators. She is an adjunct professor at the University of Winnipeg, a member of Women and Health Care Reform, and a student in Community Health Sciences at the University of Manitoba.

Barbara M. Heather teaches in the Department of Sociology, Grant MacEwan University. Her current research projects include stress and gender in farm families, and the experience of migrant university students. She is co-author of 'Women's Identities and the Restructuring of Rural Alberta' (*Sociologia Ruralis*, April 2005) and 'Reflections of Rural Alberta Women: Work, Health and Restructuring' (in P.Van Esterik, ed., *Head, Heart and Hand: Partnerships for Women's Health in Canadian Environments*, 2005). She has given conference presentations on rural issues at the annual meetings of Canadian Sociology Association, Western Social Sciences Association.

Dawn Hemingway has been a resident and activist in northern British Columbia for more than seventeen years. She is associate professor and chair of the School of Social Work at the University of Northern British Columbia (UNBC) and adjunct professor in community health sciences and gender studies. Her teaching/research interests include northern/rural community–based research, organizing, and policy development; northern/rural health/quality of life, particularly women's health and aging issues. Dawn is a director with Women North Network/Northern FIRE: The Centre for Women's Health Research at UNBC and plays a leadership role in a variety of local and regional organizations, including Stand Up for the North, Northern Women's Forum, and Active Voice Coalition. In recognition of her work, Dawn has received the Northern BC Today's Woman: Leader in Knowledge Advancement and Forging our Future with Education Awards, the Bridget Moran Advancement of Social Work in Northern Communities Award, and the Canadian Association of Social Workers 2009 Distinguished Service Award.

Beverly Illauq is the mother of an Inuit family and was the founding coordinator and director of Ilisaqsivik Family Resource Centre, in Clyde River, Baffin Region, Nunavut. Working first as a teacher and wellness coordinator with First Nations and Inuit students in community schools in northern Quebec and the Northwest Territories (Nunavut), she became more fully engaged in community development and healing projects in response to meeting the wellness needs of her own community. She remains committed to Aboriginal healing issues and initiatives, particularly in the areas of trauma recovery and the development of cultural competence.

Harpa Isfeld is a senior researcher with Prairie Women's Health Centre of Excellence, whose recent work has focused on the application of gender-based analysis to indicators of women's health, which contributed to the development of *A Profile of Women's Health in Manitoba* and to training resources delivered to health planning and programming staff in several rural (and urban) health regions throughout Manitoba. She holds a master of arts degree with specialization in medical anthropology and has mainly worked in applied, community-based research and social policy development settings. Her areas of research have included capacity-building approaches to chronic disease prevention in low-income neighbourhoods, participatory research supporting return-to-work and adjustment by farmers with a disability, and the relationship between social inclusion and the health of children and families living in poverty.

Noreen Johns farms with her family near the community of Zelma, Saskatchewan. She has long been an activist on behalf of agriculture and rural community. Over the years Noreen has served on several health-related boards, including the Provincial Health Council, Saskatchewan

Health Information Network (SHIN), District 4 Saskatoon Health Region Advisory Network, Agriculture Health and Safety Network, and the Heart and Stroke Foundation of Saskatchewan, and was the Saskatchewan representative to the Heart and Stroke Foundation of Canada. She is currently a board member of Prairie Women's Health Centre of Excellence.

Barb Keith, MSW, RSW, is a clinical supervisor for Addiction Services at Vancouver Coastal Health, and has been a part-time instructor at the University of Northern British Columbia. Previously she lived for twenty-six years in the North, working primarily with substance-using women and Aboriginal populations. Her research background (mainly institutional ethnography) includes health care and access, substance use and problem gambling, and the rural/urban divide.

Margaret Keith is an adjunct assistant professor with the Department of Sociology, Anthropology and Criminology at the University of Windsor and is affiliated with the University of Stirling and the University of York. She earned her PhD from the University of Stirling. She has advanced the use of mapping techniques for conducting qualitative research and has co-authored several journal articles describing their applications. Her current research focus is on occupational and environmental risk factors for breast cancer. She is currently employed by the National Network on Environments and Women's Health at York University. She is an international board member for *New Solutions: A Journal of Environmental and Occupational Health Policy* and an editorial board member for the *Journal of Risk and Governance*. She co-authored, along with James Brophy and others, two books: *Workplace Roulette: Gambling with Cancer* and *Barefoot Research: A Worker's Manual for Organizing On Work Security.*

Wendee Kubik is an associate professor of women's and gender studies at Brock University. Her master's degree focused on farm stress in Saskatchewan and her PhD on the changing roles of farm women and the consequences for their health, well-being, and quality of life. Recent publications include *Torn from Our Midst: Voices of Grief, Healing and Action from the Missing Indigenous Women's Conference, 2008*, edited with Brenda Anderson and Mary Hampton; and *Rural Communities Adapting to Climate-Induced Water Stress*, edited with Darrell Corkal, Alejandro Rojas, and David Sauchyn. Her recent research includes a five-year project funded from the SSHRC Community-University

Research Alliance program (CURA) entitled "Rural and Northern Response to Intimate Partner Violence" on behalf of the RESOLVE (Research and Education for Solutions to Violence and Abuse) Tri-provincial Research Network.

Tamara Landry is a PhD candidate in health and rehabilitation sciences, health promotion field, in the Faculty of Health Sciences at Western University. Tamara completed her MA in sociology from the University of Windsor and her BA (Hons) in anthropology from Western University.

Belinda Leach is professor in the Department of Sociology and Anthropology and associate dean (research) in the College of Social and Applied Human Sciences at the University of Guelph. She held a University Research Chair in Rural Gender Studies between 2004 and 2009 and led a Community-University Research Alliance, Rural Women Making Change. Her research investigates gender, livelihoods, and economic restructuring in Canada. She is co-editor with Winnie Lem of *Culture, Economy, Power: Anthropology as Critique, Anthropology as Praxis* (2002), and co-author with Tony Winson of *Contingent Work, Disrupted Lives: Labour and Community in the New Rural Economy* (2002), which was awarded the John Porter Award of the Canadian Sociology and Anthropology Association. She also co-authored, with Charlotte Yates and Holly Gibbs, *Negotiating Risk, Seeking Security, Eroding Solidarity* (2012) and co-edited, with Barbara Pini, *Reshaping Gender and Class in Rural Spaces* (2011).

Beverly D. Leipert is an associate professor in the Arthur Labatt Family School of Nursing at Western University. From 2003 to 2009 she held the first and only research chair in North America in rural women's health. She grew up on a farm in rural Saskatchewan. She received BA and BSc in nursing degrees from the University of Saskatchewan in 1977, the MSc in nursing degree from the University of British Columbia in 1992, and the PhD in nursing degree from the University of Alberta in 2002. Her research focuses on the determinants of rural women's health, rural women's empowerment, community health nursing, and qualitative methodologies, particularly photovoice. She has conducted several research studies and written and published extensively in the field of rural women's health and community health nursing. Previous to her academic career, she was a public health nurse for ten years in rural and remote Saskatchewan, a staff nurse at Vancouver General

Hospital, and a community health nurse in Vancouver. She was also one of the founding faculty members of the University of Northern British Columbia, where she assisted in the development of three nursing programs, including the Certificate in Rural and Northern Nursing. She also conducted some of the first research that explored the health of women in northern Canada and rural and northern public health nursing practice.

Jo Little is professor of gender and geography at the University of Exeter in the UK. She has published extensively on rural gender issues within Western economies. Her early work explored rural women's labour market participation and gendered constructions of community, while more recently her research has focused on rural gender identities, sexuality, and embodiment. As part of the study of the rural body, Jo's work has considered practices of well-being and the importance of therapeutic landscapes. Her books include *Contested Countryside Cultures* (1997, with Paul Cloke), *Gender and Rural Geography* (2002), and *Critical Issues in Rural Gender Studies* (2005, with Carol Morris).

Diane Martz is the director of the Research Ethics Office and Research Faculty with the Saskatchewan Population Health and Evaluation Research Unit at the University of Saskatchewan. Previously she was the research manager for the Prairie Women's Health Centre of Excellence in Saskatoon and the director of the Centre for Rural Studies and Enrichment at St. Peters College in Muenster, Saskatchewan.

Lynn McIntyre is professor and Canadian Institutes of Health Research Chair in Gender and Health in the Department of Community Health Sciences, Faculty of Medicine, University of Calgary. She holds a medical degree, a master's degree in community health and epidemiology, and is a fellow of the Royal College of Physicians of Canada in public health and preventive medicine. Dr McIntyre's research is focused on hunger and food insecurity issues both domestically and in lower- and middle-income countries, with a particular interest in women. Her research with Canadian farm women has examined the use of food provisioning practices as a lens for understanding the social context of food behaviours and the health status of farm families. In addition, she has investigated the daily food provisioning experiences of ultra poor, head-of-household women in Bangladesh in both rural and urban settings.

Christina McLennan is with the Thompson Rivers University School of Social Work and Human Service in Kamloops, BC. Her research interests are primarily focused on the social determinants of women's health, women-centred approaches to creating healthy communities, and building social work approaches to online information and resource networks. Christina is a coordinator with the Women North Network/Northern FIRE at the University of Northern BC and is also a community activist working towards women's equality.

Pertice Moffitt is manager, Health Research Programs, Aurora Research Institute/Aurora College; adjunct professor, MN program, Dalhousie University; and sessional instructor, MN program, Athabasca University. Her research and teaching interests include nursing philosophy and science, nursing ethics, women's health, culture and health, scholarship of teaching, evaluation, and health promotion. She has worked closely with the community of Behchoko and the Tlicho people. She is currently working on a multidisciplinary SSHRC-funded project entitled 'Rural and Northern Response to Intimate Partner Violence' in the Northwest Territories and partnered with researchers and community partners from the Prairie provinces.

Phyllis Montgomery is an advanced practice nurse, educator, and researcher in the area of psychiatric mental health nursing. She received her master of science in nursing from the University of Toronto and her doctorate from McMaster University. Many of her research projects focus on women's efforts to craft a life in the presence of challenging circumstances.

Nuelle Novik is an assistant professor with the Faculty of Social Work at the University of Regina. She is currently chair of the Standards of Practice Committee with the Saskatchewan Association of Social Workers (SASW) and is a board member with the Canadian Mental Health Association. She continues to maintain a counselling practice, counselling part time out of a community agency in Regina. Her research interests include rural and remote social work practice and healthy aging, social work practice with seniors, mental health practice, palliative care, and issues related to food security.

Heather Peters is associate professor with the School of Social Work at the University of Northern British Columbia and holds a PhD in social work from the University of British Columbia. Her research interests include social policy and housing policy with specific attention to the effects of policy on women, care givers, vulnerable populations, and northern and rural communities. She has also completed research and published articles that explore access by marginalized populations to social and health services, including an examination of the role of policy in facilitating or impeding such access.

Barbara Pini is professor of sociology in the School of Humanities at Griffith University, Australia. She has an extensive publication record in the fields of gender studies, rural sociology, employment, public policy, and politics. Recent papers have appeared in *Gender, Work and Organisation; Policy and Politics; Work, Employment and Society; Journal of Rural Studies; Sociologia Ruralis;* and *Telecommunications Policy.* Her first book, *Masculinities and Management in Agri-political Organisations Worldwide,* was published in 2008. She is co-editor with Belinda Leach of *Reshaping Gender and Class in Rural Spaces* (2011) and of *Women and Local Government: International Case Studies* with Paula McDonald (2011).

Marilyn Porter was born and brought up on a sheep farm in North Wales, UK. She moved to Canada in 1980 and has taught and researched at Memorial University in St. John's, Newfoundland, ever since. Much of her research has focused on women in Newfoundland, and especially rural women's economic lives. She has published many articles on aspects of this topic, and one book, *Place and Persistence in the Lives of Newfoundland Women* (1993), as well as co-editing the readers *Their Lives and Times – Women in Newfoundland and Labrador: A Collage* (1995) and *Weather's Edge: A Compendium of Women's Lives in Newfoundland and Labrador* (2006). Her most recent project was a team interdisciplinary, cross-cultural narrative study entitled *Women's Experience of Their Reproductive Lives in Pakistan, Indonesia and Canada,* which collected narratives from three-generational families of women in diverse situations.

Krista Rondeau is a registered dietitian and holds a master's degree in health promotion studies. For her thesis, she conducted qualitative research on how farm women in Canada conceptualized food safety within the context of their daily food provisioning practices. She is currently a research associate with the Department of Community Health Sciences at the University of Calgary, where she works on both domestic and international-focused household food insecurity and food provisioning research projects.

Lynn Scruby holds a BN degree from McGill University, an MS degree in public health from the University of Minnesota, Minneapolis, and a PhD in interdisciplinary studies from the University of Manitoba. In her position as assistant professor in the Faculty of Nursing at the University of Manitoba she teaches community health in both the undergraduate and graduate programs. Her areas of teaching expertise include health promotion, population health, knowledge translation, and health policy. She has conducted research with vulnerable populations in both urban and rural contexts, including program and policy directions. Her research program utilizes the lens of equity and social justice and includes the study of organizational collaboration for population health promotion in inner-city neighbourhoods. She serves as prairie region research coordinator and co-investigator for a national study exploring social support and rural women's health; is a research associate with the Manitoba Centre for Nursing and Health Research; and is a member of the Qualitative Research Group at the University of Manitoba. In addition to her work on several community boards of directors and foundations, she is a member of the National Research Panel for Family Resource Programs Canada.

D. Lynn Skillen is a professor emerital sessional instructor in the Faculty of Nursing, University of Alberta and a published writer of creative non-fiction. She worked as a public health nurse and nurse practitioner in Canada and as a nurse researcher (community development) and regional nursing officer (public health services) in Colombia, South America. Related research focused on the health, safety, and wellness of rural and urban women in paid and unpaid work environments from the perspective of recipients and providers of health care. Her research interests included the organizational factors that underlie work hazards, the cross-cultural factors that influence workplace health and safety, and the influence of professional ideologies on actions taken in the workplace to reduce health and safety risks. When not teaching after-degree nursing students, she cycles, hikes, skis, travels, and writes.

Karen Soldatic is currently based at the School of Social Sciences, University of New South Wales, Sydney, Australia. Her main area of research interest focuses on the global restructuring of disability welfare and social provisioning measures and the differential impact on intersecting disabled identities in varying spaces and places.

Kelly Stickle recently completed a master's degree in psychology through the University of Northern British Columbia. His employment history ranges from commercial fishing along the British Columbia coast to serving as a residence hall dean at a private boarding academy. He is currently working in the central Alberta social services field with at-risk adolescents.

Deborah Stiles, Steven Dukeshire, and **Kenneth Paulsen** are, respectively, director and team members of the Nova Scotia Agricultural College's Rural Research Centre. Stiles holds a PhD in history and a master's degree in English, and writes non-fiction, fiction, and poetry. She also does research in social history, agricultural policy, and rural gender and culture studies. Dukeshire holds a PhD in psychology and researches in the areas of rural women's health and decision-making behaviour. Paulsen holds a PhD in history and researches and writes in the fields of community studies, eighteenth-century Nova Scotia history, and genealogy. Co-authors/students Melanie Goodridge, David Hobson, Jamie MacLaughlin, Katriona MacNeil, and Christian Rangel were employed by the Women's Health in Rural Communities project at the Rural Research Centre, and contributed to research and writing during the five-year tenure of this Canadian Institutes of Health Research–funded research project.

Rebecca Sutherns holds a PhD in rural studies from the University of Guelph and a master's in public administration from Queen's University. Her research has focused on issues of gender, place, and health, with particular emphasis on maternity care. She has worked in international community development and is active in local health and social service planning and advocacy. She is a professional facilitator who runs a strategic planning and policy analysis consulting firm in Guelph, Ontario.

Deborah Thien is associate professor of geography at California State University, Long Beach, USA. Originally from Vancouver Island, BC, she is a feminist geographer whose research examines the juxtaposition of emotion, health, and well-being with gender and in rural and remote places. She holds a PhD in feminist geography from the University of Edinburgh, Scotland. She has conducted fieldwork in Canada, Scotland, New Zealand, and the United States and published the resulting research in journals that include *Emotion, Society and Space*; *Gender, Place and Culture*; and *The Canadian Journal of Public Health*. She has also authored or co-authored several book chapters, for example, in *Emotion, Place & Culture* (2009). She is currently working on a book about posttraumatic stress disorder and the militarization of trauma.

Wilfreda E. (Billie) Thurston is a professor in the Department of Community Health Sciences, Faculty of Medicine, and the Department of Ecosystem and Public Health, Faculty of Veterinary Medicine; an adjunct professor in the Faculty of Nursing; and a member of the Institute for Public Health, University of Calgary. She grew up on a farm on the coast of Nova Scotia when hay was still stowed loose. She received a BA in psychology from Acadia University in 1974, an MSc from Memorial University of Newfoundland in community medicine in 1986, and a PhD in health research from the University of Calgary in 1991. Her research has included the determinants of health with a focus on gender and other social institutions that marginalize populations and the development and evaluation of programs and policies. This has included the health impacts of and health system roles in preventing gender-based violence. More recently she has been studying the determinants of Aboriginal people's health. Between 1974 and 1986 she worked in child welfare, was an addiction counsellor, worked in a women's centre, and was director of a shelter for women leaving family violence. Involvement in the women's movement included policy advocacy at all levels of government. As an academic she has taught graduate courses in health promotion, evaluation research, and gender and women's health. She has supervised numerous honours and master's theses and doctoral dissertations.

Anita Vaillancourt is assistant professor in the social work program at Algoma University and a PhD candidate in the Factor-Inwentash Faculty of Social Work at the University of Toronto. In addition to completing her doctoral research on welfare reform in northern rural and non-metropolitan settings, Anita also conducts research in the areas of women's addiction, family violence, social exclusion, social policy, and critical pedagogy. Anita's teaching, practice, and research endeavours are informed by over ten years of experience working with chemically dependent women, working with women who experienced and/or witnessed violence, and working in the areas of social policy, community development, and child welfare. Anita's work is further shaped by her community work as an anti-poverty and women's rights activist.

Theresa Vladicka has an MA in sociology from the University of Victoria (2007). She is currently working with the Government of Alberta, Advanced Education and Technology, as a research and policy analyst.

Andrew Watterson is a professor of health, director of the Centre for Public Health and Population Health, and head of the University of Stirling's interdepartmental Occupational and Environmental Health Research Group. Previously, he was professor of occupational and environmental health at De Montfort University, Leicester, UK. He is a chartered fellow of the Institution of Occupational Safety and Health and holds a PhD in social sciences from Bristol University. He was a founder of the UK Pesticides Trust (now PAN UK) and sat on the HSC Chemicals in Agriculture Working Group for many years. He has published widely on agricultural health and safety in general and pesticides in particular, including *The Pesticide Users' Health and Safety Handbook: An International Guide* and *Pesticides and Your Food*. His current research interests relate to the interface between science, policy, regulation, and civil society.

Jayne Whyte grew up on a farm in rural Saskatchewan but recently moved into seniors' housing in Regina. As an independent contractor since 1996, she uses qualitative research to publicize issues of women, poverty, intercultural learning, and mental health. Jayne advocates the use of gender-place analysis and disability awareness in research and decision making.

Juliana Wiens holds a master's degree in women's studies from Dalhousie University. She has a qualitative research background in women's health, and has conducted research in a variety of areas, including black women's health, mental health and depression, professional boundaries in the workplace, and addictions. Her employment history includes both research and social service work. Currently, she works full time as an employment counsellor and is in the process of completing a master's of education degree in counselling.

Susan Wismer is recently retired from her positions as associate professor in the Department of Environment and Resource Studies and director of independent studies at the University of Waterloo. She has long-term research interests in environmental and social justice, rural development, gender, and environment. Currently she is on contract as the University Community Outreach Advisor for a CIDA-funded development project in Indonesia, working with Islamic universities on gender-sensitive socially inclusive forms of community engagement.

Alanah Woodland holds a master's of community health sciences from the University of Calgary. Her master's research was entitled 'Sexual Health: Engaging Urban Indigenous Youth.' She has conducted research in the areas of Aboriginal homelessness, primary care evaluation, and Aboriginal youth health. She is a St'at'imc/(Irish/English) woman committed to indigenous rights and indigenous health. She has recently moved to St'at'imc territory and is enjoying spending time with the St'at'imc elders and her family. She is enjoying the opportunity to explore the application of community health science knowledge and skills in rural community-based programming and projects. She maintains an avid interest in population health interventions, leadership, community-based evaluation, ethics, primary health care, and eco-health. She has also taken up cedar bark weaving, ayuverdic head massage, and healing touch techniques. She currently works as a full-time Aboriginal patient navigator, a part-time community development coordinator, and an occasional marriage commissioner. In her spare time, you'll find her somewhere exploring, learning, fishing, singing, drumming, and enjoying being home.